Studies in the Psychosocial

Studies in the Psychosocial seeks to investigate the ways in which psychic and social processes demand to be understood as always implicated in each other, as mutually constitutive, co-produced, or abstracted levels of a single dialectical process. As such it can be understood as an interdisciplinary field in search of transdisciplinary objects of knowledge. Studies in the Psychosocial is also distinguished by its emphasis on affect, the irrational and unconscious processes, often, but not necessarily, understood psychoanalytically. Studies in the Psychosocial aims to foster the development of this field by publishing high quality and innovative monographs and edited collections. The series welcomes submissions from a range of theoretical perspectives and disciplinary orientations, including sociology, social and critical psychology, political science, postcolonial studies, feminist studies, queer studies, management and organization studies, cultural and media studies and psychoanalysis. However, in keeping with the inter- or transdisciplinary character of psychosocial analysis, books in the series will generally pass beyond their points of origin to generate concepts, understandings and forms of investigation that are distinctively psychosocial in character.

Guilaine Kinouani
Hannah Reeves • Clau Di Gianfrancesco
Editors

Creative Disruption

Psychosocial Scholarship as Praxis

palgrave
macmillan

Editors
Guilaine Kinouani
School of Social Sciences
Race Reflections, Birkbeck, University of London
London, UK

Hannah Reeves
School of Social Sciences
Birkbeck, University of London
London, UK

Clau Di Gianfrancesco
School of Social Sciences
Birkbeck, University of London
London, UK

ISSN 2662-2629 ISSN 2662-2637 (electronic)
Studies in the Psychosocial
ISBN 978-3-031-63663-9 ISBN 978-3-031-63661-5 (eBook)
https://doi.org/10.1007/978-3-031-63661-5

This Palgrave Macmillan imprint is published by the registered company Springer Nature Switzerland AG.
The registered company address is: Gewerbestrasse 11, 6330 Cham, Switzerland

Acknowledgements

We would like to warmly thank our colleagues, the teaching and non-teaching staff, mainly from within the Department of Psychosocial Studies at Birkbeck, University of London, for having helped with the realisation of this project since before its conception as a book. Particularly, we would like to thank Professor Stephen Frosh for his support and guidance throughout and for his helpful comments on much of the writing. We also wish to give our thanks to our peers and fellow psychosocial studies PhD students. You made our time at Birkbeck stimulating. Our ongoing conversations and exchanges continue to enrich us as scholars. While the department no longer endures as a distinct entity, its work will persist. Finally, we would like to express our deep gratitude to the authors whose work we have included in the volume, as well as the authors who expressed an interest in contributing but whose excellent proposals we were unable to include due to pragmatic constraints. Engaging with this breadth of intellectual work has galvanised our own excitement for and commitment to psychosocial studies.

Contents

Notes on Contributors

John Adlam is a group psychotherapist and independent researcher. He works for the most part in the National Health Service. He is a co-founder of the Reflective Practice Research Network; a founder member of the Association for Psychosocial Studies and the Henderson Heritage Group; and former vice-president of the International Association for Forensic Psychotherapy. His book with Christopher Scanlon—*Psycho-social Explorations of Trauma, Exclusion and Violence: Un-housed Minds and Inhospitable Environments*—was published by Routledge in 2022. He is also co-editor of three books, most recently *Violent States and Creative States: From the Global to the Individual* (2018, Jessica Kingsley Publishers).

Iris Aleida Pinzón Arteaga is a psychologist and social researcher. Member of the interdisciplinary research group 'Violence, Language, and Cultural Studies' of the Autonomous University of Bucaramanga (Colombia). Her research involves the deployment of psychoanalytic concepts and critical approaches to reflect upon psychosocial phenomena. Her areas of interest fall generally within the areas of culture, collective memory, epistemology, and knowledge production. Her latest article (with researcher Arturo Bandinelli), titled "Knowledge and Truth in Contemporary Society: A Psychoanalytic Investigation of the 'Post-Truth Era'" (Awry, 2022), interrogates the relationship between truth and knowledge in the so-called post-truth era by means of Lacanian psychoanalysis.

Arturo Bandinelli is a London-based filmmaker, independent researcher, and psychoanalyst in formation at Centre for Freudian Analysis and Research. In his creative and research practice, he explores the relationship between desire and technology, body and language, and psychoanalysis and epistemology. His written publications include "What Does the App Want? A Psychoanalytic Interpretation of Dating App's Libidinal Economy" (*Psychoanalysis, Culture and Society*, 2021, co-authored with Carolina Bandinelli) and "Knowledge and Truth in Contemporary Society: A Psychoanalytic Investigation of the 'Post-Truth Era'" (Awry: *Journal of Critical Psychology*, 2022, co-authored with Iris Aleida Pinzón Arteaga).

Sasha Bergstrom-Katz is an artist and a researcher. She completed her practice-based PhD co-supervised across Psychosocial Studies and the History of Psychology at Birkbeck, University of London, in 2023. Her PhD thesis, *On Intelligence Tests: Psychological Objects and their Subjects*, makes an aesthetic enquiry into the material cultures and history of American intelligence tests. In January 2024, she began a Leverhulme Trust–funded postdoctoral fellowship jointly at the Max Planck Institute for the History of Science and the University of Bielefeld. She has exhibited her artwork internationally and holds an MFA from the University of California, Irvine.

Nancy Blair is an environmentalist, social justice activist and psychotherapist with a Master's Degree in Environmental Studies from Dalhousie University, and a Master's Degree in Education (Counselling) from Acadia University. She works from her private practice, Nancy Blair Counselling, in Nova Scotia, Canada—individual, group work, presentations and media. A major influence is her work in Animal Assisted Therapy in Counselling and Pet Loss and Bereavement Counselling.

Rayann Bryan is a PhD student at the University of Greenwich, investigating the experiences of Black Caribbean mothers and daughters who migrated to the UK during the Windrush era (1950s to 1960s). Beyond the academia, Rayann is the driving force behind the Thelma Matilda

Alves Foundation, a Black women's mental health charity. As the founder and CEO, Rayann strategically applies Black feminist theory, providing a vital platform for support and empowerment for Black women in England. In both academia and advocacy, Rayann weaves a narrative of resilience and positive change.

Robert Chapman (they/them) is currently Assistant Professor of Critical Neurodiversity Studies at Durham University.

Clau Di Gianfrancesco is a PhD candidate at Birkbeck, University of London. Their research focuses on gender, sexuality and interactive theatre practices, particularly those derived from Theatre of the Oppressed. Since 2016, they have collaborated with various Theatre of the Oppressed companies worldwide. Their work explores the potential of this theatrical practice to drive social change.

Tom Fielder is a PhD researcher in Psychosocial Studies at Birkbeck College, University of London. His thesis is titled "Admitting Demons: Brexit and Psychoanalysis". He has published scholarly articles in *History of the Human Sciences* and the *Journal of Psychosocial Studies.*

Micha Frazer-Carroll is an author, journalist, and editor living in London. Micha is committed to challenging systems of oppression and supporting social justice movements in building towards a liberated future. Writing is one technique Micha uses in order to do this. She is the author of *Mad World: The Politics of Mental Health* (Pluto, 2023).

Elena Gkivisi is a PhD researcher at Birkbeck College, University of London. Her research focuses on psychoanalysis, literature, cultural studies, feminism and philosophy; it investigates paradigms of subjectivity in contemporary writing. She is the author of two critically acclaimed novels in the Greek language as well as of short stories, reviews and essays. She has also studied law and has trained and worked as a Barrister.

Rebecca Esho Greenslade (she/her) is an existential-feminist psychotherapist, supervisor and writer, currently living between London and Virginia. She is the founder of the Feminist Therapy Network. Alongside her therapeutic practice, Rebecca is a faculty member of The Minster Centre, London, and is currently undertaking PhD research with the

Department of Psychosocial Studies at Birkbeck University, London. Her research re-conceptualises a contemporary feminist psychotherapy via an ethos characterised by 'technologies of the self', or *askesis*. Rebecca is a Zen student and practitioner in the White Plum Lineage and is currently undertaking Buddhist Chaplaincy training with Upaya Zen Center.

Ayelen Hamity is a graduate in Psychology and Philosophy from the University of Pretoria, with a Master's in Critical Diversity Studies from the University of Witwatersrand and a Master's in Psychoanalytic Studies from Birkbeck College. Currently pursuing a PhD at University College London, her research delves into the intersections of psychoanalytic theory and migration studies, focusing on the experiences of psychoanalysts from Buenos Aires residing in London. She is actively engaged in human rights work within London and contributes to understanding diverse perspectives in the realm of subjectivity, neocolonial dynamics, and psychoanalytically informed political interventions.

Guilaine Kinouani is an award-winning writer, psychologist, group analyst and thinker. She is the founder of Race Reflections. She taught critical psychology, social sciences and black studies at Syracuse before her PhD at Birkbeck. Her first book *Living While Black* (2021) exposes the impact of racism on black minds and bodies. Her second book *White Minds* (2023) is a psychosocial exploration of the quotidian workings of whiteness. Her thesis examines whiteness and the afterlives of colonialism and enslavement in the clinic using Afro-analytics, a frame she is developing to rethink racial trauma, inheritance, transmission and associated issues of communication and embodiment within the black diaspora.

Daniela Larraín-Salas is a clinical psychologist, at Universidad Católica de Chile, and holds an MA in Social Psychology, Universidad Diego Portales, Chile. Currently, she is a PhD researcher in Psychosocial Studies at Birkbeck College. Her investigation explores the construction of the figure of the perpetrator through legal archives regarding political violence during the Chilean dictatorship. Her research interests are political violence in Latin America, memory, archives, and practices of recording through the lens of psychoanalysis, feminism, psychosocial studies, and aesthetics. She is also a Member of the Red Interamericana de investigación en Psicoanálisis y Política (RedIPPol) and of the Centre for Iberian and Latin American Visual Studies (CILAVS).

Leila Lawton passion for people and inclusive clinical and research practice has been cultivated through 19 years of combined experience working with culturally diverse groups within primary and secondary care and the third sector—ranging from community mental health, learning disability and youth offending teams, memory clinics, in-patients wards and NHS talking therapies. Leila has lived experience of mental health difficulties as well as being a carer for others with mental health needs. Her research interests include racial trauma, reflexivity, PTSD, anti-racism and intersectionality. She contributes to the evidence-base and policy to empower communities to inform the systems response towards their healing. Leila is committed to developing solutions through education to address systemic and structural racism.

Jane Ribbens McCarthy, PhD is a sociologist at The Open University, Milton Keynes, UK, holding various honorary and voluntary roles, including visiting professor at the University of Bath. Particular themes have included family troubles, meanings of 'family' and understandings of 'relationality,' including work in China and Senegal. She is currently focused on antiracist work in the bereavement sector, alongside decolonising the aftermath of death and its significance for the climate and ecological emergency. Her work is published extensively as Jane Ribbens McCarthy. Jane.McCarthy@open.ac.uk https://www.open.ac.uk/people/jcrm2 Existential Dis/Connections (open.ac.uk).

Michelle Michael is a forensic psychologist working for the National Health Service.

Halina Pytlasinska runs a private therapeutic practice for individuals, couples and supervisees in Buckinghamshire, UK. Pytlasinska has worked as a lecturer, training counsellors for Abingdon and Witney College and as a freelance consultant trainer in all sectors on teamwork, leadership and innovation. Creative and performance arts are integrated into her clinical work. Pytlasinska is trained as an actor and has worked as a jazz singer. She is a member of the Climate Psychology Alliance. Her current interests include social dreaming, LGBTQ+ issues, neurodiversity, creativity in workplace settings, decolonisation and climate change.

Jennifer Ramsay is a Scottish storyteller living in Spain. She works with fairy tales in private practice and as a creative group facilitator. Ramsay facilitates a course called 'Dancing with Death' and is presently writing a book on this subject. She holds a Degree in Biological Sciences and incorporates the Celtic wheel of the year into her work. Ramsay is the founder of Story Arte, a centre for Personal Development and Storytelling in Madrid.

Hannah Reeves is a transdisciplinary scholar working across psychosocial studies, sociology, anthropology, and environmental humanities; her long-term commitments are to exploring human-nonhuman relations in sites of anthropogenic disturbance ethnographically, particularly in urban settings. Hannah is passionate about fostering collaboration within and beyond academia, including with collaborators based in visual arts, archaeology, and the natural sciences.

Janedra Sykes is a certified Equity, Diversity, and Inclusion (EDI), organizational development coach, and consultant. She is a partner at Arboreta Group, LLC, a San Diego-based consulting firm serving non-profits, governments, and businesses, offering strategic planning, training, evaluation, and facilitation services. Janedra is an International Coaching Federation-certified organizational development coach. She holds a Master of Arts in Nonprofit Leadership and Management from the University of San Diego and a Bachelor of Arts in History from the University of California, Los Angeles.

Dwight Turner is Course Leader on the Humanistic Psychotherapy Course at the University of Brighton, and a psychotherapist and supervisor in private practice. He wrote *The Psychology of Supremacy* (2023) and *Intersections of Privilege and Otherness in Counselling and Psychotherapy* (2021), both published by Routledge, together with chapters in anthologies, and over 50 academic papers on everything from intersectionality in psychotherapy to dreamwork, to Afrocentric spirituality. An Intersectional Psychotherapist, Dr Turner is an experienced conference speaker and can be contacted via his website www.dwightturnercounselling.co.uk or on social media on LinkedIn, Threads, or on Twitter at @dturner300.

Els van Ooijen is a retired integrative-relational psychotherapist and Ex Visiting Lecturer in Counselling and Supervision at the University of South Wales, UK. Recently Ooijen joined the editorial board of *Explorations* (the online *Journal of the Climate Psychology Alliance*). Her books include *Integrative Counselling and Psychotherapy* (co-written with Ariana Faris, 2012) and *Clinical Supervision Made Easy*, 2003, 2013 (2nd ed.). Ooijen's current interests and activities include social dreaming, decolonisation, climate activism, shamanic practice and Zen Buddhism.

List of Figures

1

Introduction

Hannah Reeves, Clau Di Gianfrancesco, and Guilaine Kinouani

The Twist in the Möbius Strip

Within the field of psychosocial studies, reflexivity has served to trouble artificial boundaries between research/life, researcher/researched, inside/outside, and thus to foster the creation of a Möbius strip-like space. Similarly, artistic formulations of reflexivity have contributed to the formation of such a space from which "the dominant, entrenched academic community and its claims to scientific ways of knowing" can be critiqued and disrupted (Finley, 2008, p. 72) (Fig. 1.1).

Attempting to trace a straightforward path around the outside of a Möbius strip seems like an impossible task. Every apparently external surface leads inside, and every apparently internal surface leads outside. Every possible path subverts the notion of internality and externality as

H. Reeves • C. Di Gianfrancesco
School of Social Sciences, Birkbeck University, London, UK
e-mail: hreeve03@mail.bbk.ac.uk; cdigia02@mail.bbk.ac.uk

G. Kinouani (✉)
School of Social Sciences, Race Reflections, Birkbeck University, London, UK

G. Kinouani et al. (eds.), *Creative Disruption*, Studies in the Psychosocial,
https://doi.org/10.1007/978-3-031-63661-5_1

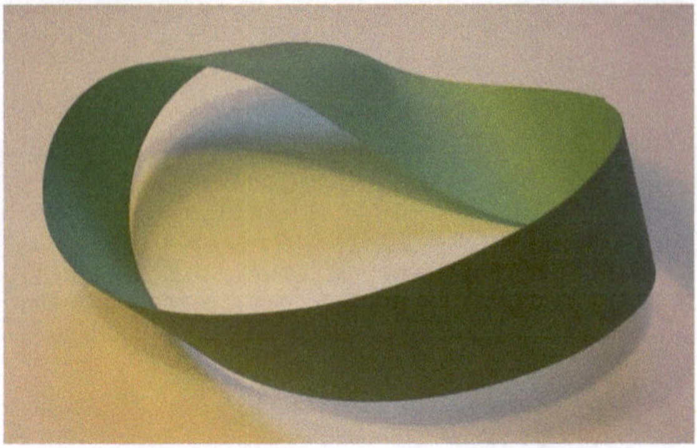

Fig. 1.1 A mathematically accurate Möbius strip

fixed, just as the ostensibly internal world of the psyche is continually bound up with, flows into, and constitutes the ostensibly external realm of the social.

Everyday life moves along habitual paths. From the bodily routines through which we maintain ourselves and others, as we navigate our way through physical and virtual spaces (from the domestic through to institutions of every scale), social reproduction is sustained by lives lived along lines (Ingold, 2015, 2011/2022). Often, that we are moving along a particular trajectory only becomes palpable when the path is disrupted: when some obstacle gets in the way; when the path is damaged, becomes impassable, or falls out from under us.

Faced with disruption, a previously unremarkable backdrop draws sharply into focus. We might suddenly realise we are following a path that was laid out for us by one or many others; perhaps we are being pulled or pushed along it. That path allowed us to see, hear, feel, live, know *something*, yet clouded something else: "[W]hen we follow specific lines, some things become reachable and others remain or even become out of reach" (Ahmed, 2006, p. 14). Disruption asks us to find another way: over or under, double back and find another way, or diverge entirely. What queer possibilities might we happen upon—and generate—in the overgrown surround? What friction might we encounter along the way? (feministkilljoys, 2018).

The twist in the Möbius strip reminds us that attempting to trace a line through psychosocial topographies calls for perpetual reorientation. If we choose to stay with a particular path, it will lead us from inside to outside, upside to underside, and back again: eventually, we realise we are on a non-orientable surface. The psychosocial will not stay still, yet doing psychosocial scholarship demands finding ways to stay with the paths that constitute it. Orientations "take time and require giving up time" (Ahmed, 2006, p. 20). A psychosocial praxis asks us to stay with "some worlds and not others" (Haraway, 2016, p. 165) while we continue to adapt: to orientate and reorientate, even to purposefully disorientate. As Sara Ahmed has argued, the loss of a sense of aim, purpose, or even of who one is "can be converted into the joy of a future that has been opened up" (Ahmed, 2006, p. 20).

As authors, we acknowledge that our positionalities profoundly shape our orientations, including our respective orientations towards the psychosocial. In different and intersecting ways, we cannot afford—and cannot be afforded—the hubris of *zero point* epistemology (Castro-Gómez, 2021; Mignolo, 2009). Doing psychosocial scholarship is as much a personal praxis as an intellectual-political praxis. As such, we posit this introduction as a Möbius strip-like space, leading us from one dimension of psychosocial praxis into another and back again. While the emphasis or orientation of this praxis shifts and transmutes throughout the sections and chapters that follow, others are never far away: mutually articulated on the reverse surface, close behind and always approaching (Fig. 1.2).

Guilaine: Too Sociological or Too Black?

In order to share my psychosocial studies story, I need to start with my scholarly journey, and to start with my scholarly journey, I need to take you through parts of my journey through life. I am a psychologist by background and group analyst. A Parisian born, inner-cities-bred French woman. I grew up poor, I am the child of Congolese "immigrants" who were born colonial subjects and have genocidal histories. Although I completed a literary baccalaureate, which had heavy doses of languages, literature, and philosophy, my first degree in England was a kind of "pick and mix" bag of sociology, cultural studies, language, and literature. Wherever I could, I would focus my work on inequalities, migration,

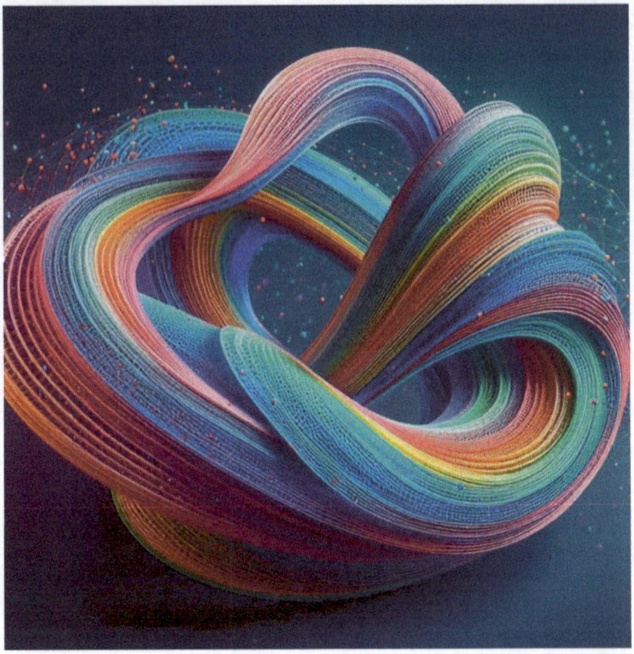

Fig. 1.2 A composite Möbius strip-like form generated by Bing's Image Creator. While no longer mathematically accurate, it holds together more or less coherently

blackness, the afterlives of colonialism, enslavement, and historical atrocities.

After further engagement in cultural studies this time as related to mental health and in psychology, I got into clinical psychology. Despite choosing a contextually focused course which I thought was going to be aligned with my critical thinking and the integrative essence of my worldview, I realised very quickly all that I knew, had experienced, and thought about the world was deemed too radical, not sufficiently psychological and simply too sociological. This was a turning point for me. And it was a painful one.

Repeatedly I heard that my thinking was out of place. Once, I was warned that insisting on wanting to study whiteness amounted to committing career suicide. I often say that my years in academic psychology have been the most distressing period of my adult life. I am still trying to make meaning out of this experience. At that time, I met a white South African Psychology Professor who had said to me, she had been struck by the number of black African students within higher education institutions, who had compared their experience of psychology training to that of an amputation, before she had left her post on the continent.

As someone of Congolese descent, her words resonated then. And they resonate even more now. The amputatory imagery and symbolism brought me a sense of recognition of what I was encountering with the discipline of psychology and its disciplinary encounters. I have continued to ask myself what limb(s) or other body parts these students imagined were being forcefully extracted from their body, in the process of their professional socialisation. I thought about who they needed to become to survive these brutal spaces.

Today, I think about these fantasies as forced splitting. As a form of psychic amputation whereby the black subject must split off from their blackness, the history of psychology, and their historicised lived experience. As an expectation of dissociation from what they know, from how they make sense of social and structural realities. Amputation as alienation in the Fanonian sense. Amputation therefore of the black subject, of their subjectivity. But I also imagine these amputations, as punishment for "transgression"—punishment for daring to be or think "differently." For challenging established orthodoxies and systems of thought, white, male, colonial, Western, modern. Some might say, for challenging the Master. Recently, my work has got into conversation with post-colonial haunting (Coly, 2019) which made visible these ghosts and shadows I had viscerally felt and witnessed but which had until then remained obscure, unnamed, and unnameable.

I got into analytic studies largely to make sense of my psychology experience. It helped. I intuitively knew there were group forces at play. I knew without knowing that what was going on was not only about me, my history, or even that of those involved. I was desperate to grasp the invisible forces I saw enfolding when racialised social actors come together. And it is through group analysis' interests in social and historical phenomena, in group trauma and consequent conceptualisations of the psyche as a collective entity, that I discovered psychosocial thinking. I came across Professor Stephen Frosh's (2013) article: "Psychoanalysis,

Colonialism, Racism." I had not heard of him. Nor heard of the psychosocial. I got intrigued and read more of his work. Then … I discovered there had always been elements of psychosocial analytics in my thinking. The familiarity of the ideas created a sense of homeness. I understood a bit more about my out-of-placeness within "traditional" psychology and its continuing gaze on my blackness. I approached Professor Frosh, who supervised the first part of my PhD before his retirement. The part I like to refer to as the pre-Congo disruption. A period of transition which coincided with a trip to my ancestral land. Palestine, Sudan, and the D.R. Congo, in particular, burst onto our collective consciousness. With that, mass suffering and trauma, genocidal conflicts, displacement from ancestral lands, collective states of homelessness are issues which sit at the core of my thinking. I was forced to rethink who and what I wanted to be in the world and if/how the psychosocial may support me to get there. The psychosocial is not to be idealised. There are no ideas and theories that can be expressed outside the murky matrices of power relations, historical repetitions, or geopolitics. As a black woman body few are the spaces that I can occupy and be free of violence. When I started my PhD, psychosocial studies represented fundamentally a meeting point for all my learning. A space which echoed all that I was, or at least how I viewed myself. Hybrid, transgressive, bold, rebellious, creative, and disruptive simply by virtue of my insistence on being free. Free to think, to move, and to be. A place where I could bring the complexities of my existence and all I had learnt about the world. As I progressed through my research, it became clear that a large part of my academic journey had been about trying to find a home, in the epistemic sense as I say, in a way that echoes my lived reality as a migrant who is, as I stated, a child of "migrants" and has displacement as a core feature of her history. And that the resonance that I had felt spoke to something much deeper, something which cannot be understood by intellectual means alone. Something that I carry within. The deep forests of the Congo. Metaphorically, epistemically, and ancestrally. The psychosocial created a path for me to find that home, or at least to plant seeds of a home to come: Afro-analytics. A space where we start by reclaiming the discarded within ourselves and with that, the African roots of ideas whitewashed as Western which are uncritically accepted as white. This is necessary to recognise the sophisticated metaphysics of the so-called primitive. To imagine spaces of healing, feeling, and thinking for our black minds and bodies centred on unconscious or invisible group phenomena and felt embodied experiences that honour African cosmologies and onto-epistemologies while archiving and witnessing the phenomenology of being racialised as black in a white supremacist world. I hope this collection gives something of the flavour of my academic journey through the psychosocial and where it has taken me: home. I hope it helps to demonstrate the potential of thinking and feeling beyond borders and that through the words of others too, demonstrates the fundamental and dangerous illusions that are disciplinary boundaries as colonial borders which only split us from parts of who we are and who we can be, if we make space for disruption.

Psychosocial Junctures

Moments of disruption—planned and unplanned—are everywhere in the fragile terrain of the social world, from micro-level gestures of resistance and refusal at the local scale to globally disruptive phenomena such as climate and ecological breakdown and pandemic. Disruption often precipitates discomfort, along with the temptation towards containing and smoothing out disruption as we meet it in the field and in the academy. In their historical concern with classification, coding, neat trajectories, and conclusions, the white, cisheteropatriarchal ways of knowing that dominate the academy's epistemic space mandate precisely this regulation of disruption. And yet, moments of disruption also present junctures from which we might cultivate *response-ability* (Haraway, 2016), eliciting ethical psychosocial engagements with our disrupted world.

Responding to the disruption we inevitably meet demands methodological creativity and epistemological criticality. Yet the modes of thought and practice enabled by this kind of intellectual labour have often been figured as antithetical to science (perhaps then even to Knowledge itself) in the Western academe. The scientific method is figured as offering a privileged access to a "reality," to which other ways of knowing are considered supplementary at best. Writing on physics, Isabelle Stengers (2005, p. 184) rejects the idea that physics is equivalent to reason itself *and* the idea that physics is "just like any other" social practice. No practice, Stengers argues, can be defined as "like any other": "just as no living species is like any other" (Ibid.). This recognition, for Stengers, is the first step towards realising an *ecology of practices* (Ibid.). Taking seriously the distinct contributions of different knowledge practices—especially in their generative confluences and frictions—helps us to understand the world in its complexity and multiplicity.

As a field founded on transdisciplinarity, perhaps psychosocial studies is already an ecology of practices. The entrenched separation of the psyche and the social pervades any discipline concerned with subjectivity and/or sociality: as such, the psycho/social binary permeates diffusely through the arts, humanities, social sciences, and natural sciences, as well as our day-to-day *habits of being* (hooks, 1990, p. 25). Scholars and practitioners from across diverse fields of knowledge production frequently find themselves navigating psychosocial problematics, whether overtly or implicitly. As an emergent field, psychosocial studies thus offers a meeting place for a diverse range of scholars and practitioners. Yet, thinking generatively together between and across epistemologies does not happen automatically. It takes work: a psychosocial praxis.

The psychosocial—as a field, as an analytic, and as praxis—is, in a sense, built on creative disruption. Its very existence disrupts the entrenched, Eurocentric separation of the "individual" psyche from the social, challenging the underpinnings of a number of established disciplines. Psychosocial studies therefore offers a particularly potent nexus from which to creatively respond to—and perhaps purposefully harness and refigure—the inevitable disruption we encounter. In meeting at the psychosocial, we collectively tend fertile ground from which to navigate transdisciplinarity, explore capacious subject matter, and deepen our ethical commitments. A psychosocial praxis implores us to create and hold space for forms of knowledge that the Western academe might otherwise construe as contentious, invalid, or contaminating. A psychosocial praxis asks us to stay disruptive; to stay true to the field's disruptive foundations.

But has this provocation been taken up with the commitment it requires thus far? (Fig. 1.3).

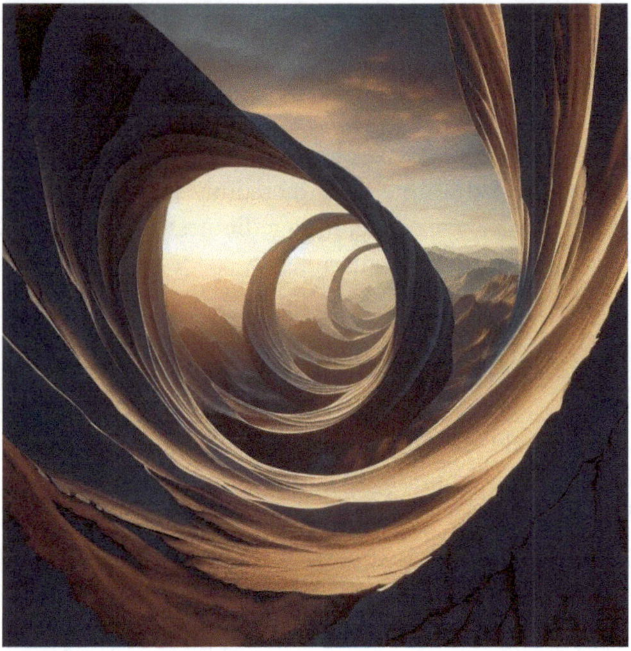

Fig. 1.3 A Möbius strip-like form winding its way through the landscape. Generated with Bing's Image Creator

Clau: Psychosocial Cracks

> [...] but the world doesn't so much stop as it cracks. What cracked is our perception of the world, how we relate to it, how we engage with it. Afterward we view reality differently—we see through its *rendijas* (holes) to the illusion of consensual reality. The world as we know it "ends." We experience a radical shift in perception, otra forma de ver. (Anzaldúa, 2015, p. 15)

Dominant systems make so much and so many impossible. We have to fight for some of us to be possible. So much that has come to wrapped in fatalism—gender fatalism, institutional fatalism: girls will be girls; boys, boys; institutions, institutions. [...] Possibility can take the longest time because to make something possible requires dismantling what makes it

> not so. This is why possibility is not plucked out of thin air. Possibility comes from intimacy with what has thickened in time, the walls, the doors, how rooms are occupied, making it hard to breathe. (Ahmed, 2023, p. 210)

Perhaps paradoxically, the psychosocial is, for me, something that is quite concrete and, at the same time, incredibly slippery. I experience the psychosocial as a space to explore, in togetherness, ambiguities, frictions, and hopes. In the liminal, transdisciplinary space that psychosocial studies offers, where different theories and praxes come together, I found room to *stay with the trouble* (Haraway, 2016) of my questions and to observe how these were not just the fruit of an academic interest detached from myself. Rather, what I have been asking myself has increasingly revealed itself to hold deep psychosocial embroilment with intimate and personal conundrums around gender, masculinities, collectivity, and utopia. Oscillating between personal-academic-political, the psychosocial offered a theoretical, but also very tangible, space for me to move across disciplines and through different non-academic spaces (theatre companies, activist collectives, etc.). In this transdisciplinary wandering, at times deeply focused but mostly aimless and loopy, I have met thinkers, colleagues, activists, artists (also *artartivist*), and friends whose work prompted a need—or rather a recognition of an already present desire—to think-do in togetherness more than in any other more "traditional" and "proper" academic format. My longing for being with others while asking myself questions bigger than myself and greater than my research has been accompanied by a simultaneous suspension of the need to produce and excel in my studies. I have increasingly opted for collective, participatory, and caring ways of learning-practicing together.

Yet, while suggesting, with these paragraphs, that such research is profoundly different from positivist, traditional, neoliberal, and individualistic ways of researching, it is also not a new way of doing research. Researching is always relational. And while some universalistic epistemologies still claim a view from nowhere, we are always situated. Our assumptions, ideas, and insights always stem from the time and space we move through. We are never alone when we ask questions. Accompanied by the words of authors who before us have sought to explore similar fields, we move along intertwined paths, assuming the responsibilities that come with these inheritances. We are guided by supervisors and mentors and inspired by friends, flatmates, colleagues, participants, and many others who touch our work in more or less tangible ways. As we think with past and present collaborators, we create the space for further collaborations with our potential future readers.

This rich non-linear temporality also prompted me to start this personal reflection with the words of thinkers who have deeply inspired my thinking these past years. Their words point to a need to crack, fight against, and undo oppressive systems that produce universalistic knowledges, which violently define our bodies in terms that don't suit us; regulate our wishes, desires, and relationships; truncate and eradicate ourselves from complex ecologies made up of human and non-human relations.

Leaving my BA in Psychology wounded—seeing, together with three other colleagues, my BA thesis rejected as it was deemed not psychological enough—I continued my studies with a need for redemption. I wanted to prove that I wasn't the diligent but unclever student I was often told I was. Yet, I found that this brought only sporadic and short-lived "satisfaction" and mainly an insurmountable amount of anxiety, burnout, and isolation.

Now, as I write this somewhat messy reflection on what the psychosocial means to me, I feel that those who mostly helped me to move away from those experiences of unworthiness, anxiety, and desire to succeed were those I encountered through/in the psychosocial. They were authors like Gloria Anzaldúa, Sara Ahmed, Jack Halberstam, and Judith Butler, but also my teachers, lecturers, and colleagues. To the latter, I feel profoundly indebted, as they have continued to show me that there are other ways of researching—with their projects, their enriching critiques, and insights while reading together/researching or offering feedback on my thinking. While such collegial relationships are often fraught with competition and rivalry, I mostly encountered supporting and nurturing environments.

So, in asking myself once more: what does the psychosocial mean to me? I wonder whether the psychosocial is a space where we gather after cracks and disruptions emerge. A space from which we might begin to unpick the unquestionable Truths that Knowledge in Academia promotes. A space to remain with what has been splintered, snapped, and broken and where we might be capable of withstanding (and look for) tensions and ambiguities. If so, might it be that psychosocial ways of coming together as researchers/artists/activists/therapists/etc. are also informed by the intolerable institutional and academic restrictions and wounds we have accumulated and actively sought to tend to and heal? Could the psychosocial be a space where we labour to collectively imagine, create, and enact different possibilities in our wounded selves, communities, and times?

Disrupting Destruction

The theme of creative disruption emerged in conversation while planning a conference as part of the Department of Psychosocial Studies at Birkbeck, University of London. We were brought together by our interest in exploring the potential of non-traditional methodologies and toyed with the idea of having either "creative" or "disruptive" in the conference title: *creative disruption* emerged as a hybrid term which went on to pose further analytical questions. Only later did we learn that creative disruption is an established concept in the marketing world, itself following the Marx-derived concept of *creative destruction,* popularised by Joseph Schumpeter (1942/2003).

According to Schumpeter (1942/2003, pp. 82–83), "[T]he fundamental impulse that sets and keeps the capitalist engine in motion comes from the new consumers' goods, the new methods of production or transportation, the new markets, the new forms of industrial organization that capitalist enterprise creates." Capitalism sweeps up the old as it generates the new, clearing the ground as if life and death were its own inventions. More recently, marketing professionals have reimagined creative destruction as creative *disruption* (Dru, 1996). As a technique, this refers to purposeful attempts to break conventional patterns of behaviour (in the market or within businesses) to accelerate sales or growth; proponents claim that disruptive advertising campaigns are "more effective, more intrusive because they represent a profound break with the status quo" (Dru, 1996, p. vii). Writing on his *disruption* methodology, marketing executive Jean-Marie Dru argues that "companies must create new worlds. They must constantly do, undo and redo" (Ibid.). While disruption puts a palatable spin on destruction, the theoretical and ethical orientations of these conceptualisations are aligned. The older, less technologically sophisticated, or less marketable paradigm is destroyed or disrupted, and displaced with a more "advanced" set of market relations or consumer trend. The teleological trajectory is a relentless onward march to progress.

As David Harvey (2007, p. 35) has noted, neoliberal cycles of creative destruction are only possible through "the wholesale commodification of nature in all its forms." Capitalism's creative destruction incessantly cycles through new industrial paradigms of efficiency and intensification. Often, this depends on extracting natural resources more quickly and more violently. In the Western academy, we frequently see this same extractive impulse applied as research practice (Cruz & Luke, 2020; Szeman & Wenzel, 2021). Participants are seen from a distance as sources of extractable data rather than as collaborators to co-create with in proximity.

Our psychosocial commitments prompt us, the authors, to resist capitalism's pervasive hold on life itself: on the psyche and the (more-than-human) social. As Walter Mignolo (2009, p. 161) has highlighted, "[D]ecolonial options start from the principle that the *regeneration* of life shall prevail over primacy of the *production and reproduction* of goods at the cost of life." How, we wonder, might we carve out space to create that does not depend on violently displacing what is already there—epistemologically and materially? How can we generate "work" that feeds something other than the market? From where do we feed that work? What resources do we have—and what resources do we need?

This volume tentatively attempts to reclaim creative disruption. Rather than reducing the creative to a tool for capitalist "innovation," and disruption to an instrumentalising device that makes this possible, we attempt to gather the remnant threads of radical possibility that creative disruption might offer. Whereas a special issue of the *Journal of Arts Management, Law, and Society* leant into creative disruption as "incessantly destroying the old while incessantly creating the new" (Borrup, 2018, p. 226), we ask after a different ethical and temporal orientation. The various contributions twist, fray, and reweave these into a different kind of disruptive gesture. Rather than hurtling ever faster to the future, could we generatively inhabit multiple temporalities which creatively disrupt the former? How might creative disruption draw us instead into *relations of care* in which "the present is dense, thickened with a multiplicity of entangled and involved timelines rather than compressed and subordinated to the linear achievement of future output"? (Puig de la Bellacasa, 2017, 203). How can we do justice to our psycho/social inheritances, while staying with—and creatively responding to—the trouble they carry with them?

Here, we name the relentless *hegemonic timescape* of progressivist timelines (Puig de la Bellacasa, 2017, p. 174)—and its epistemological underpinnings—as an object of *our* creative disruption. Stengers (Stengers, 2005, p. 185) has highlighted the shared underpinnings of capitalism's relentless clearing of the ground (for itself) and epistemological movements towards clearing the ground for specific disciplines and concepts to dominate. Conversely, attuning to the transdisciplinarity of psychosocial studies asks us to stay with the problem of how each practice might "foster its own force, make present what causes practitioners to think and feel and act" (Stengers, 2005, pp. 186, 195). At the same time, psychosocial transdisciplinarity asks us to embrace those moments when boundaries dissolve, to let practices mingle, to reconstitute each other, sometimes even to become unmappable within a more established disciplinary schema.

Whereas the hegemonic timescape demands that we don't "waste time" pondering epistemological concerns and simply get on with being productive, we insist that unpacking different knowledge practices, and the ways in which they intersect, is necessary—and takes time. In staying with the challenge of forging transdisciplinary epistemological space, the contributors to this volume variously experiment with an ethics of creative disruption that moves at speeds at which *multispecies knots of ethical time* (Rose, 2012) can flourish. Across and in the cracks between these contributions, this volume begins to realise creative disruption as an ethical psychosocial praxis (Fig. 1.4).

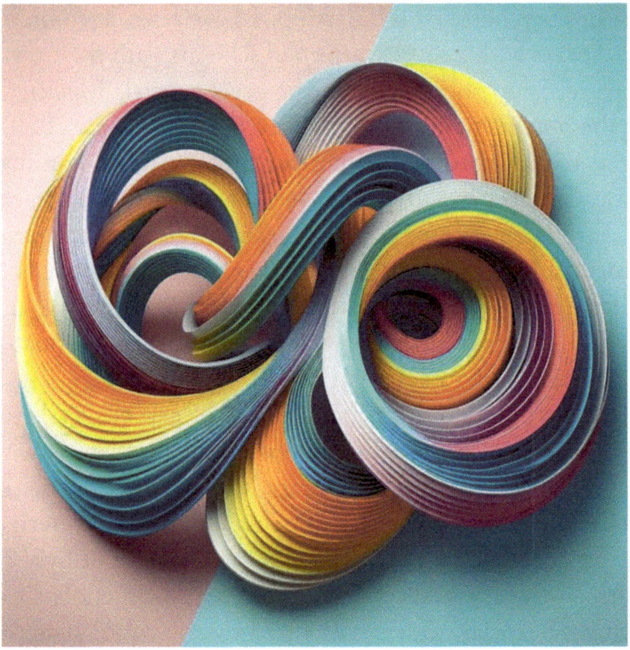

Fig. 1.4 A Möbius strip-like shape winds incessantly into itself. Generated with Bing's Image Creator

Hannah: An Endless Loop?

For me, the draw of psychosocial studies was the way in which the field's very existence already implies a critique and mode of analysis. As a queer and neurodivergent woman who has felt utterly let down by the individualising mode of Western psychiatry, psychosocial studies offered a ground from which to reclaim some critical agency. How different the world looks when internal (psyche) and external (social) are no longer a given. How radically different do our ethical obligations to each other look when we interrogate this entrenched binary? What tools do we need to make sense of such a world that are not yet, or not fully, available to us? Naming the psychosocial offers a point around which such burgeoning or overlooked practices—and those who are committed to developing them—can gravitate.

In pursuing psychosocial scholarship, I have been honoured to share intellectual spaces with a diverse group of scholars with their own distinct connections to, and conceptions of, the psychosocial. Together, we have inhabited the *productive frictions* (Jokinen & Nordstrom, 2020) that the psychosocial makes possible. Often, we find ourselves communicating across vast differences in our respective subject matter and in the bodies of theory that inform our various approaches. Yet, what the psychosocial tends to inevitably foreground is collective attention to issues of ethics, positionality, justice—and subtlety. Here, it feels, is where we most often find our common ground, from which we cultivate personal-political-intellectual solidarity across difference.

For all the disruptive potential and praxis of psychosocial studies as a transdisciplinary space, I nonetheless stew on the problem of whether the field can ever really transgress the binary it seeks to challenge. I wonder, does the term "psychosocial" itself somehow imply some eternal reiteration of the psycho/social binary, even without the slash or hyphen? In the Möbius strip, we see inside/outside surfaces flowing endlessly into one another. Is psychosocial studies structured this way too? If so, how far is psychosocial studies capable of thinking liminally *between* the psycho/social? What constitutes this liminal space from within and *outside* the psycho/social? What (and how many) other "surfaces" might be possible, necessary, or already nascent? Might we need to think with additional dimensions to truly overturn the psycho/social binary? If so, what are they and where might they lead us?

Psychosocial studies already attracts and is constituted by scholars from a range of disciplinary backgrounds, not just psychology and sociology, as the name might suggest. The "psy" in psychosocial directs me to foreground the production of subjectivity in my work; it asks me to attend to the "contact zones" (Haraway, 2008) through which I navigate the field. More broadly, though, the "psy" in psychosocial does seem to ensure that psychosocial thinking remains in some way bound to the "psy" disciplines and theories: psychology, psychiatry, psychoanalysis. These are areas of study I do not directly engage with in my own work; often, their practices sit uncomfortably with me for intellectual and personal reasons. Perhaps this discomfort is the psychosocial provocation I have, as yet, neglected to stay with. On the other hand, I remain committed to forging out more space for thinking subjectivity and sociality without the psy-disciplines.

All this said, aligning oneself with psychosocial studies is also riddled with the pragmatic constraints. If we think psychosocially but not with the psy-disciplines, where will our work be recognised and who will employ us? This question now takes on an additional urgency with the dissolution of the Department of Psychosocial Studies at Birkbeck, which provided a hub for psychosocial thinking that was, perhaps, unparalleled in its commitment to the transdisciplinarity of the field (Fig. 1.5).[1]

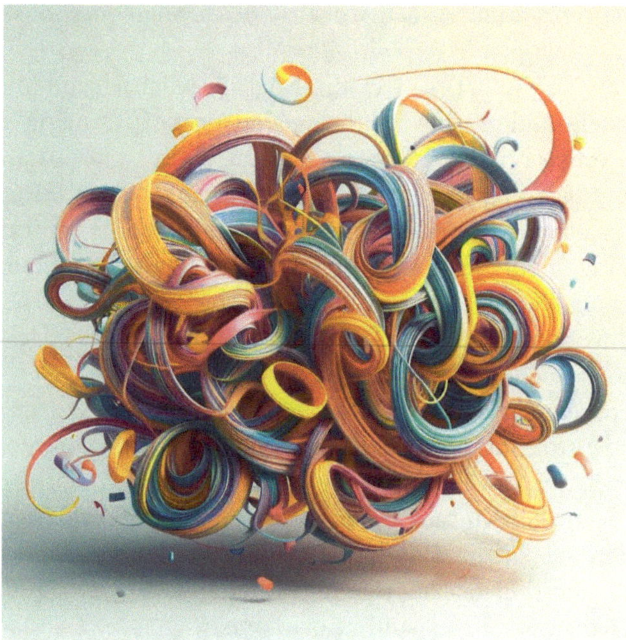

Fig. 1.5 The form of the Möbius strip pushed to its limits. Generated with Bing's Image Creator

[1] In 2023, Birkbeck underwent a college-level restructure, resulting in the Department of Psychosocial Studies (along with a number of other previously distinct departments) being absorbed into the new School of Social Sciences. In preparation for the restructure, in 2022, Birkbeck's senior management announced 140 proposed job cuts (Weale, 2023), triggering large numbers of academic and administrative staff to take voluntary redundancy.

Overview of Chapters: (Un)tracing Creative Disruption

This collection introduces new and emerging voices in psychosocial scholarship, from within and beyond academia and the clinic. Collectively, the authors offer a frame of reference through which creative disruption can be realised as psychosocial praxis. Their contributions grapple with moments of disruption as sites of discomfort, discontent, and dis-ease. Working across queer theory, disability studies, psychoanalysis, postcolonial studies, black feminism, whiteness studies, and anti-racist critique, the authors explore creative disruption through questions of power, knowledge, allyship, and responsibility.

To begin, in Chap. 2 Leila Lawton, Michelle Michael, and John Adlam performatively guide us through their experiences of "Dancing the Dance of Disruption" as NHS workers in a structurally racist healthcare system. Yet, as the authors highlight, while their chapter plays with language as a means of creatively disrupting white dominance and its institutionalisation, nothing about this play with language is "for pleasure or leisure" (Lawton et al., see Chap. 2). The authors unpack what it is to take on the emotional work of anti-racism "from inside, but from the edge" (Lawton et al., see Chap. 2) of the institution.

Chapter 3, co-authored by Ayelen Hamity and Daniela Larraín-Salas, invites readers to consider "Echoes of the Other Language," interrogating power, translation, and liminality by placing ideas and theories emerging from the South (specifically, Latin America) into dialogue with others developed in the North. In so doing, Hamity and Larraín-Salas (re)examine the (dis)location of language and geographies from a psychosocial perspective that seeks to expand its own praxis.

From here, the volume shifts to Dwight Turner's Chap. 4, "Being Black Freud." Turner foregrounds the work of the black activists within psychology, counselling, and psychotherapy who have escalated their struggle against white supremacy in their professions since the murder of George Floyd in 2020. Offering a heuristic exploration of the responsibilities, pitfalls, and pain of being a black activist, Turner considers the role of community, colonial ideas of the individual, and the experience of imposed and internalised hate that comes with being a black activist.

The next contribution (Chap. 5), from Rayann Bryan, takes a turn in affective emphasis, instead calling readers to consider the possibilities and challenges of "Doing Love in Research." Elaborating bell hooks' (2018) work on love, Bryan argues for black feminist research as an act of love—an exploration of personal identity, healing, and transformation—while staying with the question of how far it is truly possible to do love within the institutional constraints of academia.

In Chap. 6, "Playing with Brexit," Tom Fielder explores creative praxis as a way to elaborate psychosocial thinking about Brexit. By engaging with notions of performance, theatricality, and play through different writing registers, Fielder poses questions about knowledge production in psychosocial studies, drawing attention to the limitations of more conventional modes of academic "performance."

Offering a sometimes overlapping, sometimes divergent consideration of play, Chap. 7, "On Creative Destruction," by Sasha Bergstrom-Katz stretches Donald Winnicott's (2010) theory of "object relating," to work with play, destruction, and creation, as a research methodology: in this case, to study an intelligence test kit. Specifically, Bergstrom-Katz illuminates two practice-based projects staged in the hope of "getting to understand" the tests by playing with others: firstly, through an immersive exhibition display wherein guests were invited to explore and play-with a series of games and tests; and secondly, in one-on-one interviews wherein the test objects were made responsible for directing the form of the conversation.

Chapter 8, by Robert Chapman and Micha Frazer-Carroll, unpacks "Long Covid and the Politics of Disablement." Considering the mass disabling caused by the emergence and prevalence of long Covid, the chapter contends that this can also be understood as a mass neurodivergifying event. While emphasising that this has been destructive for many, the authors also consider that this mass neurodivergifying might open up creative possibilities for a new politics of disablement.

Further unpacking the potential of neurodiversity, Chap. 9, "Involuntary Attention as Creative Disruption," from Hannah Reeves, offers a contemplation on the implications of neurodiverse sociality for psychosocial studies, arguing that a neurodiverse sociality is already a more-than-human sociality. Drawing on her experience of doing auto/ethnography at a burial ground and "wild" garden of remembrance as a neurodivergent researcher, Reeves problematises neurotypically humanist paradigms of social research and makes tentative gestures towards materialising neurodivergent strategies.

Chapter 10, "The Clinician as Killjoy (Without Killing Joy)," from Rebecca Esho Greenslade brings us back to a perhaps more typical site of psychosocial struggle: the clinic. Drawing on Sara Ahmed's (2017) figure of the feminist killjoy, Esho Greenslade examines both the ethical urgency and the challenges of killjoy work within clinical practice. Esho Greenslade investigates the role of killjoy clinicians in making room for alternative therapeutic possibilities of solidarity aimed at disrupting the legacies of harm and dehumanisation that continue to haunt the psy-disciplines, going on to articulate the ethical, therapeutic, and revolutionary potential of a clinical killjoy praxis.

Staying with the clinic, Chap. 11, "Creative Disruptions with/in Psychoanalysis," by Arturo Bandinelli and Iris Aleida Pinzón Arteaga interrogates the potentials and limitations of psychoanalysis as a creatively disruptive psychosocial theory and practice in the context of late neoliberal societies. Considering the work of Jack Halberstam—both his *Queer Art of Failure* (2011) and his conversation with Marie-Hélène Brousse (Halberstam & Brousse, 2016), the authors engage with forgetting and stupidity to explore the disruptive potential of psychoanalytic praxis.

Shifting gears into a radically different mode of analysis, in Chap. 12, "The Heart of Rhythm: Congolese Music as Creative Disruption," Guilaine Kinouani foregrounds the disruptive potential of Congolese rhythms and dancing, arguing that their sensuality has the potential to make space within psychosocial studies for alternative imaginaries and onto-epistemological practices. Exploring this disruptive space through poetic and analytical writing, Kinouani asserts the power of Congolese rhythms in challenging modernist, masculinist, and Eurocentric ways of being in the word.

Chapter 13, "Nonprofits, Black and White Women's Power Dynamics Through an Antebellum Lens," from Janedra Sykes, uses critical fabulation (Hartman, 2008) to unpack the "Mammy and Mistress trope," a power dynamic present in black, white, cis-gendered female relationships in American nonprofit workplaces. Drawing on the author's professional experience and research in American nonprofit organisations, the chapter explores a scene from an American melodrama, *Imitation of Life*, made in 1934, considering the overt and covert mechanisms through which black women in nonprofits are required to perform as the Mammy for white women.

Adding another layer of critical consideration of racialised dynamics, in Chap. 14, "Waking Up from Whiteness," Nancy Blair, Els van Ooijen, Halina Pytlasinska, Jennifer Ramsay, and Jane Ribbens McCarthy collectively explore their whiteness and the cisheteropatriarchal, racialised systems within which their whiteness occurs. Aiming to creatively disturb their whiteness, the authors set to investigate this topic collectively, experimenting with creativity and other dreamwork methods from psychotherapy and counselling. They remember, share, analyse, and build on their dreams, so as to seek new possibilities beyond the individual preoccupations of their Anglophone worldviews.

Picking up various orientations touched upon throughout the volume, in Chap. 15, "Collaborative Fragmentation," Clau di Gianfrancesco and Elena Gkivisi read Bracha Ettinger's (2006, 2020) matrixial theory with and through queer and anti-racist theories and practices. In so doing, the authors investigate the points of connection, friction, and creative potentiality running through these theories. Through their engagements, di Francesco and Gkivisi offer a matrixially informed style of writing where moments of creative disruption can be collectively practised and where rigid and oppressive definitions of subjectivity may be subverted.

Finally, as Guilaine Kinouani draws the volume to a close with her Afterword on "Epistemic Disruption, the Creative and Liberation," she draws the reader in the disturbance which permeated the project, requiring of us to leave the encounter as disturbed witnesses. We are forced to rethink ideas we may have taken for granted, the "trans" aspiration of the psychosocial, the possibility of being free from "the past" and of disrupting the very systems we have so passionately critiqued. Haunted by what has been, Kinouani observes a profound liberatory paradox: the need to bear witness thus to confront suffering and death to be able to draw from the forces of life to theorise, resist, and experience joy. A duality which is at the core, thus, of creative disruption.

References

Ahmed, S. (2006). *Queer Phenomenology: Orientations, Objects, Others*. Duke University Press. Retrieved from http://ebookcentral.proquest.com/lib/bbk/detail.action?docID=1169326

Ahmed, S. (2017). *Living A Feminist Life*. Duke University Press.

Ahmed, S. (2023). *The Feminist Killjoy Handbook*. Allen Lane.

Anzaldúa, G. (2015). *Light in the Dark/Luz en lo Oscuro: Rewriting Identity, Spirituality, Reality*. Duke University Press.

Borrup, T. (2018). Creative Disruption in the Arts-Special Issue Introduction. *The Journal of Arts Management, Law, and Society, 48*(4), 223–226. https://doi.org/10.1080/10632921.2018.1497392

Castro-Gómez, S. (2021). *Zero-Point Hubris: Science, Race, and Enlightenment in Eighteenth-Century Latin America*. Rowman & Littlefield.

Coly, A. A. (2019). *Postcolonial Hauntologies: African Women's Discourses of the Female Body*. University of Nebraska Press.

Cruz, M., & Luke, D. (2020). Methodology and Academic Extractivism: The Neo-colonialism of the British University. *Third World Thematics: A TWQ Journal, 5*(1–2), 154–170. https://doi.org/10.1080/23802014.2020.1798275

Dru, J.-M. (1996). *Disruption: Overturning Conventions and Shaking Up the Marketplace*. Wiley.

Ettinger, B. (2020). *Matrixial Subjectivity, Aesthetics, Ethics, Volume I 1990–2000*. Palgrave Macmillan.

Ettinger, B., & Ettinger, B. (2006). *The Matrixial Borderspace*. University of Minnesota Press.

feministkilljoys. (2018, November 8). Queer Use. *Feministkilljoys*. Retrieved from https://feministkilljoys.com/2018/11/08/queer-use/

Finley, S. (2008). Arts-Based Research. In J. G. Knowles & A. L. Cole (Eds.), *Handbook of the Arts in Qualitative Research: Perspectives, Methodologies, Examples, and Issues*. Sage. https://doi.org/10.4135/9781452226545

Frosh, S. (2013). Psychoanalysis, Colonialism, Racism. *Journal of Theoretical and Philosophical Psychology, 33*(3), 141–154. https://doi.org/10.1037/a0033398

Halberstam, J. (2011). *The Queer Art of Failure*. Duke University Press.

Halberstam, J., & Brousse, M.-H. (2016). Queering Psychoanalysis: A Dialogue Between Jack Halberstam and Marie-Hélène Brousse. *The Lacanian Review, 2*, 2–29.

Haraway, D. (2008). *When Species Meet*. University of Minnesota Press.
Haraway, D. (2016). *Staying with the Trouble: Making Kin in the Chthulucene*. Duke University Press.
Hartman, S. (2008). Venus in Two Acts. *Small Axe, 12*(2), 1–14.
Harvey, D. (2007). Neoliberalism as Creative Destruction. *The Annals of the American Academy of Political and Social Science, 610*, 22–44.
hooks, b. (1990). *YEARNING: Race, Gender and Cultural Politics*. South End Press.
hooks, b. (2018). *All About Love: New Visions*. William Morrow.
Ingold, T. (2015). *The Life of Lines*. Routledge.
Ingold, T. (2022). *Being Alive: Essays on Movement, Knowledge and Description*. Routledge.
Jokinen, P., & Nordstrom, S. (2020). A Queer Cyborg Ethnographer in the Performative Friction of Dissenting Ontologies. *Qualitative Inquiry, 26*(6), 1077800420912796. https://doi.org/10.1177/1077800420912796
Mignolo, W. D. (2009). Epistemic Disobedience, Independent Thought and Decolonial Freedom—Walter D. Mignolo, 2009. *Theory, Culture and Society, 26*(2–8), 159–181.
Puig de la Bellacasa, M. (2017). *Matters of Care*. University of Minnesota Press.
Rose, D. B. (2012). Multispecies Knots of Ethical Time. *Environmental Philosophy, 9*(1), 127–140.
Schumpeter, J. A. (2003). *Capitalism, Socialism and Democracy*. Routledge. (Original work published 1942).
Stengers, I. (2005). Introductory Notes on an Ecology of Practices. *Cultural Studies Review, 11*(1), 1. https://doi.org/10.5130/csr.v11i1.3459
Szeman, I., & Wenzel, J. (2021). What Do We Talk about When We Talk about Extractivism? *Textual Practice, 35*(3), 505–523. https://doi.org/10.1080/0950236X.2021.1889829
Weale, S. (2023, November 13). Dismay at Threat of 'Devastating' Job Cuts at Birkbeck, University of London. *The Guardian*. Retrieved from https://www.theguardian.com/education/2022/nov/13/dismay-at-threat-of-devastating-job-cuts-at-birkbeck-university-of-london
Winnicott, D. W. (2010). *Playing and Reality* (Reprint). Routledge.

2

Dancing the Dance of Disruption

Leila Lawton, Michelle Michael, and John Adlam

Introduction

We-the-authors (respectively, a female Ugandan British psychotherapist, a female working-class British-Jamaican psychologist (awaiting registration) and a privately educated White European male) work in the UK National Health Service (NHS) in a multicultural urban setting. To this statement of our positionality, we would add that we operate as agents of the State—we draw a salary from the State, implement or enforce its laws and reproduce its discourses—in a structurally racist healthcare system.[1]

[1] By "structurally racist" we specifically mean that the organisational structures and operation of power and force within the NHS discriminate against and oppress racially minoritised people. Ethnic inequalities and structural racism in mental health care generally are now well documented (see e.g. Lawrence, 2020; NHS Race and Health Observatory, 2023; Aiyegbusi, 2023). This chapter has racism and racialisation as its focus—this is not to disregard other intersectionalities and oppressions, for example, along axes of gender or class.

L. Lawton • M. Michael • J. Adlam (✉)
NHS, London, UK

G. Kinouani et al. (eds.), *Creative Disruption*, Studies in the Psychosocial,
https://doi.org/10.1007/978-3-031-63661-5_2

In this chapter we interrogate the ethical challenges involved both in representing such systems in the culturally diverse communities we serve and in seeking to disrupt—from inside, but from the edge—the dominant discourses of the organisation which employs us. NHS workplaces are "dilemmatic spaces" (Honig, 1996) which contain inherent contradictions and antinomies (the NHS being socialistic in conception and capitalistic in implementation; egalitarian in its offer to be free at the point of access to all parts of a vast and diverse community, yet hierarchical in structure, racialised and toxically othering in practice). They are therefore psychosocial settings that are frequently experienced as *hostile environments* (Lawton & Adlam, 2021; Scanlon & Adlam, 2022). In such circumstances, *anti-racist* practices (Kendi, 2019) of creative disruption become *necessary*.

bell hooks ([1994] 2006, p. 105), discussing the anti-feminist backlash of the late 1980s and early 1990s, argued that "[t]he time has come to interrupt, intervene, and change the channel"; she wrote vividly of her fear of punishment, censorship, and ostracism from both Left and Right for speaking out on the intersections of race and gender and class and power. In our own discussions we foreground the intense emotional work of what we think of as "dancing the dance of disruption," and we attempt to map some of the challenges and surprises of staying in the dance. We note that a little hope can sometimes be a dangerous thing.

Finding your voice in the rubble of sorrow and grief whilst fighting a battle you didn't choose is no small feat. Speaking out in "vulnerable spaces" evokes extreme emotional responses and pressure either to appease, smooth over and disperse fragile "awkwardness" or to allow yourself to be silenced (Eddo-Lodge, 2018). Examining and unpicking your own survival strategies highlights how you have moulded yourself to be able to cope (Snyder, 2016). In challenging these ways of keeping safe, it makes it imaginable that you might be able to navigate the shark-infested waters of a racialised society while incorporating your true authentic self within the work role—and inviting others to do the same.

Mbembe urges that "in a contemporary neoliberal order that claims to have gone beyond the racial, the struggle for racial justice must take new forms" (Mbembe [2010] 2021, p. 41). The top-down, corporatist roll-out of policies promoting the anti-racist practice in the organisation needs to be creatively disrupted "from the edge" to give it bite and meaning, lest it become just another move that reproduces Whiteness. This said, we also ask how we may credit ourselves with *actual or effective* practices of "creative disruption," when there is no tangible evidence that structural racism in the NHS has been meaningfully disrupted. In the spirit of ethical consistency, we aim to see if we can also creatively disrupt the conventions and structures of how chapters in books such as this one ordinarily get written.

We discuss various experiences of working within a loose grouping of activist colleagues. These are experiences of making moves to disrupt discourses and reproductions of Whiteness embedded in the structures and practices which sustain racism and racialisation within the organisation. Some of these steps in the dance have "landed" and had a significant impact; many have been pushed back against. In order to maintain confidentiality, and with one eye on those pushbacks, we have chosen not to spell out the particular initiatives we have in mind.

The durability of reproductions of Whiteness—in Kinouani's words, "the production and reproduction of the dominance, and privileges of people racialized as white" (Kinouani, 2019, p. 62)—may partly stem from the ruthlessness with which the in-group acts in one of two directions. Either it incorporates by offering honorary membership (brings into the fold, White-washes) or it scapegoats, marginalises or expels would-be disruptors so that they can no longer disrupt (and here the ancient and dreadful dynamics of "Field" and "House" from the times of slavery and the plantations are still active and operative).[2] How therefore do we know that we are being disruptive, or how disruptive we are being? We glimpse here an underlying tension: we may need to sustain our sense of having been and continually being disrupted, in order to be and to remain disruptive.

Throughout this chapter, we play with the languages of the dance. However, in case there is any doubt in the reader's mind, nothing about

---

[2] The French anthropologist Claude Lévi-Strauss identified two violent societal defensive responses to difference and the fear of difference: the "anthropophagic," in which the feared difference is eliminated by violently swallowing up the Other within the body of the in-group; and the "anthropoemic," in which the feared difference is evacuated or expelled beyond the borders (Levi-Strauss, 1955; Scanlon & Adlam, 2022, pp. 105–107).

it is for pleasure or leisure. The dance of anti-racist disruption is potentially a lethal one: the consequences of any mis-steps are often much more like *Squid Games* (2021) than *Saturday Night Fever* (1977).[3]

First Dance

When dancing the dance of disruption, watch where you place your feet. When you feel the flow and the rhythm; best you make subtle suggestions; in how you change your position so that your oppressor doesn't slow … you down.

Ensure that your partner doesn't see you as too powerful or too opinionated, so at times put your head down and let them take the lead.

Whom to trust? Keep your eyes open at all times, watch your step and don't talk too much. On the dance floor be mindful of others who may be watching, reviewing your moves, even those who smile may not be your allies.

Consider where you place your back, so that your view is not restricted, best to avoid gliding; in favour of keeping your back against the wall.

You can fail to keep your balance in the face of a key protagonist's indirect request to remove yourself from the dancefloor. This is metamorphosed by heated communications, the firm application of pressure through carefully constructed letters and forceful words. You can be forced to change your position; stop moving to your own rhythm.

However, there is strength in a pause which cultivates skill in artfully executed moves, strategic tools in allies. You have to rest, recuperate and revive. Then take up your position once more. There must always be an encore.

The Dance of Creative Disruption

Toni Morrison stated that "[t]he world does not become raceless or will not become unracialized by assertion. The act of enforcing racelessness … is itself a racial act" (Morrison, 1992, p. 46). She adds that

[3] In the television series *Squid Games*, would-be gameshow winners in search of a bonanza prize discover that the losers at each stage of the contest are instantly killed. We would like to report that we have all the dancefloor moves of a Travolta—or that we float like butterflies and sting like bees, as Muhammad Ali used to dance—but the reality is altogether different.

> the slave's own narrative, while freeing the narrator in many ways, did not destroy the master narrative. The master narrative could make any number of adjustments to keep itself intact. (1992, pp. 50–51)

Manifestations of the transgenerational transmission of racialisation and racial trauma are viscerally present across the organisation and embodied in every encounter, and molecules of projected shame and aggression are the air that we breathe.

Make your point, by all means (thus runs the messaging), about "cultural diversity"—we the oh-so-enlightened liberal "civilised" in-group give you our blessing and are all ears—just don't make it "aggressively." "We" do not care to be reminded of our own violence. We will turn on you in a flash to remind you of our own limitless capacity for fear-fuelled hatred, if you should presume to break those unwritten rules of the dance that we have set for you. You can play for "our" football team; but miss a penalty and our teeth get bared very quickly (see e.g. Guardian, 2021).

For half a millennium, "we" have been terrified of the possibility that you might in your righteous wrath seek a just revenge (after all, chip away only a thin layer of veneer, you will remember that we always found you savage)—"we" therefore strike pre-emptively whenever "we" can. And at the same time "we" can be (sort of) subtle about it: we've been developing our power retention skills base for centuries now. There's no power play quite like an apparently "power-sharing," "co-producing" power play:

> We will incorporate color-ed folks into our fold, whenever possible and at our own pace, provided they're team players, speak highly of us, pretend to care what we're thinking, are highly qualified … but, and this is key, *we won't entertain the rancour which shits on our fantasy space.* (Wilderson III [2008] 2015, p. 409 [our italics])

Whiteness, as Kinouani shows, is "woven into the fabric" of societies such as the UK and "all aspects of 'our' culture, norms, and values centre and privilege white people," although White people may often not be consciously witting to these psychosocial realities (Kinouani, 2019, pp. 62–63).[4]

In short, the dominant discourse of Whiteness is *received*: a given; "common sense" (to deploy a term often lethally weaponised by our political classes in this country to wage racial war upon its citizens). Wilderson III describes

> a way of being in the world which legitimises institutional practices … accepts, and promotes, them as timeless—without origin, consequence, interest, or allegiance—natural and inevitable. (Wilderson III [2008] 2015, p. 407)

This very same Whiteness, which Toni Morrison described as "mute, meaningless, unfathomable, pointless, frozen, veiled, curtained, dreaded, senseless, implacable" (Morrison, 1992, p. 59), is therefore to be understood as the *necessary* object of creative disruption.

Necessity requires us to dig deep, brace ourselves and be courageous. Yet personal life experience teaches us that conversations around oppression and White "supremacism" (indeed, bell hooks' "white supremacist capitalist patriarchy" [hooks [1994] 2006, p. 231])[5] do not come with ease. The thirst for activism has increased; yet "permission" given to discuss race in White spaces has consequences. Fighting for a place at the table only to find that the gatekeepers have given you a low stool. Craning your neck to get peek-a-boo glimpses of policy while your influence is circumscribed to ensure that it fits the dominant agenda. Raising your head to speak and finding it metaphorically patted, invited to be satisfied with the White in-group's ideas about promoting anti-racism.

Formal yet voluntary roles promoting racial justice create visibility within organisations with false implications of power. The role itself speaks to the lack of power experienced across the workforce and the difficulty that established power has in acknowledging the needs of racially

---

[4] We do not mean to suggest that White people are not conscious of their racism. The term "unconscious bias" is used to White-wash many a racialised aggression.

[5] We put this word in inverted commas because its iteration otherwise risks reinforcing the received, transgenerationally transmitted racism inherent in the idea that there could possibly be anything supreme or superior attached to the relative melanin-recessiveness of one's skin (see Brissett, 2023).

minoritised groups within the workforce and the communities that the organisation is there to serve.

When you're in that position of perceived power, this creates visibility on the dance floor. This attracts others to reach out to you because of your visibility and express challenges that they are experiencing, rather than use the mechanisms that are there within the organisation for them to use, because sometimes those mechanisms aren't really fit for purpose. That in itself causes a problem for the people who have and hold and wield the power.

They might attempt to silence you or reduce the level of influence that you have because that wasn't in the script; you weren't supposed to have the influence you now wield. Yes, go and set up that group, but please, don't challenge, don't question, don't raise your voice too loud, lest you be considered to be punching above your weight, going above your station, not knowing your place:

> … many Africans are convinced … that the sort of African that Europe tolerates and accepts is the African whose energies it continually captures and hijacks, one who obeys with the docile fidelity of an animal able to recognize its master once and for all. (Mbembe [2010] 2021, p. 167)

And that in itself is the challenge of the dance, that in itself is the challenge of the contact, and that in itself is the challenge that speaks to racial battle fatigue, that sense of being silenced, that sense of a reality experienced, being denied, doubted, or minimised. People can get tired or burned out and step away from the work that it represents for fear of reprisals, repercussions and lack of security in their day-to-day lives and professional roles. There are all sorts of different ways in which you can be squeezed or squeezed out (Rhead et al. 2020).

So again: how do you do that dance of disruption, or how do you keep up the energy, the flow and the rhythm to stay in step? On the other hand, sometimes you're called to not do what's expected and to not just toe the line: to maintain a dynamic movement seeking to address the issues impacting disparity that have yet to be translated into actions. Advocating for inclusive ways of working, or amplifying voices that are most marginalised—voiceless, unseen, unheard, demoralised and unvalued—can get you a mark put on your back.

How do you attempt to address racism whilst still sustaining raw wounds experienced due to racism; hands and legs again (metaphorically?) tied; your work, intent and passion blocked by sequences of well-rehearsed moves? How do you stay safe, rest, recuperate or revive? You may more than once have to retreat from the dance floor—recognising the requirement to make oneself small in the intervals, to present as though you lack rhythm or flow until once again you can speak out with all the force and pace that is within you.

Is there strength to push back in the face of such limitation and unspoken compromise, to disrupt those well-rehearsed, stately formations that threaten to squeeze you and your demoralised comrades out of the conversation altogether? You are brimful with ideas about infrastructure and operational strategy that are grounded in your long experience of working within the sector. Isn't that bigger than all the egos and corporate power plays? Feedback has been invited—it has been given freely—it has been grudgingly received—but it has not been welcomed. And yet, at the core of it, all we want to do is improve experience, outcomes and access to good mental health provision for the communities that we serve. If that threatens to upset the applecart and disrupt those courtly dances so profoundly, then mastering some new steps becomes imperative.

Second Dance

The favourites on this dance floor stride out confidently and effortlessly and begin their choreographed sequence. The troupe perform their smoothly rehearsed flowing shapes of anti-racist initiatives and rhythmical upcycled policies with an air of concealed triumph and centuries of experience. The professionalism with which they execute such movements and deliver their performance leaves the other(ed) contenders breathless. Even to the disadvantage of an away crowd, they exude a (cultural) competence that is strong and feels risky to rival. The promise of the moves and the hope of the beat momentarily storm up collaborative enthusiasm within the crowd.

The crescendo hits, and the dancefloor ignites and becomes like fire as it becomes enriched by the rhythm of crowd participation. The carnival of lengthy consultations, with staff, patients and carers baring souls, lives lost, vulnerably sharing their tears and pain. The tempo slows and the lights dim, and the troupe ease to a sorrowful pace as they regroup and reform as if in humble reflection.

The finale comes as a surprise (to some), a rather magical illusion of sorts with some smoke and a few mirrors. As the sequence concludes, the troupe offers up a formation created to be seen but not felt. It deftly swirls around and does not disturb the racialised flow, although it can be skilfully moved and displayed where necessary but ingeniously has no lasting trace. It manages to bring about little or no change and mostly (racially) exhausts and silences those it claims to want to protect. The cries of betrayal and protest are silenced with tones of ingratitude and an unwillingness to tune in to the reality. The following act tries not to let the chilling performance, the show of strength, perturb them, and they courageously find their places centre stage.

Footsteps on the Dance Floor

Wilderson III aptly summarises the drive and the dilemma that the organisation we work for pursues and is beset by:

> White people … are guilty of asking themselves the question, How can we maintain the maximum amount of order, with the minimum amount of change, while presenting ourselves … as having the best of all possible intentions. (Wilderson III [2008] 2015, p. 408)

Your presence alone is an act of disruption. To dare to be black or brown and take up White space in White departments is out/cou-rageous (Fields et al. 1998). Unwittingly you have stumbled onto the dancefloor—your disruption: being a minority. You quickly realise that the first dance you're entered into, and find your rhythm to, is the "cultural assimilation fandango." Do you awkwardly but authentically hold your space whilst bearing witness to the White lens of care provided to the Black patients, or do you learn to shimmy off your identity on the dancefloor? While learning the steps of this dance you contemplate the cost to your career (if you don't), and to your developing professional integrity and soul (if you do). Either way, there is no choice but to embark on your career with your dancing shoes on.

Expect your supervisor, your first dance partner, who's supposed to coach and promote your growth, to quickly inform you that your life as a trainee will be more challenging due to being a "person of colour." A pre-dance pep talk perhaps, before they proceed to provide a painful placement experience that adopts an angry and contemptuous supervisory style. Where rehearsal dances swiftly turn into live performances, requests for feedback are labelled "needy" and an inability to work and learn under their intense hostility is labelled a "learning disability." As their disdain for you grows, so do the decorative hives that creep up their necks and become a part of their supervision costume. Nevertheless, they will be delighted in the "elite" placement provision they are providing you and will demand expressions of gratitude for allowing you to dance with them in what they have entitled, "Your baptism of fire."

During these dances, you know that you are defenceless; you are already on the back foot, feared and mistrusted, so there is no choice but to try to keep up and appease. No one will believe you, and they know it. This is the dance. They have the power professionally and intersectionally and know the words to use to annihilate your character. They know the system and the tolerance of the powers backing them. It only takes a few placed moves that easily conjure up Black stereotypes that will see you cast out. As you dance on the eggshells, in your heeled shoes you might wish you had a bodycam to witness your innocence, and the flickers of fear, hatred and contempt in the face of the Other. The perpetrators will gaslight you as their victimiser. Like any narcissistic relationship you cannot react because your reaction will then be the problem and the proof of the problem. As the bullets of truth are shot at your feet, you dance like your career depends upon it.

The setup is like agreeing to play, dance along, and believe in the Emperor's new clothes. So, choosing not always to and holding onto your identity in these White spaces can be viewed as quite affronting, uncooperative and lacking in professionalism. It would mean to metaphorically point out the Emperor's nakedness and induce White shame, fragility and its resulting wrath (Di Angelo, 2011). To echo the patients' experience and corroborate their stories of having to comply or continue to be feared (Rudder, 2023) is a dangerous dance to execute in itself. To further dare to try to address these things for the patients, carers or the staff is another level of madness altogether.

Saidiya Hartman describes a different, but related, kind of dance: a dance she likened to a New York street hustle in which a combination of factors would

> convince you that you had a chance after all and that you were not predator and prey but somehow all in it together. You'd participate in the game knowing that the odds were stacked against you and that in all likelihood you'd walk away having lost what you staked. (Hartman [2007] 2021, p. 88)

In the dance of disruption we are depicting here, the dancers are bravely willing to go over the parapet and pool together to create their own othered and bottom-up dance. Frightened but lionhearted we carve out the embodiment of cultural moves, capturing the roots of ancestral rhythm and tempo. Moves that soothe, that sing of healing and offer a moment of peace and freedom. You hoped to have danced well enough previously with bowed heads and well-placed feet (that colonist-imposed dance of "compromise between constraint and collaboration" (Mbembe [2010] 2021, p. 102)) to be permitted to perform this short dance, a moment's reprieve.

However, despite your elegance, flexibility and poise, your ideas are knee-jerk resisted, kicked into the long grass or shut down shortly after starting. The mere mention of Othered-owed initiatives triggers the frenzied White dance of hysteria and the booming of their quickened heartbeats sets the beat and the resounding bass of their battle dance.

Fanon taught that "[d]ecolonization, which sets out to change the order of the world, is, obviously, a programme of complete disorder" (Fanon, 1961, p. 27). War cries of anxiety and anticipated uprising and violence, an assumed result of empowerment and enough space to draw a good long breath. The pejorative reaction of the Whites having imagined taking their knee off the Othered neck (Apata, 2020). A condition you might like to refer to as *equalophobia*: an extreme fear of acknowledging the truth of racism, its barbaric history, owning one's privilege because of it, acknowledgement of wanting to retain the status quo and fear of retaliation and *disorder* if the oppression is dismantled.

Last Dance

Picture this: light streams in through open windows. An uneasy group of potential partners are assembled for the dance. On one side of the ballroom: senior representatives of the organisation, signed up for the masquerade in advance. Power and privilege are present and palpable.

Facing them across the floor, we shuffle anxiously—a cluster of wallflowers. We have positioned and prepared, pressed our case, practised our steps; right now, it's showtime. We are also not without power, both individually and collectively, and not only because some of us are White; and we are determined, but we are certainly at a disadvantage, up against a differential.

Introductions are made, cards are marked; the music begins. We are not slick: we are dispersed, and we do this work off the clock. We have come with specific proposals in mind, but we are suddenly feeling awkward, on the back foot. There's a sleepy feeling in the air. Maybe we should sit this waltz out after all—regroup, book the band for another time.

But what's this? A slide glimmers on the screen: nicely formatted, of course; plausible, even compelling. Guys, chill, be at peace, it whispers—we are already right on the case. Together we can do the Powerpoint shuffle! Here are the workstreams, the metrics, the agreed outputs. Here's the five-year plan—and look, it's all been properly rolled out for consultation, and here are some inspirational quotes. A (Micro)soft landing into a snowy blanket of discourse and corporate-speak.

All of a sudden it's manifest: a shroud of Whiteness has descended. We've each put our best foot forward, popped our heads above the parapet, and here it is, we're going to be buried beneath an avalanche of bullet-points, just like (it now becomes clear) we always feared we would…

The Beat Goes on

We have tried to convey something of the difficulty and dangerousness of the dance, the twist or the two-step of creative disruption in anti-racist practice: an awareness brilliantly captured by bell hooks, when she wrote of the great Black American artist Jean-Michel Basquiat that he

> journeyed into the heart of whiteness. White territory he named as a savage and brutal place. The journey is embarked upon with no certainty of return. Nor is there any way to know what you will find or who you will be at journey's end. (hooks [1994] 2006, p. 36)

We have commented on how adept the White in-group is at smothering dissent by incorporating and neutralising Otherness. We should also note that dances of *destructive* racist disruption of the moderate reformist agenda, in contrast, are much more likely to flow unchecked, tacitly endorsed by the in-group. Such dances and dancers are only ever shut down if their bops and pogos become so flagrant—and therefore bring the organisation explicitly into open "disrepute"—that the tacit endorsement is exposed to the light and can no longer merely hide in plain view.

Meantime, the only protection for Black colleagues from barrages of racial and racialised sexual abuse comes in the (literally paper-thin) form of fading posters on the wall, vapidly proclaiming zero tolerance policies that are never enforced. You will search in vain for a meaningful position statement on racial abuse from the old professional guilds and royal colleges in the UK (Aiyegbusi, 2023) or for prosecutions of racial abuse initiated by healthcare provider organisations.

What chance does the creative dance have in such circumstances? Maybe we only ever know we've been disruptive when we get shut down. Achille Mbembe observes that "[b]ehind the veil of neutrality and impartiality, racial power still structurally depends on various legal regimes for its reproduction" (Mbembe [2010] 2021, p. 40) and asks a question with which we emphatically join: "How do we radically transform the law?" (ibid.).

Mbembe describes racism as "fundamentally a technology of dispossession" (Mbembe [2010] 2021, p. 53). The structural violence of unequal access to opportunity kills. We labour to dismantle racist structures: however, creative disruption requires a charming dance, and racial battle fatigue can be disabling. You have to choose to retreat—to pause the dance, take a seat: to let go from time to time. Otherwise, hope is lost, and we crumble, and flop to the floor in a heap.

Even in the course of drafting this chapter through the spring and summer of 2023, we three all have witnessed, experienced and been exposed to dispiriting and disturbing pushback on some of the "moves in the dance" we have been speaking to. One thing we can always rely upon: in the morning, racism will still be there. We wake to another day of deciding which battles to fight, which to retreat from; dodging bullets on the societal dancefloor where racially minoritised people are constantly positioned, where to question the rhythm is to risk never getting another chance to dance.

Acknowledgements We want to express clearly that the kind of work we have been discussing in this chapter does not rest with individuals so much as with groups and coalitions of groups of colleagues and comrades. If there is credit to be claimed for any particular move in the dance we three have been involved in, the credit does not lie with us three, but with those groups and with the generations that have gone before. Although much of what we have written has to do with the dangerousness of the dance of disruption, we also say thank you to all those individuals (who here shall be nameless but are not forgotten) who have at different moments lent a hand, cleared a path or opened a door.

References

Aiyegbusi, A. (2023). *Mental Health Care and the Enduring Challenge of Racial Trauma*. Eileen Skellern Lecture. Cardiff University. Retrieved July 20, 2023, from https://www.youtube.com/watch?v=eKaphoN1RXU

Apata, O. G. (2020). I Can't Breathe: The Suffocating Nature of Racism. *Theory, Culture and Society, 37*, 241–254. https://doi.org/10.1177/0263276420957718

Brissett, L. B. (2023). Dark Beam of Light: What Covid is Telling us About Race Relations. In H. Brunning & O. Khaleelee (Eds.), *The Covid Trail: Psychodynamic Explorations* (pp. 233–250). Phoenix.

Di Angelo, R. (2011). White Fragility. *International Journal of Critical Pedagogy, 3*(3), 54–70.

Eddo-Lodge, R. (2018). *Why I am No Longer Talking to White People about Race*. Bloomsbury.

Fanon, F. (1961). *The Wretched of the Earth* (C. Farrington, Trans., 2001). Penguin Modern Classics.

Fields, B., Reesman, K., Robinson, C., Sims, A., Edwards, K., McCall, B., Short, B., & Thomas, S. (1998). Anger of African American Women in the South. *Issues in Mental Health Nursing, 19*(4), 353–373. https://doi.org/10.1080/016128498248980

Guardian. (2021). *"Unforgivable": Gareth Southgate on Racist Abuse of England Players*. Retrieved July 1, 2023, from https://www.theguardian.com/football/2021/jul/12/gareth-southgate-racist-abuse-of-england-players-unforgiveable

Hartman, S. ([2007] 2021). *Lose Your Mother: A Journey Along the Atlantic Slave Route*. Serpent's Tail.

Honig, B. (1996). Difference, Dilemmas, and the Politics of Home. In S. Benhabib (Ed.), *Democracy and Difference: Contesting the Boundaries of the Political* (pp. 257–277). Princeton University Press.

hooks, b. ([1994] 2006). *Outlaw Culture*. Routledge Classics.

Kendi, I. X. ([2019] 2023). *How To Be An Anti-Racist*. Vintage.

Kinouani, G. (2019). Difference, Whiteness and the Group Analytic Matrix: An Integrated Formulation. *Group Analysis, 53*(1), 60–74.

Lawrence, D. (2020). *An Avoidable Crisis: The Disproportionate Impact of Covid-19 on Black, Asian and Minority Ethnic Communities*. The Doreen Lawrence Review. Retrieved from https://www.lawrencereview.co.uk/

Lawton, L., & Adlam, J. (2021). *Reflecting on 'Race': Responses to Psychosocial Retraumatisation in the Workplace*. Retrieved from https://slam.newsweaver.com/Monthly/gywf3e5n78a

Levi-Strauss, C. (1955). *Tristes Tropiques* (J. Weightman & D. Weightman, Trans., 1973). Reprinted 2011. Penguin Classics.

Mbembe, A. ([2010] 2021). *Out of the Dark Night: Essays on Decolonization*. Columbia University Press.

Morrison, T. (1992). *Playing in the Dark: Whiteness and the Literary Imagination*. Picador.

NHS Race and Health Observatory. (2023). *Open Statement from the NHS Race and Health Observatory to the Healthcare System on Addressing Racism in the Workplace*. Retrieved June 4, 2023, from https://www.nhsrho.org/news/open-statement-from-the-nhs-race-and-health-observatory-to-the-healthcare-system-on-addressing-racism-in-the-workplace/

Rhead, R., Chui, Z., Gazard, B., MacCrimmon, S., Woodhead, C., & Hatch, S. L. (2020). The Impact of Workplace Discrimination and Harassment among NHS Staff Working in London Trusts: Results from the TIDES Study. *British Journal of Psychiatry Open, 7*, e10. https://doi.org/10.1192/bjo.2020.137

Rudder, S. (2023). *Black Men's Minds*. Bethlem Gallery, Bethlem Royal Hospital, Beckenham, UK April 27–May 7, 2022. Retrieved August 15, 2023, from https://bethlemgallery.com/whats-on/black-mens-minds/?ct=t()

Saturday Night Fever. (1977). Paramount Films.

Scanlon, C., & Adlam, J. (2022). *Psycho-social Explorations of Trauma, Exclusion and Violence: Un-housed Minds and Inhospitable Environments*. Routledge.

Snyder, C. Y. (2016). Navigating in Murky Waters: How Multiracial Black Individuals Cope With Racism. *American Orthopsychiatric Association, 86*(3), 265–276. https://doi.org/10.1037/ort0000148

Squid Games. (2021). Netflix.

Wilderson III, F. B. ([2008] 2015). *Incognegro: A Memoir of Exile and Apartheid.* Duke University Press.

3

Echoes of the *Other* Language: Responding from Another Place

Ayelen Hamity and Daniela Larraín-Salas

As we write, we think about how it would be if this essay were done as a told story—not writing it but narrating it aloud. An essay populated with hesitations, pronunciations that deceive, strong accents, words in English and Spanish—Spanglish some might say—and a collective of voices working things out as they go along. We would be within another language traversed by a particular way of inhabiting space—where forms of saying, thinking, telling stories, and embodying histories and territories are all intertwined.

> Verónica: It's very hard to translate your own work, I realised that. I've got a story that is published both in English and in Spanish. And I tried to translate it, it was originally in English. And then I thought, enough, I

A. Hamity (✉)
University College London, London, UK

D. Larraín-Salas
Birkbeck University, London, UK

G. Kinouani et al. (eds.), *Creative Disruption*, Studies in the Psychosocial,
https://doi.org/10.1007/978-3-031-63661-5_3

> can't, I won't. It just doesn't look right. I have to write it again (.) In the other language.[1]

The above words emerged during a study on the transatlantic movement of psychoanalysts from Buenos Aires to London. In them, we hear Verónica's experience of translation. Her words subvert the order of things: the 'original' language she referred to was not her mother tongue, and so, her words are emblematic of a postcolonial subject—there can be no place of origin after imperial expansion. The mother tongue is always already the other language—a relic of histories of violent (dis)location and a marker of loss and alienation. But there is something else that is happening in the above quote, an intervention that resonated as something familiar:

> "I tried…enough, I can't, I won't",
> *Traté… suficiente, no puedo, no lo haré.*

Verónica's body spoke an impasse in the possibilities of translation and a resolution in the act of writing again. From this, we pose the question, how can we understand the act of 'writing again' as different from the process of translation? With which vocabulary, from which location, and through whom might we make sense of the above impasse and its resolution?

Through a series of other voices,[2] including our own, we explore the difficulties and complexities of translation, a complexity housed in the paradigm of loss and alienation, and prompted by the context of postcolonialism. We push against the conventions of Eurocentric academic discourse by taking this context for granted. It is expected that postcolonialism be *argued for* and that what we mean by loss and alienation be *elaborated on.* In the former case, convincing assumes the reader has ignored a whole field of writers, thinkers, activists, and, of course, history-in-the-present,

[1] This quote emerged in Hamity's (2024) doctoral research. During this project, Verónica was invited to choose the language she would like to be interviewed in.

[2] Our profound and warm thanks to Valentina Zurob, Javiera Martínez, Claudia Mohor, Mercedes Crisóstomo, Mónica Adriana Hamity, Okito 'V' Wedi, and Bárbara Berger—as well as Daniela Belmar for reading multiple drafts of this text and for her comments.

and in the latter case, *elaborating on* is simply showcasing our indebtedness and knowledge of certain Western icons and their ideas.

Instead, prompted by this feeling of familiarity, we invited dear friends to share their experiences and intimate musings about living in another territory and reckoning with *another* language. We were also accompanied by the words of scholars: Silvia Rivera Cusicanqui, María Lugones, and Gloria Anzaldúa. From different geographies, these scholars explore the *other* language and provide us with insights into what we call the act of writing again.

As we heard, read, and discussed these voices, we found our restlessness quietened through moments of resonance, while always staying attuned to the singularity of their voice, reckoning with the particularities of their embodied experiences; the questions they addressed; the (dis)locations from which they wrote. The possibility of continuing to reach an answer to the previous questions thus did not depend on finding a univocal response. But on the deferred juxtaposition of our voices, which met only when we accepted that speaking in unison always retained a remnant of distinction, interruption, and undefinition. They coexist.

This approach led us to the notion of 'writing again' as an ethics of coexistence, a concept we will present in the body of this text. Writing from within the ethical possibilities of the psychosocial, we open the space to reflect on what coexistence as juxtaposition might do to the concept of liminal space. Our intention is not to answer these questions, but to take seriously the call for a creative disruption and, so, present our initial thoughts.

Mezclando Lenguas

Every time we sat down to write this text, we took turns in reading its paragraphs out loud, *en voz alta.* Interruptions happened often, mid-sentence—*¿está bien? ¿Se dice así?* The answer that followed was uncertain—*no sé, pero me parece que sí.* We then repeated the words out loud, creating an echo, until we lost interest in whether it was right or wrong. The reading continued until the question came again: *¿está bien?* We realised that the seemingly spontaneous presence of English and Spanish was inevitable and informed our approach to writing this text, as well as how we would incorporate the voices of others.

What emerged as unplanned, carries an ethical and political practice, as is evident in the writing of scholars like María Lugones and Gloria Anzaldúa. 'Bi-lingual' writing and poli-vocality—speaking-in-writing—emerges as a political tool in the writing of Lugones, as a response to ethnocentric racism within academia in the United States. She moves between Spanish and English to unmute "everyone in the learning place", by acknowledging the wall that exists between You and I (Lugones, 2003, p. 60). This is, not because Spanish is any less laden with power, but because its presence in the context from which she writes democratises discomfort, forcing the reader to reckon with that language that is often ignored through the comfortable position of white-English academia.

There's a thick wall that must be recognised. María Lugones writes,

> as I speak to you in the many incarnations of my native tongue, one of the live tongues of this country, I feel isolated from you as if by a thick wall. *Pero no lo hago para romper la pared, lo hago para reconocerla.* My intention is not to break the wall down, just to recognise it. This recognition is a first step to an honest understanding of ethnocentric racism. (ibid. 2003, p. 60)

Gloria Anzaldúa extends this further, reminding us how writing that is populated by multiple languages serves to disrupt the authority of a particular knowledge or form of speaking. Her writing reflects a cartography that is constantly moving, "Chicano Spanish is a border tongue which developed naturally. Change, *evolución, enriquecimiento de palabras nuevas por invención o adopción* have created variants of Chicano Spanish, *un nuevo lenguaje. Un lenguaje que corresponde a un modo de vivir*", she says (1987, p. 55). Her Chicano writing is her way of inhabiting the borders that have defined her experience and many others—Mexico and Texas-US Southwest borders, but also racial, spiritual, and sexual borders that produce contradictions and multiple identities; moving from one way to another through languages, stories, songs, symbols, and testimonies she shows the bodily experience of living within these borders challenging the stasis and dispossession that the territory has produced.

> I'm almost finished writing, I see a mosaic pattern (Aztec-like) emerging, a weaving pattern, thin here, thick there. I see a preoccupation with the deep structure, the underlying structure, with the gesso underpainting that is red earth, black earth. [...] Numerous overlays of paint, rough surfaces, and smooth surfaces make me realize I am preoccupied with texture as well. Too, I see the barely contained color threatening to spill over the boundaries of the object it represents and into other 'objects' and over the borders of the frame. (ibid., p. 66)

Considering the above, a single language is insufficient to give an account of the experience of moving between (dis)locations. The move between languages offers an alternative form of relation that dethrones colonial monolingualism and considers plurality.

To account for the plurality of languages, and the poli-vocal tone of these pages, we moved from 'bi-lingual talk' to the practice of *mezclando lenguas:* a messy practice where another language seeps in to interrupt the easy flow of information by the presence of a wall or a colour that threatens to spill over the boundaries of something already known, where the reader can be discomforted, left indifferent, or moved to understand.

The Cracks in Translation

> I invite you to read practically, in the spirit of disruption, taking up the non-scripted possibilities in the cracks of domination. (Lugones, 2003, p. 45)

What unscripted possibilities lie within the cracks of translation?

Both 'translation' and 'writing again' involve the move between English and Spanish, or English and 'the other language'. Yet, the former is associated with an arduous task that may be abandoned, and the latter is the very condition for a text to come into being. The difficulty associated with translation may signal towards its relation to language and meaning. In these instances, translation emerges as a seemingly straightforward process of going sentence by sentence, from one language to the other. It points towards an understanding of languages as temporally linear and spatially flat. Words move along a start-end order and do not belong to any geography; they are simply reflections of ideas that exist in the other language without nuances or subtleties, *sin matices*. Framed in this way, the difficulty of translating language extends the idea of false equivalences between words, or the ontological position that there does not exist a comfortable relationship between words and their meaning to begin with, let alone when we cross languages.

The act of traversing between languages and encountering impasses, as witnessed in Verónica's attempts to translate, reverberated through various voices in the context of this text. These voices, while attempting translation, eventually found themselves at an impasse, and their efforts halted.

> *"No entiendo, ¿pregunto de nuevo? Ya pregunté dos veces… como si 'dos' fuera un límite establecido. Finjo frecuentemente entender. Mi traicionero recurso, el silencio".*

In the face of the above, the presence of an other emerged, transcending personal frustrations and giving rise to the imagined frustration experienced by a listener. When this presence is encountered, the impossibility of continuing, the reverberation of the "enough, I can't", or the unintended presence of silence points us to the same relationship to words and their meaning. In the context of confronting the extractivist industry based in Latin America and financed in London, a voice highlighted the impossibility of posing demands:

> *¿Cómo traducir la importancia espiritual, que las comunidades en Latinoamérica tienen con el territorio?*

Though the demands posed to the transnational companies appeared in English, the only language they would respond to, there was no possibility of being heard.

"Enough, I can't, I won't"
suficiente, no puedo, no lo haré.

What should be a dispassionate act of selecting words, asking someone to repeat themselves, or having demands met becomes situated. Situated listening, writing, and speaking are intruded by the presence of histories, geographies, and the body. One possible reading is that the difficulty associated with translation attunes us to the power dynamics embedded in language. In the cases we explored, these webs involved English and Spanish; the West and Latin America; the centre and its counterpart. Impasses may be interpreted as remnants of the postcolonial condition that imbued space with historical and textual dynamics.

Verónica's attempt to transition from English, her second language, back to Spanish, her home language/mother tongue, reinforces this condition by disrupting the notion of the 'original'. Here lies the paradoxical yet constitutive idea that the 'original' language loses its claim to a place. As Gayatri Spivak (1993) warns, there is no such thing as an original language in the catachresis that is the postcolonial condition. The structural differences between languages, and what has been termed monolingual habitus, attune us to the ways the past is in the present.

Highlighting the changing power imbalances and structural orderings of languages helps to expose historical and political orders; however further erases as new imbalances are produced, the moment dichotomies are announced. This is because, *otras lenguas, historias y cuerpos siguen siendo borrados al solo mapear esa dicotomía entre Español e Inglés*, continue being erased when only the dichotomy between Spanish and English is traced. Each identified relation of power always pushes something out in a perpetual *différance*—other languages, histories, and bodies. For the purposes of this text, this mapping also prevents us from attending to the writing again.

'Writing again' implies the possibility of something different and, so, suggests a distinct relationship with language. What if 'writing again,' instead of being a belated consequence of the intrusion of another language, becomes the very means of coexisting with other languages—*su propia posibilidad de coexistencia con otras lenguas?* Or if 'writing again' becomes a creative gesture that, while acknowledging the inevitable disruption, simultaneously allows that interruption to surface?

From Translation to Writing-Again

"I have to write it again (.) In the other language".
Lo tengo que escribir de nuevo, en la otra lengua

Resonances with impasses in translation and inhabiting *another* place move us to understand Verónica's act of 'writing again' from its creative potential. It evokes a gesture of writing without an accurate script as no words in the 'original' language could entirely predict what story was about to come in the *other* language. Writing again thus echoes a form of relation, one that recognises multiple situated stories that are ingrained in the words and the body. Stories that permeate so also brought into the present through accents, memories, silences, forms of moving, thinking, and writing, and give an account of broader stories that took place in different locations.

Writing it again means inhabiting different temporalities and territories, creating a mobile cartography as Anzaldúa suggests, that assumes that each word and grammatical configuration sediment several stories about past, present, and future experiences. Although stories could resemble those from other latitudes, they acquire multiple forms according to the situated experience. Therefore, once spoken, only an act of imagination can prevent the words from being emptied of all the significations they inherently convey. The active act of imagining a heterogeneous space where voices, memories, and contested histories could take place.

In this sense, we propose 'writing again' as holding all the modalities of language—spoken; written; visual and gestured—as carrying an alternative ethic of relation between people, languages, and territories. A question recurs: What epistemology could provide us insight into this form of relation? The Aymara metaphor of ch'ixi brought us closer to exploring these nuances through its distinct way of inhabiting time and space. We came to this metaphor through the writings and dialogues of Silvia Rivera Cusicanqui, and we introduce it here as it has helped give form to our thinking.

Silvia Rivera explains that the notion of ch'ixi sheds light on a heterogeneous world. In a ch'ixi world, instead of considering a linear or singular time, temporality is multiple and multidimensional—where past, present, and future remain connected; furthermore, multiple geographies interact and, therefore, rather than a single language, diverse languages coexist. For her, it illuminates how the *mundo indio* as well as its opposite mix without merging while simultaneously antagonising and complementing each other. It may be better grasped in relation to colours rather than words,

> [I]t is a color that is the product of juxtaposition, in small points or spots, of opposed or contrasting colors: black and white, red and green, and so on. It is this gray *jaspeado* that comes from the imperceptible mixing of black and white, which are confused by perception, without ever being completely mixed. (2012, p. 105)

By emphasising what ch'ixi represents in the Aymara worldwide, Silvia Rivera claims for a decolonial practice. According to her, the metaphor ch'ixi as an epistemology allows us to understand the heterogeneous dimension of colonial societies while also tracing the path for ethics of coexistence. It leads us to approach stories, forms of thinking and relations as coexisting without one being subsumed into the other. To explain this, Silvia Rivera recalls René Zabaleta's ideas about Bolivian society. For him, Bolivia is a *sociedad abigarrada*, where both indigenous and colonial history moves us to inhabit simultaneity from the heterogeneous. That is, different temporalities, forms of production, and understandings of the world remain intertwined and shape one another in a society marked by colonisation and *mestizaje*.

Here we must introduce another impasse, or at the very least an interlude in the current discussion. Bringing the term 'ch'ixi' complicates our writing. The idea of the ch'ixi emerged in a different (dis)location, another language, one which is not ours. But this is precisely the implication of adopting its ethic. We present the metaphor ch'ixi precisely as ch'ixi, in an antagonistic and complementary relationship with our writing and thinking. It is a concept that pushed us along as we thought about the act of writing again in relation to a territory constituted by necessary irregularities. The writing, once again seen and heard through the lens of ch'ixi, produces not a setting aside of language but rather sitting alongside language. There exists a creative potential in this, which we found in the words of another voice:

> I needed to find a way to open it to a multiplicity of meaning, there is when I found that this slash/union allowed me to retain some of the ungraspable, some of the tone that made me comfortable with the sound/image of the sentence.

The above alludes to the ch'ixi, which represents a dialectic of worlds that are subversive and mutually influential but never culminate in a blending. Blending, as we know, leads to erasure and forgetting reflecting the colonial gesture of erasing the plural configuration of territories. Instead, as Silvia Rivera highlights, ch'ixi assumes the contentious history of a territory that endured a process of domination and resistance and the equivalence between different cultures.

This kind of ethics transforms the dynamics between the speaker and listener, the writer and reader, emphasising the importance of patience and imagination: patience for the utterance which carries a singular and collective story, and imagination not as an act of figuring the other out but as an act of curiosity that asks questions about the histories, geographies, and their embodiment within the words of others.

Verónica's writing again, as distinct from the act of translation, signals towards a new, situated, story to emerge.

Responding from Another Place

What language do we use when we respond from another place? Verónica's words demand a creative gesture and an act of imagination. We do not currently live in Latin America but are from there. We write from a language that is not our mother tongue, but our conversations and writings are coloured by words and scenes that come from other places. To move from one language to another, from one place to another, one has to look at the geography of the words and how they are shaped according to the places, subjects, and stories that gave rise to them. This movement is not achieved through a process of translation, but through writing again, which makes the speaker move across languages and the listener open to plurality. It thus implies being aware, rather than of the limits of language, of the transformation of these borders every time a word is said—altering what was taken for granted without erasing what had been previously told.

Feminist scholars' reflections on the cracks of translation and the experience of inhabiting the other place resonated alongside the stories of others. Gloria Anzaldúa and María Lugones illuminated the subversive and creative power of writing in another language and raised questions as to how we may approach those languages, and Silvia Rivera Cusicanqui, how that writing could emerge as a complement and antagonism and, so, never erases.

They show us that heterogeneous space, where opposites coexist without one being subsumed into another can expand our ethical relation towards the other. This is not an intervention on the level of discourse but must be embodied. To the enigma of 'writing again' we gave form to our thinking through an epistemology that allowed us to inhabit a space that condenses histories, geographies, and corporality, which, as long as it enables us to imagine other possible relations, gives rise to an ethics of coexistence.

This chapter emerged as an attempt to articulate the ideas of familiarity with Verónica's words, which for us unfold within the psychosocial field. However, as we elaborate on them, questions with a slightly different nuance concerning the very field from which we write appear: What is the language of psychosocial? How does the 'psychosocial' make sense of the above ethics of coexistence? As psychosocial studies propose approaching phenomena from the borders of the social and subjective space, it embraces a method that questions the understanding of different worlds from defined or fragmented narratives. As Stephen Frosh (2007) says, approaching from the liminal implies being aware of the polymorphous character of the margins that accounts for the multiple layers that each situation or enunciation holds. Is the language of the liminal the language of the psychosocial?

Rivera Cusicanqui's articulation on ch'ixi, Lugone's recognition of the wall, and poli-vocal musings open methodological and theoretical challenges to the field. It certainly does not avoid the "polymorphism of marginal" (ibid., p. 644). Yet, other worlds of knowledge, other signifiers, and enunciations, indeed, inhabiting an other space, make us permanently ask what the language of the psychosocial is and, importantly, what is the status of this language. Does sustaining the language of the liminal erase the possibilities of seeing a "mosaic pattern" emerge (Anzaldúa, 1987, p. 66)? The language within this chapter suspends our possibilities of giving a definitive answer to this question, foregrounding an act of critical imagination that not only questions where we speak from but stands for being open to new creative gestures.

References

Anzaldúa, G. (1987). *Borderlands/La Frontera: The new mestiza*. Aunt Lute Book Company.

Frosh, S. (2007). Disintegrating Qualitative Research. *Theory & Psychology, 17*(5), 635–653. https://doi.org/10.1177/0959354307081621

Hamity, A. (2024). *Migrating Analysts, Analysing Migration: Tracing Signifiers of People, Places, and Movement* [Unpublished doctoral dissertation]. University College London.

Lugones, M. (2003). *Pilgrimages: Peregrinajes: Theorizing Coalition Against Multiple Oppressions*. Rowman & Littlefield.

Rivera Cusicanqui, S. (2012). Ch'ixinakax utxiwa: A Reflection on the Practices and Discourses of Decolonization. *South Atlantic Quarterly, 111*(1), 95–109. https://doi.org/10.1215/00382876-1472612

Spivak, G. C. (1993). *Outside in the Teaching Machine*. Taylor and Francis. Retrieved from http://www.123library.org/book_details/?id=60050

4

Being Black Freud: A Creative Heuristic Exploration of the Psychological Impact of Black Activism

Dwight Turner

Black Activism Rising

Since the murder of George Floyd in 2020, a number of black activists have risen to centre stage and taken their places within the world of psychology, counselling, and psychotherapy (BBC News Online 2020). Their positioning as a new age of black activist standard bearers has led to them taking on the struggle against the levels of racism and white supremacy which permeate our professions. Much like any other activist I, Dr Dwight Turner, have played a role in this vanguard movement and yet there has been an impact. I know from my own experience of the personal cost of being a black activist within our professions, and I have come across a number of stories of fellow activists whose mental health has been impacted by the levels of vitriol and hatred meted out against them, both from within and without our professions.

D. Turner (✉)
University of Brighton, Brighton, UK
e-mail: Info@dwightturnercounselling.co.uk

G. Kinouani et al. (eds.), *Creative Disruption*, Studies in the Psychosocial,
https://doi.org/10.1007/978-3-031-63661-5_4

I recall in the days after George Floyd's murder how hard it was for me to not only look at the YouTube clips of his destruction at the hands of those Minneapolis policemen, but also how much of a struggle it was to know not only what to say, not only what to do, but also did I have the right to say and do anything? The voice of blackness, the ability to stand for one's rights within a white, capitalist, patriarchal structure is often the voice of silence, is often the voice of compliance. It often has to struggle against the internalised script that should one speak up, that not only will one be labelled as a troublemaker, but that one could actually lose one's life and be destroyed by the forces which maintain the systems of oppression around us. That I, on that one night, could not sleep meant that I found myself in the days afterwards at 4.00 am writing 2000 words on my impressions of George Floyd's murder. That I published these words with the help of friends, an action which led me to find a way of expressing my rage, my sadness, my grief, and my hope that this would lead to some sort of change. These internalised messages are a massive facet in the work that black activists have to undertake to be free, and it is no coincidence that in my writings post Black Steel in the Hour of Chaos (Turner, 2020) that the thing that moves most readers or those who hear my words is that they are spoken from a place of authenticity, of pain, of depth, and of reflection.

This chapter, which is in part a heuristic exploration of this experience of being a black activist, will be using creative means designed by Moustakas (1990) as a means of understanding the unconscious internalised messages which have been taken in to the psyche of the blackness as a means of silencing and disabling the inner activist. These messages which would mean the activist has become lost within. Silenced in into a space of colonised compliance, the residue of which is the type of colonial performativity that holds echoes of the systemic ideas of Butler and others (Butler, 1988). This chapter will then consider how, when we reconnect with our inner activist, this could be used as a weapon to continue the methods of creative disruption necessary for the systemic separation and therefore cultural growth, thereby moving towards the kind of inner decolonisation necessary for the benefit of all our professions.

That this research has utilised creative methods is a massively important facet in diverting our understanding and knowledge making away from the hetero-normative white methodologies of the past and thereby utilising some of the more creative indigenous and inclusive means at our disposal. This chapter will therefore begin with the idea that even the originators of our profession were activists after some means, whilst also preparing the way to an understanding of how these disruptors had their ideas co-opted and commodified within systems of oppression, meaning that their voices were silenced.

The Colonisation of the Activist

When Edward Said (1989) wrote his paper called "Representing the Colonised," there was a recognition on the page that the activist could take many different forms. What was important for Said (1993), in his talks as part of the Reith Lecture series on BBC radio, was that the intellectual as an activist recognises the importance of the position it holds. His meanings here being that the intellectual has a strong role to play in revealing to culture what it both is and is not, where its flaws are, where its promises are. Yet, also where its actions may need to be challenged and where elements of shame and distress recognised, experienced, and learned from. For Said, the intellectual as an other or as an outsider is a form of disruption of said cultural construct. The intellectual here is as much there to cause trouble as it is to re-affirm the positives within said cultural construct.

This is no different to the works and the early writings of the likes of Sigmund Freud (1930; Jacobs, 2003). In understanding some of Freud's earlier works, we need to reconsider how many of which were political, together with how they were created and derived during a time of major cultural upheaval in Europe and across the global north, the attempts of such a man to create a diatribe of dissonance was often met with accusations and marginalisations that these ideas presented were detrimental to the German cultural construct (Frosh, 2005).

Both Freud and Said endured difficult times as activists within their fields. For Freud, his flight out from Germany and Austria because of the rise of Nazism, which was then followed by his subsequent distress and sad collapse due to cancer, contrasts similarly with Said's later cancer illness and his struggles to gain entry to America for treatment. In many ways, their struggles and their fights to be seen and acknowledged cost them both their lives; and yet in many ways both activists, both men of intellect, took on routes and passageways that challenged and changed the cultural environments around them.

The importance for this literature review in recognising the intellectual and creative capabilities of persons such as these is the reason why this chapter holds such importance and yet what is missing in some ways is the deeper cultural roots, both persons would have engaged within in order to gather and obtain the ideas and structures that they presented to the world. Alongside this, and as such this is the reason for this chapter, is a lack of understanding of just what it was that Said was accessing, or that Freud was provoked into providing, and where these ideas ultimately may have come from.

By way of understanding some of this material and some of this need and drive that sat within both of them, we need to understand the idea of civilisation. In this instance, civilisation becomes the set of criteria by which we are all deemed to live by Rousseau (1998). We are told what it is to be civilised, be it that we are informed that we need to dress a certain way, act a certain way, be a certain type of man, woman, or child. We are given roles and prescribed positions within said construct of civilisation. Even our morality is defined within this construction, and we often feel shame or guilt or are marginalised should we choose to step outside of cultural construct accordingly.

So, for example, ideas presented in the social contract highlight just what it is to be working class and French in the seventeenth century (Rousseau, 1984, 1998). Whereas, more contemporary visions represented through the work of Butler (1988) and her ideas about performativity explore the nature of performance and how a woman's position performed within the patriarchal construct of culture and civilisation marks her out as therefore civilised.

That morality, personality, and vitality are then co-opted and defined from within said structure of civilisation, ties civilisation itself to something built out of the patriarchal, while supremacist, capitalist, intersectional triumvirate (Collins, 2019; Turner, 2023). So, any sort of decolonial rebelliousness or activism that challenges any of these positions of systemic supremacy therefore will lead to the other being a gendered, racialised, or of a sexual orientation etc., to be marked out as troublesome, so much so that they may become marginalised, imprisoned, or even murdered (Cooke & Halberstadt, 2021). This builds upon the ideas presented by theorists such as Mbembe (2016, 2017) whose works centred on decolonisation being essential for any movement away from the neo-liberal, fascist, othering environments we have today, and recognises that to achieve this there has to be an internal decolonisation of the systemic ideas and structures which have co-opted so many of us who identify as the Other.

To build upon my idea, the activist, be they decolonial, racial, feminist, or otherwise, is often though working from a different form of morality to that systemically constructed. One, which is internally driven, I would argue, and which is necessary for culture to recognise and see its flaws etc., but also for it to grow and become more inclusive of other groupings accordingly (Sudbury, 2001). The cost though, on activists of colour, has traditionally been incredibly high; the murders of Martin Luther King and Malcom X being huge examples (Harvey, 2022; Hayley, 1965). These are also though obvious examples where the activism of those pair also led to their loss of life, and yet it has not stopped them any, many others, from taking up the mantel and striding forwards.

Angela Davis (1983), in her writings around racial activism, talks about the fight as being one which one undertakes on a daily basis. This contrasts with more contemporary British activists who have written about the passion and power that it takes to keep on going and how even acts such as love and self-love hold within them at their core activism and a striding away from, or outside of, the system constructs which define whether one is civilised or not (Hall, 1996; Lorde, 1984). This chapter though looks to explore those inner reaches that many of us reach when we decide to take up the mantel and become decolonial activists and looks to explore and understand the deeper psychological nay archetypal embers which we light when we fight for us all.

Indigenous Methodological Approaches to Decolonisation

To understand the methodology chosen, it is worth recognising that traditional western versions of western research methods were not going to be particularly useful in this instance. Having used grounded theory, phenomenology, and interpersonal phenomenological analysis, in the past, it became obvious that these ways of understanding the experience of the other, in particular the internalised experience of other, revolved around a very western colonised angle. That within these the other was an object to be studied, an externalised aspect which needed to be understood but which left no mark upon the researcher themselves (Charmaz, 2006; Moustakas, 1994).

One of the most interesting things though, in any sort of journey towards activism, is actually the change wrought by the process of becoming an activist within the person, the individual, the man, the woman, the LGBTQ person themselves. This was particularly important in my selection of a methodology which, although written from a more western angle, also held huge units of understanding from different cultural backgrounds. I also wanted to construct a narrative which would allow me to work with not just internalised and unconscious aspects of my experience but would also allow me the space to explore and ask questions of those intergenerational, if not archetypal or ancestral, parts of the experience of becoming said decolonial activist.

In her paper on intergenerational wounds, Brewster (2019), who although a Jungian analyst, recognised that she had the chance to use her skills to access parts of the unconscious relevant from her own cultural background, that of being an African American woman. This also gave her the chance to decolonise her understanding of herself and to build into practice a way of exploring the self which sat outside of the westernised paradigm. This, although Jungian angle, steps outside of a traditional Jungian perspective say as designed by Carl Jung, whereby his experience of travelling around more Afrocentric countries was built upon the idea of his being from a colonial background (his travels through Africa were conducted during a time where Germany was trying to establish its own colonial project in East Africa) (Burleson, 2005). His research, although incredibly useful in understanding the notion of archetypes and the collective unconscious, did little to bring to the fore the role and perspective and meaning making and guidance of the ancestors through the collective unconscious that is real and inhabited in more transpersonal theories (Antsyferova, 2000; Valley, 1991).

The importance of understanding the ancestral lineage of an individual or a collective and accessing that lineage became essential in trying to understand one's position as an activist. It was hoped this would give me the chance to align myself with knowledge, experience, and wisdom which I may have distanced myself from in allowing myself to be colonised within a western research framework. This deeper exploration also needed to involve the recognition and re-experiencing of its generational wounds, blocks, and defences that may also have become part of the barrier between my own western identity and that which sits outside in the cultural unconscious. The idea here was therefore to always look at the role that the ancestors would play in my experience.

Another core part of this chapter involves the use of creativity to access unconscious material which might ascertain the qualities and experience which might allow this researcher to explore the experiences of being an activist as well as look at the qualities necessary in order to maintain said position. This was felt to be important as utilising the creative therefore would give voice to the more indigenous, internalised, and symbolic messages residing within the unconscious shadow of my colonised self (Bauman, 2023; Tonkinson, 2013; Walter & Suina, 2019).

For this research, heuristics was chosen as the main means of exploring the unconscious experience of the activist. Heuristic research is actually derived from the ancient Greeks who used their moments, days, weeks, and months of introversion as a means of trying to understand the world around themselves. Although this method can be seen as perhaps not necessarily scientifically rigorous enough, one of the pluses in an exploration such as this one is that it brings the researcher directly into that particular scenario and experience which is being explored. This contrasts greatly amongst a good deal of quantitative and some qualitative research methods which very much place the researcher outside of the data collection process, thereby leaving an enormous hole in said research. The other part to it is that in any sort of heuristic research, it also recognises that heuristic research also challenges the power dynamics inherent within most other forms of research whereby the researcher hovers above that which is being explored, their mere presence distorting very much the elements which are uncovered.

In this instance, this recognition of the power structures inherent within research, and the attempts here to utilise a heuristic exploration to challenge these, also mirrored the challenging of internalised power systemic structures of whiteness which may preclude a researcher of colour from expressing themselves through research.

So, for example, in Drotner's (2000) research about difference and otherness, the fact that this research was conducted by a white researcher formed within a quantitative and qualitative background, and that they left themselves out of said research, would have had a deeply inbuilt impact upon the data collected and therefore the results gained. By actually placing myself at the centre of this experience which I am seeking to understand, I am therefore looking to disrupt and challenge the cultural narrative of objectifying experiences by ploughing a solo furrow through to an unconscious process in order for us to start and begin to understand it.

The hypothesis behind this was that actually being an activist is a phenomenological experience rooted in the unconscious, to borrow a term from Carl Jung (1972), and that the activist, the fighter, is actually an archetype with which if we are willing, we can access at any time. That this archetype has enacted its qualities through so many prominent persons across generations suggests that it has an awful lot to say about the direction our cultures need to follow and also a lot to uncover about the floors and problems our cultures have riddled within them.

That this exploration also holds a phenomenological angle also needs to be included. Borrowing from the work of Merleau-Ponty (1962), the idea that there is a separation between body and mind, removes much of our research and understanding from an enormous resource which holds a lot of information which we can all benefit from. The idea here is to move beyond a purely cognitive understanding of what it is to be an activist, but to delve that bit deeper into the felt experience of activism and then bring that to the surface for a great understanding of what it is to be an actual activist.

Moustakas's research takes into account six main stages. These are:

1. Initial Engagement
2. Immersion
3. Incubation
4. Illumination
5. Explication
6. Creative Synthesis

Initial Engagement

The first stage involves the correct formation of the question which needs to be explored. This formulation of a question involved a period of indwelling and meditation common to numerous indigenous groups who have used that internal exploration to understand and at times come to a recognition of the question which needs to be explored (Botha, 2011).

Immersion

The second stage involved an intense reading around this topic area; what material is there around being activist? Who has written about this? Much of this material is presented in the literature review already explored and would have influenced my meaning making accordingly.

Incubation

The third stage of this process involved regular creative dialogue with the question. In my experience, what I undertook was two hours a week on different days where I sat and I journaled and I drew and I meditated upon the experience of being an activist. What does it mean to be an activist? How did I define being an activist? What songs or music came up which represented being an activist? Looking at this and staying with this process over a month period gave me an understanding hopefully of some of the strengths, recognitions, and pitfalls of what it is to be a black activist.

This stage also involved the writing of regular rituals which were performed by myself, where I would ask questions of the ancestors in the hope of gaining some form of guidance in the forms of dreams, coincidences, and synchronicities. An example of one of these messages is written below:

> Creative disruption prayer Friday 17 February 2023 to my ancestors. Today I am giving thanks to you dear ancestors for the support you have given me, my daughter, to my colleagues at the University and in my private practice. I love how you have supported me in your work and take your guidance very seriously, especially given the challenges the world faces right now. I have a special favour to ask of you. I am conducting research into what it is to be an activist for the black community for a paper you have placed in my path. I have already had several dreams which have been incredibly informative of my process in this regard. As this research is not just about me, as it is also about you and your guidance, I would like to ask you for your help and wisdom in seeing just what it is to be a black activist. Any help, any guidance, any synchronicities, any dreams would be useful in my process. Please help me with your wisdom in this process and as always thank you. With love always. Dwight.

Illumination

The fourth stage involved me actually putting this material down, stepping away from it all, clearing my head, allowing the unconscious process to actually settle, and also creating a boundary between my own research and an ongoing personal process of exploration. What I mean by this is any sort of heuristic understanding does not end because the research has been written up and published somewhere. That process will continue within the psyche of the researcher as long as they are willing to explore and investigate said experience.

Explication

Everything which had come up through these earlier stages would now require refining and a regular relating back to the initial question, together with a cross-referencing with the edict of this book, which was to design ways and means to challenge the heteronormative, Eurocentric understandings of research into our psychologies. This process of explication involved not only moments of analysis and comparison with the source data but also some time for indwelling and self-explication, going inwards as well as going outwards until the new awareness had become properly formed.

Creative Synthesis

The next stages involve a creative synthesis in bringing all this together; the images, the songs, the ways of understanding this experience are recorded, explored, and published.

That this process took place over a short period of time is not so much of an issue. What is more important is the intensity, the depth, and the willingness to open oneself up to such an experience of research.

Creative Disruption: Discovering the Decolonial Activist

Throughout the data collection period, some 30 dreams were recorded, and diary entries kept as well. All of this data was closely considered as I sought to either confirm or deny my hypothesis that activism is an activity open to all of us, and in particular those of us of colour who seek to create better systems, and a better world.

On the gathering of this data, I was though left with a query about how best to present it, in what forms and in how much detail. One means of presenting this data was through the lens of alchemy, but my resistance was that to do so would bring with it a more Eurocentric angle to understanding this experience (Marlan, 2005). The best way to present the data was therefore just as it occurred. This is not to say that this process was a linear one, but it is to show that there were differing stages to this process. This process was difficult, circular, and led to numerous sleepless nights, and challenging emotions coming to the surface.

The dreams and diary entries were analysed and four main themes emerged out of this process. These were:

1. The Colonised Double
2. The Internalised Coloniser
3. Uncovering the Intuitive Self
4. Meeting the Ancestors

The Colonised Double

> Dream 1. I am in my parents' house and I am demanding to leave. My brother though is in the dream and he is very upset and will not let me go because if I leave I will talk about difference etc. and help find peace in the world. I want to go outside and get in my car so I can actually go out to the station and catch my train. He tries to follow me out of the house, crying so I double back on myself and I go down into the basement where I hide. I see him go around the front of the house trying to find me. As I pass my mother in the basement though, I then try to leave but my brother comes downstairs and finds me. We scuffle in the basement together.

This dream very much speaks to the tension inherent within any call to activism. Whereas there are many text from the Global North which speak of the heroes' journey as a call to arms, when this is placed in a more Afrocentric context, this call is fraught with dangers which most other cultures do not have to face and encounter (Hamilton, 2014). This would be a journey where to speak up, to speak out, as a person of colour could lead to the death, the marginalisation, or the emasculation of said self. In this dream, my brother is the part which silences me, as much as a means of self-protection, as anything else.

The Internalised Coloniser

> Dream 2. On 20 February 2023, a scene where I am in a building with a wise black man. We go into the kitchen together, which is in the basement. I go to my parents' old room in the basement and the old man is then taken away and disappears. Then, two daleks appear and I have to hide behind the door to the kitchen. The daleks come through and take the wise black man. They turn off the lights so I need to sneak out and go up to the first floor which used to be my old bedroom. I sneak into my old room as I do not want XXX to see me. He is an older, white man who is coming down from the top floor but seems to follow me into my old bedroom. I hide out on the balcony to try and avoid him initially, but they decide to back inside as I want to warn them about what is coming. XXX then says that he is aware that there are daleks in the building. This is where the dream ends.
>
> Diary Entry. On 22 February 2023 I was feeling an extraordinary level of calm last night as I was awake. I realised my instincts are wobbled by madness and by the chaos of those around me and how much I have been taught to disregard a massive part of who I am as an individual and as an activist. When I listen to my instinctual part, I often find out that it was right. For example, in my relationship with white woman XX (a past relationship in 2021) I knew when the relationship was ending and when she was leaving, and although it was quite painful at the time, I was right. There were also other instances where my instincts have proven correct about people, situations and the directions I am supposed to follow.

The "beauty" of both the dream and the diary entry are that they speak closely to the tensions which meet at the doorway of me being as an activist. The instinctual part of myself mentioned in the diary entry is that which has learnt that it is to be colonised and ignored by my adapted persona, in favour of the experiences and the trusting words of whiteness, here wrestles with the script that it was right.

The brilliance of the daleks symbol is that they come straight out of the Nazi playbook. Characters created by Terry Nation, and written for the programme Doctor Who, they were portrayed as humanoids called the Kaleds, who were genetically modified by their mad creator, Davros, thereby making them devoid of all humanity, his aim being to take over the universe (Various, 2023). That this symbol speaks so much to the nazi idea of a pure species, and that this had become internalised by myself, shows how deeply felt, and experienced, systemic whiteness can run when left unnoticed. Thereby killing off that which makes myself unique, or the racial other, in favour of some kind of co-opted co-operation and assimilation of being (Turner, 2021).

Meeting the Intuitive Self

> Dream 3. On 21 February 2023 I am at a party of some kind. I am a man with a mixture of friends but there are no sort of gay or lesbian pairings at the party. I am disappointed by this last bit as everybody else seems to have fun. I go to the living room and I see a car being blown around in the darkness by the winds because there is a storm outside. It hits another car in the street and in hitting it, it takes the front bumper off. I go to the front door and I see that actually in this car is a weasley looking white man, middle aged with long, stringy, blonde hair. He looks at me and he actually brings out a set of knives in plastic which he places on the side and looks me dead in the eye as he does so. In doing so, it is as if there is a warning that I should stop talking and not say any more. My daughter then appears behind me in the corridor and he see her. I also realise then that if I don't keep quiet, that he will harm her as well as myself.

The intuitive Self though never dies. It is there, and will fight back when it can, so that it too can be present in the world. The threats though, be they real or symbolic, are also in this dream. The main difference here is that these are external threats, they are outside of the house. The threat to my child though is one which I feel every day as an activist, that she might be harmed by the work that I do. Yet, that if I do not, that she will suffer at the hands of such hatred out in the world.

Meeting the Ancestors

> Dream 4: 27th Feb 2023 myself and a South African man are in a room wrestling in preparation for the games to come. We get on well and feel the game should be combative. At the end of the evening, we are then talking

> as we prepare to go downstairs for dinner. Everyone else has already left, and we are the last. I share a joke with my friend, and even wrestle with him as we fall down the stairs. He chases me, and we are both laughing as we enter the dining room.

There is a more playful aspect to this dream. A part of me is playing with, is wrestling with, something powerful, kind, and friendly. The dream is also external to my home, my body, my construct, and is out in the world. There is safety in the strength of this colleague, this ancestor, from the diaspora.

The colonisation of the self as shown in these dreams does not just include the adaptation of behaviours designed to make myself and my ancestors subservient to the overseers in the Global North. Colonisation is also an internalised experience, where one realises that I have been taught to ignore my instinctual self, to ignore the signs and symbols that are hidden within the dreams that I have, the coincidences that I encounter, the messages that I receive and the symbols and signals that I get from the world around me. This is what it is like to be a colonised Activist of Colour (AOC). To then recover that is to find the space and time to sit within that internal space and listen to those deeper, more meaningful words.

Bringing Psychological Meaning to the Words of the Elders

These dreams highlight a process; a process activated through a deeper engagement with my own experience as an activist and as a man of colour. That last diary statement in particular recognised how disconnected I (or we?) have become as a person of colour from our willingness to fight and disrupt systems of oppression which we all reside within. The dreams speak very much to this as well and talk about the fact that systems of whiteness no longer need to actively oppress the racialised other, their work having been done from a very early age. In fact, what often happens as per the dreams presented here, reveals just how internalised this aspect of one's own psychology as the racialised other can be, has become, and may well remain if left unchecked, unrealised, unexplored, and unresolved.

There is an indirect link here to the feminist exploration of objectification in the works of Fredrickson and Harrison (2005) and their exploration of the internalised experience of objectification and how this then has an impact on the conscious neurological mind. This also has more direct links to studies by Tull et al. (1999), and their study into the internalised experience of racism and prejudice in persons of colour in the Caribbean and cross the diaspora, their ideas linking this to increased levels of obesity and diabetes. What my work here though does is show a level of combativeness, a desire to fight back against those inner layers of internalised oppression, to bring something more realistic and authentic to the surface. This process though, is not without danger. The aspect of myself presented by my brother in Dream 1 is important to also explore that level of self-hatred which sits within the colonised and allows for their recolonisation or adaptation within systems of oppression and is also a facet of all of us within the diaspora.

That this part should be played by someone who, in my real world is as loving and kind a person as I could ever have known, was as shocking for myself and will be as shocking for all of us accordingly. What this suggests is that self-hatred is not given from outside by some malevolent force, it is offered like a gift on a silver platter from those closest towards us at times. That to explore and recognise this then brings up a lot of grief and sadness at the routes that one has been misled along to remain safe and secure within systems of racialised oppression. Adaptation, code switching, performativity, are all subtle means by which we perform and find safety (Alexandrowicz, 2017; Narayanan, 2014). That they are not just based within systems of racism is an aspect which is well understood, but the subtlety within which they enact themselves upon us all is an area that needs deeper consideration and exploration.

Accessing the Ancestral Activist

One of the richest parts of this exploration was the bridge created between the prayer written to my ancestors, and the ritual performed thereafter together, with the messages that were presented and the revealing of a possible route out of the internalised systems therein. That this was fairly moving for myself is without question, and in writing this chapter, I found myself feeling at times not only the sadness but also the gratitude at having such an army of wisdom to back me up in my words, my deeds, my actions, my activism. That they are my entourage and that they are the gateway to me accessing this archetypal part of myself should not be underestimated.

The archetypal nature of the ancestral activist is therefore very important to see and experience and recognise. That it resides so deep down in the psyche, as presented through the dreams, the accessing of the lower areas of the house, the same house that I was raised within as a child, shows the direction of travel that we must all follow in order to access this archetypal energy (McMenamin, 2016; Vaughan, 2019). This is not to say that one has to go south, it is more an idea that in order to access this part of oneself, flowing down through the body into areas of the self which one has not experienced before, is hugely important. The body therefore becomes a conduit towards accessing this archetypal aspect of the self, and yet the relationship to the body for those persons of colour is often quite problematic (Bernier, 2014; van der Kolk, 2015). From those who are raised within the diaspora who have a history of slavery example, the body was something which was abused ritualistically by the owners from the moment they were captured, to the moment they were sold, to the moment they were seen to have performed some sort of misdeed. The severing of genitals, the beating of the back, the binding of breasts meant that the body became something to be abused, something to be afraid of and aspects of dissociation and de-personalisation were often the only means that persons of colour could find in order to escape the traumas wrought against the physical selves (Akbar, 1984; Brewster, 2020).

This contrasts greatly to experiences of the body if those who were raised in more Afrocentric circles, where the body is seen as something more to be revered, respected, and held in higher regard, irrespective of gender (Asante, 1998; Mazama, 2003). In the global north, the body of blackness is often only seen as something to be sexualised, that being the safest way within which whiteness may respect (or disrespect in fact) an aspect of itself that it cannot own. The projection of this negative image of its own sexuality onto the objectified black other, therefore being an experience, will resonate for many persons of colour.

This is very different to the dream and diary data presented here. Although there were other dreams, including dreams of unions of opposites, where there is a combining, a meeting, sometimes erotically between myself as experienced in the dream and the sometimes female, and occasionally male, other (Li, 2006). These are very different experiences, more loving experiences, more Conjunctio experiences than those that might have been presented through a less conscious and therefore more sexually disruptive type of imagery (Hamilton, 2014). What these sorts of unions mean, therefore, is that in order to activate and access the archetypal activist that sits within, there has to be a union of mind, body, and Afrocentric spirit which connects one to that deeper and trans-ancestral aspect, which is not lost but is just buried. The spirit that sits in the deeper depths of one's psyche and resonates out through the words and deeds of Ida B Wells, of Marcus Garvey, of Malcolm X, of James Baldwin, of Stuart Hall, of Audre Lorde, of Angela Davis, of Malidoma Some, of Sara Ahmed, and many, many, many others is what keeps us all going, moving, talking, fighting, rising to this day.

Creative Disruption as an Act of Unconscious Activism: A Summary

This heuristic exploration took a deep, shadowy, and often painful look at the archetype of the activist, recognising that this is a force which runs through so many of us who are disadvantaged, especially in this instance from within the diaspora. This chapter recognised this search to be a challenging one, and one that not many undertake for a variety of reasons. Yet, what this chapter also recognises is that there is another force residing well outside of consciousness; that there are ancestral forces at play which if one has the courage to tap in to may well guide oneself onwards and upwards to do the good work of disrupting the systems of oppression, we are all born into and moulded by.

This chapter is therefore a map. It is a doorway to a possible route forward for those who wish to follow. For those who see injustice and wish to fight, nay to struggle and wrestle away from whiteness that something more, that justice we all crave. It is not though the territory; for experiences are not universal, they are individual; this archetype of the activist is not singular, it is phenomenological in its nature. We may all walk towards it, but for those who circle it, our experiences will be markedly different.

References

Akbar, N. (1984). *Breaking the Chains of Psychological Slavery*. New Mind.

Alexandrowicz, C. (2017). 'Straight-Looking, Straight-Acting': Countering Effemiphobia in Acting Training. *Theatre, Dance and Performance Training, 8*(1), 5–18. https://doi.org/10.1080/19443927.2016.1246381

Antsyferova, L. I. (2000). Archetypical Theory of Personality Individuation of Carl Gustav Jung—(The Second Article: "The Second Half of Life Span. The Stages of Individuation, Problems of Vocation, Destiny, Sense of Life"). *Psikhologicheskii Zhurnal, 21*(3), 10–19.

Asante, M. K. (1998). *The Afrocentric Idea*. Temple University Press.

Bauman, W. A. (2023). Indigenous Methodologies, Decolonizing the Academy, and Re-connecting Stories with Planetary Places. *Religious Studies Review, 49*(2), 165–167. https://doi.org/10.1111/rsr.16544

Bernier, C.-M. (2014). "The Slave Ship Imprint": Representing the Body, Memory, and History in Contemporary African American and Black British Painting, Photography, and Installation Art. *Callaloo, 37*(4), 990–1022. https://doi.org/10.1353/cal.2014.0181

Botha, L. (2011). Mixing Methods as a Process Towards Indigenous Methodologies. *International Journal of Social Research Methodology, 14*(4), 313–325. https://doi.org/10.1080/13645579.2010.516644

Brewster, F. (2019). Binding Legacies: Ancestor, Archetype and Other. *Journal of Analytical Psychology, 64*(3), 306–319. https://doi.org/10.1111/1468-5922.12500

Brewster, F. (2020). *The Racial Complex: A Jungian Perspective on Culture and Race*. Routledge.

Burleson, B. (2005). *Jung in Africa*. Continuum.

Butler, J. (1988). Performative Acts and Gender Constitution: An Essay in Phenomenology and Feminist Theory. *Theatre Journal, 40*(4), 519. https://doi.org/10.2307/3207893

Charmaz, K. (2006). *Constructing Grounded Theory A Practical Guide Through Qualitative Analysis*. Sage Publications.

Collins, P. H. (2019). *Intersectionality as Critical Social Theory*. Duke University Press.

Cooke, A. N., & Halberstadt, A. G. (2021). Adultification, Anger Bias, and Adults' Different Perceptions of Black and White Children. *Cognition and Emotion, 35*(7), 1416–1422. https://doi.org/10.1080/02699931.2021.1950127

Davis, A. (1983). *Women Race and Class*. Ballantine Books Inc.

Drotner, K. (2000). Difference and Diversity: Trends in Young Danes' Media Uses. *Media, Culture & Society, 22*(2), 149–166. https://doi.org/10.1177/016344300022002002

Fredrickson, B. L., & Harrison, K. (2005). Throwing Like a Girl: Self-Objectification Predicts Adolescent Girls' Motor Performance. *Journal of Sport & Social Issues, 29*(1), 79–101. https://doi.org/10.1177/0193723504269878

Freud, S. (1930). *Civilisation and its Discontents*. Penguin Limited.

Frosh, S. (2005). *Hate and the 'Jewish Science'—Anti-Semitism, Nazism and Psychoanalysis*. Palgrave Macmillan.

Hall, S. (1996). *Critical Dialogues in Cultural Studies*. Routledge.

Hamilton, N. (2014). *Awakening Through Dreams: The Journey Through the Inner Landscape*. Karnac Books Ltd.

Harvey, J. (2022). 'The Kaleidoscopic Conditions' of John Akomfrah's Stuart Hall. *Transnational Screens, 13*(2), 83–95. https://doi.org/10.1080/25785273.2022.2061130

Hayley, A. (1965). *The Autobiography of Malcolm X* (q). Golden Press.

Jacobs, M. (2003). *Sigmund Freud—Key Figures in Counselling and Psychotherapy* (2nd ed.). Sage Publications.

Jung, C. G. (1972). *Four Archetypes*. Routledge.

Li, X. (2006). Becoming Taoist I and Thou: Identity-Making of Opposites. *Journal of Curriculum and Pedagogy, 3*(2), 193–216. https://doi.org/10.1080/15505170.2006.10411612

Lorde, A. (1984). Age, Race, Class and Sex: Women Redefining Difference. *Sister, Outsider*.

Marlan, S. (2005). *The Black Sun: The Alchemy and Art of Darkness*.

Mazama, A. (2003). *The Afrocentric Paradigm*. Africa World Press Inc..

Mbembe, A. (2016). *Necropolitics*. Duke University Press.

Mbembe, A. (2017). *Critique of Black Reason*. Duke University Press.

McMenamin, J. F. (2016). The Poet's Inner Child: Early Childhood and Spiritual Growth in Dante's "Commedia". *Italica, 93*(2), 225–250. Retrieved from https://www.jstor.org/stable/44504561%0A

Merleau-ponty, M. (1962). *The Phenomenology of Perception*. Routledge.

Moustakas, C. (1990). *Heuristic Research Design, Methodology and Applications*. Sage Publications.

Moustakas, C. (1994). *Phenomenological Research Methods*. Sage Publications.

Narayanan, A. (2014). Ambivalent Subjects: Psychoanalysis, Women's Sexuality in India and the Writings of Sudhir Kakar. *Psychodynamic Practice, 20*(3), 213–227. https://doi.org/10.1080/14753634.2014.916839

Rousseau, J.-J. (1984). *A Discourse on Inequality*. Penguin Books Limited.

Rousseau, J.-J. (1998). *The Social Contract*. Wordsworth Editions Limited.

Said, E. W. (1989). Representing the Colonized: Anthropology's Interlocutors. *Critical Inquiry, 15*(2), 205. https://doi.org/10.1086/448481

Said, E. (1993). Representations of an Intellectual Lecture 2: Holding Nations and Traditions at Bay. *Reith Lectures, June*, 1–8.

Sudbury, J. (2001). (Re)constructing Multiracial Blackness: Women's Activism, Difference and Collective Identity in Britain. *Ethnic and Racial Studies, 24*(1), 29–49. https://doi.org/10.1080/014198701750052488

Tonkinson, R. (2013). Dream-Spirits and Innovation in Aboriginal Australia's Western Desert. *International Journal of Transpersonal Studies, 32*(1), 127–139.

Tull, S. E., Wickramasuriya, T., Taylor, J., Smith-Burns, V., Brown, M., Champagnie, G., Daye, K., Donaldson, K., Solomon, N., Walker, S., Fraser, H., & Jordan, O. W. (1999). Relationship of Internalized Racism to Abdominal Obesity and Blood Pressure in Afro-Caribbean Women. *Journal of the National Medical Association, 91*(8), 447–452. Retrieved from http://www.pubmedcentral.nih.gov/articlerender.fcgi?artid=2608441&tool=pmcentrez&rendertype=abstract

Turner, D. D. (2020). *Black Steel in the Hour of Chaos*. BME Voices. Retrieved from https://www.bmevoices.co.uk/black-steel-in-the-hour-of-chaos/

Turner, D. D. L. (2021). *Intersections of Privilege and Otherness in Counselling and Psychotherapy* (1st ed.). Routledge.

Turner, D. D. L. (2023). *The Psychology of Supremacy*. Routledge.

Valley, M. (1991). Spiritual Issues in Psychotherapy. *The Journal of Transpersonal Psychology, 23*(2), 105–119.

van der Kolk, B. (2015). *The Body Keeps The Score: Mind, Brain and Body in the Transformation of Trauma* (1st ed.). Penguin Books Limited.

Various. (2020). *George Floyd Death*. BBC News. Retrieved from https://www.bbc.co.uk/news/topics/cv7wlylxzg1t/george-floyd-death

Various. (2023). *The Genesis of Doctor Who*. BBC Online. Retrieved from https://www.bbc.co.uk/articles/cx8rvvrej7zo

Vaughan, A. G. (2019). African American Cultural History and Reflections on Jung in the African Diaspora. *Journal of Analytical Psychology, 64*(3), 320–348. https://doi.org/10.1111/1468-5922.12501

Walter, M., & Suina, M. (2019). Indigenous Data, Indigenous Methodologies and Indigenous Data Sovereignty. *International Journal of Social Research Methodology, 22*(3), 233–243. https://doi.org/10.1080/13645579.2018.1531228

5

Doing Love in Research

Rayann Alves-Bryan

Introduction

Love is an entity that has been spoken about and explored by many writers and academics. It is widely debated whether love is an emotion, feeling or action. In *All About Love: New Visions,* bell hooks states that love is a verb, not a noun. For hooks, love must involve care, affection, recognition, respect, commitment, trust and open communication (hooks, 2018). According to Freudian psychoanalysis, love is an ever-present and an affective bond, which is crucial to the formation of subjectivity, sociality and even civilisation (Ahmed, 2014). Both definitions place the importance of connection and investment of feelings and emotions that we can have with each other. hook's understanding of love is parallel to the Merriam-Webster definition which states that love is a "strong affection for another arising out of kinship or personal ties" (*Definition of LOVE*, 2023). Moreover, Maslow's hierarchy of needs mentions love as a vital need for human development as it facilitates feelings of motivation

R. Alves-Bryan (✉)
University of Greenwich, London, UK

G. Kinouani et al. (eds.), *Creative Disruption*, Studies in the Psychosocial,
https://doi.org/10.1007/978-3-031-63661-5_5

and fulfilment. The definitions about love clarify its description as an entity because it is distinct, independent and a force that is critical to life and the needs of humans.

Love has the ability to reproduce the collective through allegiance to an ideal and creating a bond between subjects (Ahmed, 2014, p. 124). It also possesses potentially dangerous consequences as it is a way of bonding people together and allegiance in relation to an ideal. Ahmed (2014) highlights a trend amongst "hate groups" who will rename themselves as organisations of love. I would argue in these instances it isn't that love is dangerous but rather the ability for love to be easily coopted and incorrectly used to mask behaviours that come from hate instead of love. Ahmed's discussion prompts a need to highlight the various ways that love can be coopted, misunderstood and rebranded to justify abuse. bell hooks [add citation] also observes that some parents may strike or abuse their children and claim that it is a form of love. Therefore, it is important to continue to state what love is and that love should not result in the harm of others. The discourse about love indicates that love has a range of possibilities and is an action that has unlimited and transformative possibilities. Many writers have highlighted the use of love as a tool for resistance, liberation, and building communities and relationships with others (Bell & Sinclair, 2014; Fromm, 1995; hooks, 2018; Kiriakos & Tienari, 2018).

Love and Black Feminist Research

Love is not often viewed as an emotion that is commonly associated with the research process despite its ability to play a critical role in the process. Existing work written about love in research explores love as an object of research rather investigating what it can offer the researcher and the research process (Freud, 2006; Hendrick & Hendrick, 1986, 1989; Lindholm, 1998; Sternberg, 1996). Approaching love through a creative psychosocial lens helps love to be understood beyond its emotional and psychological aspects. Opening the door to a broader examination of love as a multifaceted social phenomenon which is an integral part of human experience and social interaction. Researchers are prompted to consider love not only as a subject but a driving force behind their investigations. Moreover, when incorporated into the research process love can help to guide research decisions, establish rapport with participants and facilitate collaboration. Arguably Black feminist research emphasises the possibilities for love in the research process. Perhaps, many Black feminist researchers engage with love and an ethic of love in their research and writing. Often, Black feminist research will utilise a core component of love and foster a commitment from the researcher to produce knowledge that respects and affirms others before ourselves (Burkhard, 2019; Evans-Winters, 2019; hooks, 2018). In this chapter, I explore the idea that love can and should be centred in research specifically focusing on Black feminist research. Love provides a space for the exploration of personal identity, healing and transformation through its ability to give researchers the tools to take a radical positionality within their research that is subjective and honours their emotions and parts of their identity.

I understood the need to centre and acknowledge love within research through my own. Hearing stories from Black Caribbean women helped me to connect with my grandmother, who passed away during my early childhood. As I heard Black Caribbean women share their stories about Windrush and read Black feminist writers' stories about their mothers and grandmothers, I have been able to claim and embrace the wounds of my Black female self and others (Nash, 2013; Walker, 2004).

Many Black feminists before me have engaged with love and the ethics of love to explore its possibilities for furthering the Black feminist movement and research (Burkhard, 2019; Nash, 2013; Odozor, 2022). Arguably, love in research can be a lens that supports Black feminists to move towards reclaiming the past, gaining liberation in the present and having an emancipated future (Odozor, 2022). Moreover, it raises questions about the research process, examines intentions to conduct research and asks how Black feminist researchers can honour their research participants. Research should always honour its research participants as a fundamental ethical principle as it acknowledges and respects the participants by valuing their stories and experience, and by viewing them as the experts. It requires actively seeking their input, involving them in the process and acknowledging their contributions as equal partners in research. It is a radical concept because it challenges the traditional power dynamics between the researcher and participant, emphasising equity and collaboration. Moreover, it challenges the historical legacy of exploitative research between researchers and participants that requires researchers to be at distance from the subject of their research (Burkhard, 2019; James, 2021). Ultimately, this radical shift aims to amplify voices that have been historically silenced and create research that is more meaningful, impactful and ethically grounded.

Love can guide research decisions as love for a particular topic or research question can motivate researchers to pursue a particular line of inquiry, methodology or theoretical framework. For example, love increased my motivation and engagement during the research process. Being passionate about my research topic and wanting to honour and capture the authentic stories about Black Caribbean women drove me to seek creative methodologies that were focused on showcasing the voices of Black Caribbean women while acknowledging how my own personal identity influences the project.

Black feminist theory uses an interpretive perspective and rejects the positivist approach to research. Positivism demands the researcher to be distant from the subjects of their research and remove all emotions that are attached to their project. These principles are the opposite of what is required for Black feminist research (Burkhard, 2019; Collins, 2000; Evans-Winters, 2019; James, 2021; Lincoln et al., 2003). Moreover, Black feminism asks researchers to be emotional and close to their research by encouraging researchers to be unapologetic about their ties and emotions to the research and requires all researchers to acknowledge their positionality within the research process (Evans-Winters, 2019; Lincoln et al., 2003; Nadar, 2014).

Furthermore, the overarching concepts of the ethics of care, love, personal accountability and lived experience as critical criteria for Black feminist research not only emphasise individual uniqueness but pinpoint the necessity for emotions (Collins, 2000; Lincoln et al., 2003; Nadar, 2014). It is easy to see how love underpins all of the core elements of Black feminist epistemology as it privileges care, responsibility and knowledge (Fromm, 1995). When a researcher comes from a place of love it encourages them to be authentic, honest and committed to the community that they are researching and writing about because "love is the active concern for the life and the growth of that which we love. Where this active concern is lacking, there is no love" (Fromm, 1995, p. 21). Black feminist researchers should be actively concerned about their participants and the wider collective of Black women. The knowledge that we produce should provide some sort of understanding and healing for the Black women that share their stories and those who read them.

Doing Love as a Researcher

Love can help researchers establish a rapport with their participants and the wider community by not only demonstrating empathy and understanding but also a desire to produce credible and valid research. One could argue that embracing love in research enables researchers to adopt a subjective stance, honouring their emotions and addressing aspects of their identity with a radical positionality. For example, while undertaking my doctoral research, I have indirectly explored my self-identity by connecting with literature from other Black feminists that write literature on experiences and researching topics that are close to the self and identity.

Moreover, Black feminist epistemology states that the validity and credibility of Black feminist research and truth claims come from within our communities. Therefore, all knowledge claims must be validated within the community we are researching, and less concern should be given to how outsiders receive our work (Evans-Winters, 2019; Nadar, 2014). Love encourages researchers to take action to have their work credited and validated by the community. Also, the participants and community will feel that researchers care about their experiences and are committed to understanding their perspectives. This can be illustrated briefly by my qualitative methodology, where I shared my interview notes with each participant. The notes were a collection of my thoughts and feelings during their interview, and I gave them all a chance to respond in an unstructured and informal follow-up. Not only do their responses create richer data but also demonstrate an ethics of care as I am soliciting their responses to ensure that the stories and analysis reveal their truth.

Moreover, I am incorporating them into the analytical process through their responses and the further context they may provide for their stories. In addition, it ensures that I am sharing their narratives authentically and in a way that they are comfortable with.

My interviews with Black Caribbean uncovered a number of poignant narratives about the Windrush generation that evoked a myriad of emotions within me. In each interview, I had the privilege of delving into the life story of each woman, which left me emotionally and intellectually stimulated. I wrote pages of notes capturing the raw emotions I experienced—sympathy, sadness, shock and joy—forming an integral part of the process as I navigated through these heartfelt accounts.

I made the conscious decision to share my notes with each of the interviewees, as an act that fostered an atmosphere of mutual respect and empathy. By opening up about my initial thoughts and feelings, I was able to bridge the gap between the role of a detached researcher and that of a compassionate human being. This disclosure helped validate the participants' experiences, allowing them to feel heard and understood. It was evident that my willingness to be vulnerable resonated with them, making them more receptive to the research process. Some participants responded with a desire to further clarify certain points or nuances in their stories. This exchange led to follow up informal interviews, allowing me to gain deeper insights into their experiences and feelings. This process of reciprocal dialogue evolved into a collaborative analysis, where the participants actively contributed to the interpretation of their stories. Their involvement not only enriched the research outcomes but also reinforced their agency in shaping the narrative.

At the heart of this exchange was the driving force of love. Love, not just as an abstract concept, but as a palpable connection rooted in shared experiences and genuine empathy. Love was the driving factor that prompted me to share my emotions with the participants and invited them to engage in the research process. Thus, it could be the love that I exhibited to the participants that could have encouraged them to clarify their stories and continue to actively participate in the research. Thus, the love that I exhibited to the participants may have encouraged them to clarify their stories and continue to actively participate in the research, transcending the traditional roles of researcher and subject.

Love demands the researcher openly takes a subjective position that requires acknowledgement of the thoughts and emotions tied to their chosen research topic and the process of knowledge production. In addition, love, therefore, facilitates a potential space for researchers to do reflexivity in a new way that honours, centres and acknowledges the powerful emotions tied to conducting research that involves the self.

Love, Reflexivity and the Insider/Outsider

There are five variants of reflexivity: introspection, intersubjective reflection, mutual collaboration, social critique and discursive deconstruction (Finlay, 2002, p. 212). When reflexivity is introspective the researcher examines how their own experiences and personal meanings inform understanding and interpretations of their data (Finlay, 2002, p. 214). Introspection is not used to skew or block the participant's voices but to understand and acknowledge how their own experiences and perspectives can inform the analysis of their data.

Reflexivity as mutual collaboration recognises the participant's ability to be reflexive and a co-researcher. It creates space to move past preconceived theories and stereotypes by offering the opportunity to hear multiple voices and conflicting positions (Finlay, 2002). Jennifer Elyse James (2021) provides a reflexive practice that is informed by Black feminist epistemological ethics of caring to create a collective dialogue between herself and her participants. She has formulated a methodological practice where researchers write down their thoughts and opinions on their interviewee's narrative and share the notes with the participants and give them a chance to respond (James, 2021). James' (2021) methodological practice creates an openness between the researcher and participant that displays the care and love that the researcher has for the participants. In addition, it elicits a more in-depth narrative from the participants in their responses (Burkhard, 2019; James, 2021).

Moreover, love gives researchers the ability to authentically address the "insider/outsider" dichotomy that occurs in research and explore how it can impact the researcher's relationship with their research and participants (Collins, 2000; Dwyer & Buckle, 2009; Kerstetter, 2012).

Researchers are able to view the insider positionality as complex and riddled with difficulties that can hinder the research project (Kerstetter, 2012). Instead, I argue that the ability to embed and relate my personal experiences with those of my participants is a benefit. Lines of familiarity between the stories of my Black female participants and those of my family members offer reflexive introspection and the ability to create mutual collaboration (Finlay, 2002, p. 214). I can use the stories of my participants as an anchor point for my introspection and begin to piece together the lost stories of my grandmother that I am desperately searching for. In other words, I am able to identify and find likeness to myself and others in the participants' stories. Moreover, I can become a collaborator and avoid erasing myself from the research, creating a collective dialogue between myself, my grandmother and participants (James, 2021).

Love and Knowledge Creation

Love can be a central part of a researcher's wider reflexive framework that encompasses intimacy and vulnerability. The intimacies created as part of the research process arguably help to extend any feminist reflexive practice by bringing to attention the temporal conditions of affective puncturing and the risks of wounding being equated with reflexive comprehension (Page, 2017, p. 27). Researchers, such as Fraser and Puwar (2008) and Page (2017), have argued that sensory, emotional and affective relations are central to how researchers engage, produce and understand their research.

Intimacy, love and vulnerability are produced during the course of the research as we engage and carry the smells, textures, pains, desires, sounds and visuals when we collect data, conduct analysis and present our data (Fraser & Puwar, 2008). While these insights are important to Black feminist researchers generally academia does not provide space for these insights to be featured. Fraser and Puwar (2008, p. 2) state that "the rhythm, smell, sense, tension and pleasure that go into producing what will become research and data remain largely outside of such discussions." Often sociologists and social researchers are trained to be objective, and this is jarring to the practice of love and general Black feminist theory (Collins, 2000; Taylor, 2018).

Centring love in research asks that researchers are more subjective by connecting with all elements of the research and engaging with how the research makes us feel. We may explore possible connections with our participants and use our research to engage and understand parts of our identity and lived experiences. Thus, the need for researchers to be objective can hinder the ability for love to be fully actioned within research. Researchers are constrained by the need to show a certain level of objectivity to the wider academic community. Therefore, questions remain as to whether it is truly possible for love to be fully practised in research if a certain level of distance needs to be present for research to be accepted by academic peers.

While love can provide critical observations for research and can create richer and more authentic knowledge, there may not be a language or framework within academia that is available for researchers to authentically explore the emotional ties to their research (Fraser & Puwar, 2008). Arguably Black feminist research is an act of love as it challenges and disrupts mainstream ideas about how knowledge should be produced: it offers researchers a framework that asks us to acknowledge our emotions, feelings and identity. This can be perceived as a radical act of love, especially when academia has a preference for objectivity and "real" scientific methods that create distance between the researcher and the researched which is heralded to be unbiased.

Academia overlooks Black feminism, and while inroads have been made and some Black feminist academics have received their flowers (James, 2021, p. 208), there is still a preference and privilege towards white Western schools of thought that ignore and are unable to comprehend Black women's experiences and our research (Collins, 2000; James, 2021; Lincoln et al., 2003). The exclusionary practices of academia can make it impossible for love to be fully practised in all disciplines of knowledge products. Black people and Black feminist theory are often placed in exclusionary marginalised positions where their theories and knowledge are not deemed as worthy as their counterparts (Wright et al., 2007). Thus, many Black feminists may make compromises about their research and as a result avoid embedding the core elements of love in an attempt to have their work perceived as "serious" and worthy of reward. We then have to ask how much is lost in research and the reflexive practice when researchers are unable to fully explore love within their own work. Further questions are raised about the possibility to truly practise love as a researcher when the academy marginalises and excludes minoritised groups. Exercising love demands acceptance, care, commitment and respect that the academy does not fully offer to particular communities, specifically those who are viewed as the "subaltern" (Spivak, 1988). Those who are part of the colonial populations, lower social classes and the Other are often left voiceless and are spoken for by those in positions of power (Ibid.). If academic institutions are unable to do the core elements of love, then it may not ever be able to be fully present. Thus, love in research becomes limited to the actions of the researcher and is invisible in wider academia.

Conclusion

In conclusion, love has many possibilities to enrich the research process for both researchers and participants. Love is not only an emotion but an action that sticks people together and in turn can bond the researcher to their research topic and participants. In this chapter, I have explored how Black feminist theory can be a lens for researchers to engage and use love in their research and engage more authentically to their research. I would argue that researchers should consider how intimacy, love and vulnerability are reproduced during the course of knowledge production as part of their reflexive practice to critically examine their choice of research topic, how they share their research and engage with their participants. Moreover, centring love, as Black feminist epistemology encourages, can push researchers to explore creative methodologies that honour their feelings and emotions.

References

Ahmed, S. (2014). *The Cultural Politics of Emotion* (2nd ed.). Edinburgh University Press.

Bell, E., & Sinclair, A. (2014). Reclaiming Eroticism in the Academy. *Organization, 21*(2), 268–280. https://doi.org/10.1177/1350508413493084

Burkhard, T. (2019). I Need You to Tell My Story: Qualitative Inquiry for/With Transnational Black Women. *Cultural Studies ↔ Critical Methodologies, 19*(3), 184–192. https://doi.org/10.1177/1532708618817883

Collins, P. H. (2000). Black Feminist Epistemology. In *Black Feminist Thought: Knowledge, Consciousness, and the Politics of Empowerment* (Rev. 10th anniversary ed., pp. 251–273). Routledge.

Definition of LOVE. (2023, March 23). Merriam Webster. Retrieved from https://www.merriam-webster.com/dictionary/love

Dwyer, S. C., & Buckle, J. L. (2009). The Space Between: On Being an Insider-Outsider in Qualitative Research. *International Journal of Qualitative Methods, 8*(1), 54–63. https://doi.org/10.1177/160940690900800105

Evans-Winters, V. E. (2019). *Black Feminism in Qualitative Inquiry: A Mosaic for Writing Our Daughter's Body* (1st ed.). Routledge. https://doi.org/10.4324/9781351046077

Finlay, L. (2002). Negotiating the Swamp: The Opportunity and Challenge of Reflexivity in Research Practice. *Qualitative Research, 2*(2), 209–230. https://doi.org/10.1177/146879410200200205

Fraser, M., & Puwar, N. (2008). Introduction: Intimacy in Research. *History of theHumanSciences,21*(4),1–16.https://doi.org/10.1177/0952695108095508

Freud, S. (2006). *The Psychology of Love.* Penguin Books.

Fromm, E. (1995). *The Art of Loving.* Thorsons.

Hendrick, C., & Hendrick, S. (1986). A Theory and Method of Love. *Journal of Personality and Social Psychology, 50*(2), 392–402. https://doi.org/10.1037/0022-3514.50.2.392

Hendrick, C., & Hendrick, S. S. (1989). Research on Love: Does it Measure Up? *Journal of Personality and Social Psychology, 56*(5), 784–794. https://doi.org/10.1037/0022-3514.56.5.784

hooks, bell. (2018). *All About Love: New Visions* (First William Morrow paperback ed.). William Morrow.

James, J. E. (2021). Black Feminist Epistemological Methodology: Bridging Theory and Methods to Research Health and Illness. In Z. Luna &

W. N. L. Pirtle (Eds.), *Black Feminist Sociology: Perspectives and Praxis* (1st ed.). Routledge. https://doi.org/10.4324/9781003199113

Kerstetter, K. (2012). Insider, Outsider, or Somewhere in Between: The Impact of Researchers' Identities on the Community-Based Research Process. *Journal of Rural Social Sciences, 27*, 20.

Kiriakos, C. M., & Tienari, J. (2018). Academic Writing as Love. *Management Learning, 49*(3), 263–277. https://doi.org/10.1177/1350507617753560

Lincoln, Y. S., Denzin, N. K., & Collins, P. H. (Eds.). (2003). Toward an Afrocentric Feminist Epistemology. In *Turning Points in Qualitative Research: Tying Knots in a Handkerchief* (pp. 47–67). AltaMira Press.

Lindholm, C. (1998). Love and Structure. *Theory, Culture & Society, 15*(3–4), 243–263. https://doi.org/10.1177/026327649801500301 1

Nadar, S. (2014). "Stories are Data with Soul"—Lessons from Black Feminist Epistemology. *Agenda, 28*(1), 18–28. https://doi.org/10.1080/10130950.2014.871838

Nash, J. C. (2013). Practicing Love: Black Feminism, Love-Politics, and Post-Intersectionality. *Meridians, 11*(2), 1–24. https://doi.org/10.2979/meridians.11.2.1

Odozor, E. T. (2022). A Love Ethic for Black Feminisms: The Necessity of Love in Black Feminist Discourses and Discoveries. *Hypatia, 37*(2), 241–256. https://doi.org/10.1017/hyp.2022.13

Page, T. (2017). Vulnerable Writing as a Feminist Methodological Practice. *Feminist Review, 115*(1), 13–29. https://doi.org/10.1057/s41305-017-0028-0

Spivak, G. C. (1988). Can the Subaltern Speak? In C. Nelson & L. Grossberg (Eds.), *Marxism and the Interpretation of Culture* (pp. 271–313). Macmillan Education. Retrieved from https://abahlali.org/files/Can_the_subaltern_speak.pdf

Sternberg, R. J. (1996). Love Stories. *Personal Relationships, 3*(1), 59–79. https://doi.org/10.1111/j.1475-6811.1996.tb00104.x

Taylor, B. K. D. (2018). Rejecting Objectivity: Reflections of a Black Feminist Researcher Interviewing Black Women. *A/b: Auto/Biography Studies, 33*(3), 721–726. https://doi.org/10.1080/08989575.2018.1499505

Walker, A. (2004). *In Search of Our Mothers' Gardens: Womanist Prose.* Amistad Press.

Wright, C., Thompson, S., & Channer, Y. (2007). Out of Place: Black Women Academics in British Universities. *Women's History Review, 16*(2), 145–162. https://doi.org/10.1080/09612020601048704

6

Playing with Brexit

Tom Fielder

In this chapter I have included the full script of my presentation at the 2022 Birkbeck Psychosocial Studies PhD conference, "Creative Disruption: Expanded Methods in Psychosocial Thinking and Practice", from which this volume has emerged. Or rather, I have included the full script of the presentation I had *intended* to present at the conference, but was unable to deliver, due to Covid-related illness. It was not until the end of October 2022, during one of our PhD research seminars, that I was able to give what Dr Margarita Aragon described as my "presentation/one-man play". My original presentation for the conference was titled, "A Dramatization of Brexit Psychobabble". The idea was to explore the potential of creative practice to more effectively communicate the concerns of my doctoral research, specifically through a kind of "dramatization" of my research material. I felt that the dual focus of my research—Brexit and psychoanalysis—lent itself particularly well to such a dramatization: the Hollywood fascination with the psychoanalytic encounter on the one hand, and the familiar media spectacle of Brexit

T. Fielder (✉)
Birkbeck University, London, UK

G. Kinouani et al. (eds.), *Creative Disruption*, Studies in the Psychosocial,
https://doi.org/10.1007/978-3-031-63661-5_6

and its television personalities on the other. The very first idea was to play Boris Johnson on the couch, on the morning after the referendum, swearing uncontrollably. It is only more recently, thanks to Antony Seldon's (2023) account, that we have learned the words Johnson actually used that morning: "Holy shit, fuck, what have we done?". There would be some strong language, as I have indicated, and those likely to be distressed by satirical impersonations of Boris Johnson ("gorillaesque", in the words of one comrade) were advised to prepare themselves appropriately. Yet as I began to put the script together—which involves a collage of primary research materials, together with academic commentary and creative writing—I felt that I was engaging in a process that went beyond simple amusement.

Should that be surprising? As a conference participant, the formal intention was to contribute to the creative disruption of psychosocial methods. If I was enjoying myself, I was enjoying myself as a psychosocial researcher, stimulated by the way in which the conference theme had been articulated, and unable simply to forget my concerns as a PhD researcher. The notion of irony may be helpful here: what if I separate myself, for a moment, from the routine conventions of my doctoral research to date, and try speaking like this? Psychosocial studies itself proceeds on the basis of a kind of irony: in not knowing how to authoritatively define itself as a scholarly field, or even whether it wishes to do so, psychosocial studies is free to think in new and creative ways. My own dramatization of Brexit and psychoanalysis involves accessing an alternative vision of reality, in which familiar voices speak in different ways. Such creative disruption of what is taken-for-granted opens up novel possibilities for thought, inviting us into a more creative relationship with the power structures that shape our psyches and our politics. Why should it be this way? Can we imagine and even begin to enact what Jeannete Winterson (2016), in the immediate aftermath of the referendum, called "better stories"?

I have retitled this chapter, "Playing with Brexit", to retain the reference to theatricality, but also to allow me to push a little further my sense of the kind of work involved in putting together and then performing this piece. I am indebted here to Candida Yates' immensely helpful study, *The Play of Political Culture, Emotion and Identity* (2015), which I read a couple of months after writing the script. Yates uses the idea of "play" as a metaphor with which to explore the psychodynamics of political culture in the UK's "postmodern mediatised landscape" (Yates, 2015, p. 17), as marked by "the increasingly fluid boundaries between popular and political culture" (p. 16). She identifies two "ideal types" or modes of play, "partly [reflecting] existing debates within political, cultural and media studies" (ibid., p. 16; cf. Craig, 2004; Thompson, 1995; Washbourne, 2010). "On the one hand", writes Yates (2015, p. 16), "'play' suggests a form of manipulation where members of the public are seduced and positioned as passive 'dupes' of oppressive forces of ideological governance and Machiavellian political processes." This is the negative or passive sense of being "played with" by celebrity politicians such as Boris Johnson or Nigel Farage. "Yet, on the other", she continues, "it connotes a more interactive mode of political communication and engagement, where voters may identify, contest or flirt with political parties and politicians" (Ibid.). This is the more positive possibility in which voters may experiment and "play with" their political subjectivities and identities. "Play", in this latter sense, inhabits a "transitional" space, where political identifications can be continually reworked and recreated (Winnicott, 1971). Yates (2015, p. 16) notes that less has been said about the emergence of such transitional spaces "for 'feeling-ful' modes of identification and fantasy" in the contemporary mediatized environment, and, I would add, the possibilities these spaces afford for psychosocial praxis.

Yates (2015, p. 17) writes that her approach "uses psychoanalytic ideas" to develop her twofold reading of the play metaphor, and the psychoanalyst D.W. Winnicott is the key reference. She specifically links the new "potential" spaces within what Craig (2004) has called the "mediatised political field" of political culture, to what Winnicott called "the transitional 'cultural field' of the psyche and imagination, where the ongoing engagement with transitional phenomena and fantasy take place", and through which "identity and a sense of self are also shaped" (Yates, 2015, p. 17; see also Yates & Day Sclater, 2000). Winnicott's thinking about play is closely related to his theory of transitional phenomena. The space of play, writes Winnicott (1968, p. 592), "is not inside by any use of the word … Nor is it outside, that is to say, it is not a part of the repudiated world, the not-me, that which the individual has decided to recognize (with whatever difficulty and even pain) as truly external, outside magical control." Rather, playing takes place in an intermediate zone, where some aspect of the external world can be invested with subjective meaning, and then modified or "played with" in the service of that subjective material (see also Townsend, 2019). For the Kleinian psychoanalyst Robert Caper (1996, p. 859), play is "a serious type of experimentation", "a way of externalising fantasies originating in one's inner world so they may be seen and learned about". "To control what is outside", as Winnicott (1968, p. 592) writes, "one has to do things, not simply to think or to wish, and doing things takes time. Playing is doing."

To take another example of recent psychosocial scholarly engagement with Winnicott's thinking about play, Lynn Froggett (2018) uses his ideas in her study of the "deep play" of socially engaged art. On Winnicott's account, writes Froggett, exploration in play "is stimulated by the non-identity of self and object and therefore the need to reach across a gap to find the other, who is always in some measure elusive. There is a willing disorientation or destabilisation of self in the process" (ibid., p. 28). Like Yates, Froggett distinguishes between different kinds of "play": on the one hand, the "distracting", "mimetic play of simulation" (ibid., p. 20), which she considers in relation to commercial video games; and on the other hand, "the disorienting exploration of deep play" (p. 31), which she associates with "the critical and reflective operations of art" (p. 19). It is the difference between "dancing on the surface of things" and "encountering something that stops you in your tracks, disorients you, makes you think" and which "only comes to fruition with profound emotional and aesthetic engagement" (ibid., p. 22). For Froggett, such deep play involves a willing encounter with otherness, "negotiating the strain of reconciling what appear to be inner and outer realities, in order to discover the world anew". "It is a process," she continues, "awash with affective cross-currents of love, aggression, creativity, destructiveness and care. Play is getting to know and knowing is emotional work" (p. 28). So then, playing with Brexit? By which I mean, "getting to know" Brexit through a kind of "playing with" the political identifications—including the *otherness* of those identifications—that a psychosocial researcher such as myself might associate with Brexit?

I am not sure if my conference presentation, relayed in the script below, qualifies as socially engaged art. But I would like to think of it at least as a form of play, in which I have invested an external phenomenon—namely Brexit—with what Winnicott (1968, p. 598) calls "dream meaning and feeling". Reflexivity has become a central priority within psychosocial research, and involves seeing the "resonance" that a researcher may experience with their material as a helpful source of information, rather than a problem (Frosh & Sheldon, 2019). Is there a link between reflexivity, including the construction of narrative in reflexive writing, and play? I could certainly describe the "play" that I offer here as a kind of reflexivity, in which I seek to organize my research material, and my emotional investments in that material, into a narrative arc or "drama" that deliberately flaunts its theatricality. This was a therapeutic process, in the sense that it allowed me to play with the voices that I spend so much of my time listening to, giving licence to my own ambivalence, situating those voices in the story that I found I had to tell. But I also hope it might have a wider therapeutic or even political efficacy, given the excessive familiarity of the voices involved. I am not a Brexit supporter, and yet I was going to play *as* Boris Johnson and Nigel Farage, David Cameron, and Dominic Cummings, narrowing my critical distance from these characters through my own (questionable) impersonations, risking an acutely problematic series of identifications in order to see where I could take them in theatre. I was recently able to offer an abridged version of this presentation at a PhD seminar in the Birkbeck English department. A colleague afterwards commented on my somewhat "unhinged" impersonation of Nigel Farage: "Do you think: yes, go Nigel?". Indeed, there is certainly ambivalence, but by giving ourselves permission to act out those inner voices as parts of a bigger picture, perhaps we are able to understand them in a different way, and even puncture them of their power.

A Dramatization of Brexit Psychobabble

Standing in front of audience, wearing a white shirt and blue tie. A Union-Jack headband has been placed stage right, a copy of Ali Smith's Autumn stage left. A glass of water situated somewhere behind.

When I heard the title of the conference today—creative disruption—I, of course, almost immediately, thought about Brexit.

And not only because I am a Brexit researcher, who obviously has difficulty not thinking about Brexit, but also because there did seem to be a certain kind of fit between Brexit and creative disruption.

Not a perfect fit. If Dominic Cummings is said to favour the "creative destruction" theory of politics, he has always, as the journalist Rachel Sylvester (2021) writes, "put a greater emphasis on destruction than creation".

Step to the right, gesturing quizzically.

"Is this what you wanted? This disruption?", Cummings was asked in a recent interview (Moore, 2022).

Step to the left. Looking ahead, a slight roll in the eyes and shoulders.

"There are a lot of people who think that. It's partly why a lot of people voted for Brexit. It's partly why a lot of people were happy at the thought of the Vote Leave guys going into Number 10. They thought, rightly, that we would shake that shit up and things would be very different. People like me say: all these things are rotten. They say: we are going to cause chaos" (ibid.).

Step right.

"Have you ever had therapy?"

Step left.

"I'm not interested in my own emotional state."

Step right.

"Why not?"

Step left.

"Never have been."

Step right.

"But you're interested in other people's emotional states?"

Step left.

"I've got no interest in my own emotional state. Or myself. I find my own emotional state the most boring subject I could think of."

Return to centre, academic tone.

The first rule of psychoanalytic politics is not to indulge in armchair or "wild" analysis about the inner lives of prominent political actors. I do not pretend to offer such analyses in what follows. What I have to offer is a bit of "play": a dramatization of my research—Brexit psychobabble—to explore the potential of creative practice to more effectively communicate my scholarly concerns.

I am a researcher of Brexit and psychoanalysis, of what happens when we bring these two things—Brexit and psychoanalysis—together, into the same room, or lecture theatre, the same mental and emotional world.

Creative disruption is the game today, linking creativity to disruption, seeing what we can do with psychoanalysis, and also literature in my case, to work through the violence of the world around us, and also inside us.

We listen to Boris Johnson, to Nigel Farage, perhaps a little too often if we are a Brexit researcher, and their voices become part of us, of our world. What do we do with those voices? Perhaps we can try acting out a little theatre.

That suffices for an introduction. Now, let's begin.

Pacing around in front of audience, drawing them in. Place a chair centrally, in front of the audience.

I want you to imagine you're a psychoanalyst. [*pause*] And Boris Johnson is lying on your couch [*point to the chair*]. And it's 24 June 2016, the morning after the EU referendum result. And Johnson's campaign for Vote Leave has been successful.

Sit on chair. Look menacingly at the audience, before relaxing back on the chair, hands over head. Withdraw hands.

Fuck. Fuck. Fuck, fuck, fuck, fucking fuck. Fuck.

Walk around the chair, straighten tie, raise eyebrows. Return to sit on the chair.

Silence. Look at each member of the audience in turn, as if challenging them to say something.

Fuck.

Again get up and walk around to address audience.

You're the psychoanalysts. What do you say to him? ... Hold that thought.

I want to read you an extract from David Cameron's (2020 [2019]) autobiography …

Dandyish adjustment to hair and tie. Speaking as if thinking carefully, but also staging a justification.

"What I can say is that throughout it felt as if a sort of cloud was hovering over us. Small to start with, but growing ever larger and darker. Gradually, every killer argument was being drowned out, and every advantage slowly sunk ... It wasn't that Leave was besting us in every battle. It was that the physics of politics seemed to have changed. The upper hand became the losing hand, and the higher ground—which we felt we had captured—was surrounded" (ibid., p. 658).

Sit on the chair to face the audience. Slightly mock sincerity.

"I did everything I could, taking every opportunity, deploying every reasonable, rational, persuasive line, speaking from my heart. But it was like one of those bad dreams where you're trying to shout but no sound is coming out" (ibid., p. 672).

Stand up and walk back around the chair to face audience. Academic tone.

On being asked to sum up the argument against holding a referendum by his director of communications, Craig Oliver, in 2015, David Cameron instantly responded: "you could unleash demons of which ye know not." As Oliver (2017 [2016]) reports in his inside story of Brexit, *Unleashing Demons*, those words proved prophetic, and during the run-up to the referendum and afterwards, "David Cameron's fear that he would unleash demons was fully realised."

Those two sentences I've just read out are the first lines of my thesis.

The demons have been unleashed, and what are we, what are you, what are any of us going to do about it? As scholars, as individuals, as communities?

Sudden change of pace, swinging an arm and moving quickly towards the audience.

"Fight fight, fight"… the novelist Ali Smith (2012) told her audience at a Book Festival in Edinburgh in 2012.

More restrained.

"Language is never not up for it. It's a fight to the life. All we need to do, reader or writer, from first line to final page, is be as open as a book, and be alive to the life in language – on all its levels" (Smith, 2012).

So, right here, right now, that fight for the life and death in language is still unfolding.

Drawing in the audience.

In the red corner, we have …

Go to pick up Union Jack headband, retrieve and place on head, ominously.

Nigel Farage.

Twist round chair, so that the back of the chair is facing the audience.

It's 23 November 2016, two weeks after Donald Trump has been elected President of the United States. [*place one foot on the chair, reaching towards the audience*] And Nigel Farage is at the Ritz Hotel in London, croaking his villainy over the gilded banister to his assembled muster of supporters.

Climb on chair, so standing on chair, facing audience. Very loud. Addressing audience as if they're supporters.

"There's one problem we've got. In America the revolution is total. The Obama administration, and all those ghastly people are out, the Trump people are in, and they're now in control. The problem we have in this country is that while the people have spoken, the same players have just been shuffled around the chessboard, and we're still being run by the career professional political class. And I'm not sure what's going to happen over the next couple of years, but I suspect there's another big, seismic shock in British politics, perhaps going to come at the next general election ... This is unfinished business. The people have spoken, but the establishment don't want to listen. So there are great battles to be fought, and I'm going to go on fighting those battles" (*Guardian*, 2016).

Swirl water in mouth, drink, shake head.

Can we wash this bad language out of our mouths, out of our ears, out of our minds, out of our politics? How do we begin to do so?

We can sit quietly for a moment perhaps [*sit on chair for 10–15 seconds, catch breath*], and then, in the blue corner, we find a book.

Go to pick up the copy of Ali Smith's Autumn.

Let me read you the beginning of Ali Smith's *Autumn* (2017 [2016]), widely hailed as the first post-Brexit novel:

Read very beautifully:

"It was the worst of times, it was the worst of times. Again. That's the thing about things. They fall apart, always have, always will, it's in their nature. So an old old man washes up on a shore. He looks like a punctured football with its stitching split, the leather kind that people kicked a hundred years ago. The sea's been rough. It has taken the shirt off his back; naked as the day I was born are the words in the head he moves on its neck, but it hurts to. So try not to move the head. What's this in his mouth, grit? It's sand, it's under his tongue, he can feel it, he can hear it grinding when his teeth move against each other, singing its sand-song: I'm ground so small, but in the end I'm all, I'm softer if I'm underneath you when you fall, in sun I glitter, wind heaps me over litter, put a message in a bottle, throw the bottle in the sea, the bottle's made of me, I'm the hardest grain to harvest to harvest. The words for the song trickle away. He is tired. The sand in his mouth and his eyes is the last of the grains in the neck of the sandglass. Daniel Gluck, your luck's run out at last. He prises open one stuck eye. But – Daniel sits up on the sand and the stones – is this it? really? this? is death?" (Smith, 2017 [2016], pp. 1–2)

More academic narrative tone.

Boris Johnson quickly recovered from the disappointment of winning the EU referendum. Still, he would see his therapist occasionally … [*very sudden*] "Fuck, fuck, fuck" he would say, and then "we won, we won, we won" [*again quite sudden and sharp, emphatic gesturing*] … "we are going to get Brexit done and unleash Britain's potential". [*take another sip of water*] … But he had other things to say to his therapist too, after winning the election in 2019 …

Sit on chair, faced towards audience again, as at the beginning. Subtle impersonation of Boris Johnson.

I've had a recurrent nightmare. [*rise from chair towards audience*] It's early in the morning – or earlyish – and I'm leaving Downing Street, for a jog or a walk, sometimes with the dog, sometimes without, and I go through St James Park on a familiar route, and people recognise me, smile at me, point at me, take photos [*narcissistic gestures, perhaps asking audience members if they want a selfie*], sometimes say something, and so on, err, and I'm jogging along [*gorilla-like hunched jogging motion*] … but suddenly [*genuine alarm*], my path is suspended high above the Thames [*unsteady*], and the river is gushing furiously below [*gesture below*]. And I have a terrible desire to jump, to fling myself into the air, to be swallowed up by the churning water … and I close my eyes and clutch my knees [*do so*], and yet all the people around me are going on as normal, going to work, [*building anger*] my advisors and colleagues, and they don't help me. They don't even notice me. And the dog is tugging at the lead. But I can't get up, I can't get up, I'm completely stuck … [*pause*] And then …

well, perhaps I wake up, in Downing Street [*self-satisfied*], and I beat my chest [*do so, three times, angrily*], and I shake these thoughts, away! ... [*sit down on chair to face audience, more relaxed, ironic tone*] You know, it's just a game, isn't it? [*chuckle*] Tell me, am I playing the game well? [*he thinks he is*] You know, you shouldn't believe a word I tell you …

Stand up, modestly, walk round chair to face it. Quiet, ominous. No longer impersonating Johnson.

I had a vision, watching all the people yelling and protesting outside Downing Street after the prorogation of Parliament. Johnson would not escape these furies. Sooner or later, they would come for him, they would clad him in irons, they would escort him to a dank grey cell, and he would whimper pitifully as they thrust him inside and locked the door, there to await his trial, for the terrible misuse of the freedom of his office. … [*kneel by the chair, as if to whisper in Johnson's ear*] Do you really think you'll get away with it? With all of it? Even now they are coming for you.

Walk back to face audience. More confidently.

I could read you more extracts from speeches by Farage or Johnson … Which would you prefer? [*pause*] Neither, right?

Well, how about something that Jacqueline Rose (2021) wrote for the *Guardian* last year?

Careful, reading an academic quotation.

"In my ideal scenario, social trauma and injustice would not be seen as belonging to another universe from our most wayward fears and desires. Instead, they would both find their place at the negotiating table, as we tentatively begin to draw the outlines of a better world" (Rose, 2021).

Look to audience again.

Are you sure you don't want to hear me speaking the words of Boris Johnson or Nigel Farage?

I hope this is somewhat cathartic.

Let us at least stick with our image of Boris Johnson on the couch. But [*pause, raise a finger*] let us dress him in the garb of ancient tragedy.

Moving towards audience, crouching, pointing to stage left.

Hark! The prophetic power of psychoanalysis approaches … or is it Sophocles (2015)?

As a narrator, explaining to the audience.

Tiresias the blind prophet is brought before a mighty king of the world and speaks truth to power, but Oedipus is not ready to listen.

Now as Tiresias, pointing at the chair from behind, stage left. Slight depth added to the voice.

"You have your sight, yet do not see the truth of how the place you're at is bad … Do you know what people you are from? You little realize you're an enemy to your own kin below the earth and here above. One day the fearful-footed curse from mother and from father shall with double spike expel you from this land. You see things focused now, but then you shall see dark … There is no human who shall be more harshly ground to dust than you" (Sophocles, 2015, lines 414–428).

Sit on chair as Oedipus.

"I cannot bear to listen any more to this man's raving. To hell with you … If I'd known you'd talk such lunacy, I never would have brought you near my home … You're nothing but a nuisance here" (Ibid., lines 429–447).

Rise to collect audience. Lyrically:

"Millions of characters, each with their own epic narratives singing it's hard to be an angel until you've been a demon." (Tempest, 2013, p. 2)

That's Kae Tempest (2013) in her poem *Brand New Ancients*: me and you, all of you.

Spoken again, in the same way.

"Millions of characters, each with their own epic narratives singing it's hard to be an angel until you've been a demon" (Tempest, 2013, p. 2).

Pause, more academic tone, approaching conclusion.

Oedipus is an everyman, though perhaps a better man, than Boris Johnson. I could not imagine Johnson gouging out his eyes at the end of the story.

What are we left with? How does this story end?

Looking at audience, to indicate that it is their story too.

Read as a quote:

"From someone who has sight he shall turn blind, from someone rich become a beggar, and then he'll make his way towards an alien land by probing for his footsteps with a stick" (Sophocles, 2015, lines 454–458).

Johnson has just survived a vote of confidence. Do we really imagine him—or Nigel Farage, or anyone really—abandoning wealth and status, making his way towards an alien land: France, Rwanda perhaps, without his sight, probing for his footsteps with a stick?

Perhaps it is up to us to do the work of mourning, which our political leaders are unable to do for themselves.

So let us imagine, perhaps tonight, perhaps a year hence, perhaps in the very last moments of his life, Boris Johnson is back with us on the couch.

Sit on the chair. Long pause. Eyes opening and closing. Look at audience. Look down, closing and opening eyes again.

I'm sorry. I'm sorry. I'm sorry. Forgive me. Forgive me. I'm sorry. I'm afraid. I'm afraid.

Epilogue

The transdisciplinary ethos of psychosocial studies may take the researcher where they are ill-prepared to go: exposing them to disciplinary frontiers or customs which insist on a form of recognition that the researcher may not be able immediately to afford. Conversely, the disciplinary formations that encounter such researchers may have something to learn from the creative journeys they each have taken, and the disruptive provocations they each bring with them. In this chapter, I have used psychoanalytic writing about "play" as a theoretical framework for my own journey in dramatizing my doctoral research about Brexit. The language of play appeals particularly to the context of theatrical performativity, since theatre is synonymous with "play", and acting with "playing". "If it be true that good wine needs no bush", Rosalind remarks at the end of Shakespeare's *As You Like It*, "tis true that a good play needs no epilogue" (Shakespeare, n.d., 5.5.3–5). Like "good wine", a "good play" needs no additional advertisement: as far as "playing" is concerned, it suffices unto itself. "Yet to good wine", Rosalind continues, "they do use good bushes, and good plays prove the better by the help of good epilogues" (5.5.5–7). An epilogue may be expected to improve the text. But rather than boasting of her own "good epilogue", or Shakespeare boasting through her of his own "good play", she is quick to elicit the audience's suspicion about the “case” that she is in, “that am neither a good epilogue nor cannot insinuate with you in the behalf of a good play!” (5.5.7–9).

In the context of my own scholarly considerations, I am aware that I have strayed into the dramaturgical without considering the manifold ways in which theatre and performance studies have engaged the political. In their introduction to *The Oxford Handbook of Politics and Performance*, the editors describe an emerging recognition “across the social science/humanities boundary … that politics and performance are connected intrinsically” (Gluhovic et al., 2021, p. 3). In a chapter titled “Comedy and the Performative Politics of Brexit”, James Brassett (2021, p. 579) even describes “Brexit comedy” as “a socially consequential practice that teases at the (changing) social and political consensus in ways that defy expectations, conventions, and representations”. The editors of the handbook call for “an interdisciplinary conversation in the broadest sense”, commending “a shifting and unpredictable evolution of mutual influence, borrowing and blending across disciplines toward richer and more diverse theoretical and empirical analyses” (Gluhovic et al., 2021, pp. 17–18).

In this spirit, I suggest that recent psychosocial engagements between “play” and “political culture” can benefit the study of politics and performance (Yates, 2015). In particular, psychoanalytic thinking about play—e.g., in the work of Donald Winnicott—may help scholars to articulate the complex imbrication of the psychic and the social in politically engaged art. Brassett (2021) celebrates comic play in the context of Brexit, and I might also emphasize that the language of “play” implies a lightness and degree of pleasure that is absent from the more strenuously critical vocabularies of performance. A child may chuckle at the stiffness of parental performativity—as if there was always something pretentious about the world of adult performance—but that is not to say that the child’s pleasure in play is simply naïve. I am reminded of Terry Eagleton’s (2008 [1983], p. 166) reflections on literary criticism: “The reason why the vast majority of people read poems, novels and plays is because they find them pleasurable.” “This fact is so obvious,” he continues, “that it is hardly ever mentioned in universities.” Eagleton then emphasizes, with reference to psychoanalysis, and against the “trivializing overtones” associated with the word "pleasure", that "pleasure and displeasure are extremely complex issues" (ibid.).

Acknowledgements I am grateful to the conference organizers for giving me the opportunity to develop my thinking in a more creative way, and to the editors of this volume—Guilaine, Clau, and Hannah—for accepting my contribution. Thanks especially to Clau Di Gianfrancesco for her careful reading and suggestions, which have improved this piece.

Funding Details This work was supported by the Economic and Social Research Council under Award Number ES/P000592/1.

References

Brassett, J. (2021). Comedy and the Performative Politics of Brexit. In S. Rai, M. Gluhovic, S. Jestrovic, & M. Saward (Eds.), *The Oxford Handbook of Politics and Performance*. Oxford University Press.

Cameron, D. (2020 [2019]). *For The Record*. William Collins.

Caper, R. (1996). Play, Experimentation and Creativity. *International Journal of Psychoanalysis, 77*, 859–869.

Craig, G. (2004). *The Media, Politics and Public Life*. Allen & Unwin.

Eagleton, T. (2008 [1983]). *Literary Theory: An Introduction*. Blackwell Publishing.

Froggett, L. (2018). Deep Play and Simulation in Urban Space: Of Art and Video-Games. In *Where Strangers Meet: Art in the Public Realm* (pp. 16–36). The British Council.

Frosh, S., & Sheldon, R. (2019). Transmission, Relationality, Ethnography. *Angelaki, 24*(3), 117–134.

Gluhovic, M., et al. (2021). Introduction: Politics and/as Performance, Performance and/as Politics. In S. Rai, M. Gluhovic, S. Jestrovic, & M. Saward (Eds.), *The Oxford Handbook of Politics and Performance*. Oxford University Press.

Moore, S. (2022). A Conversation with Dominic Cummings. *Letters from Suzanne*, 29 May 2022. Retrieved from https://suzannemoore.substack.com/p/a-conversation-with-dominic-cummings

Oliver, C. (2017 [2016]). *Unleashing Demons: The Inside Story of Brexit*. Hodder and Stoughton.

Rose, J. (2021). Life after Death: How the Pandemic has Transformed Our Psychic Landscape. *The Guardian*, 7 December 2021. Retrieved from https://www.theguardian.com/society/2021/dec/07/life-after-death-pandemic-transformed-psychic-landscape-jacqueline-rose

Seldon, A. (2023). *Johnson at 10: The Inside Story*. Atlantic Books.

Shakespeare, W. (n.d.). In B. Mowat, P. Werstine, M. Poston, & R. Niles (Eds.), *As You Like It*. The Folger Shakespeare. Retrieved from https://www.folger.edu/explore/shakespeares-works/as-you-like-it/read/

Smith, A. (2012). How Should Authors Approach the Task of Writing a Novel Today? *EWWC*, Aug 19, 2012. Retrieved from https://www.youtube.com/watch?v=bHOSXziim9A&t=2547s

Smith, A. (2017 [2016]). *Autumn*. Penguin.

Sophocles. (2015). *Oedipus the King*, in *Oedipus the King and Other Tragedies* (O. Taplin, Trans.). Oxford University Press.

Sylvester, R. (2021). Dominic Cummings has Nothing to Lose from a Briefing War with No 10—And Johnson Risks Losing Everything. *Prospect Magazine*, 26 April 2021. Retrieved from https://www.prospectmagazine.co.uk/politics/dominic-cummings-boris-johnson-leaks-downing-street

Tempest, K. (2013). *Brand New Ancients*. Picador.

The Guardian. (2016). Nigel Farage Hands out Ferrero Rocher at Ritz Party—Video. *The Guardian*, 24 November 2016. Retrieved from https://www.theguardian.com/politics/video/2016/nov/24/nigel-farage-at-ritz-party-another-big-seismic-shock-is-coming-video

Thompson, J. P. (1995). *The Media and Modernity: A Social Theory of the Media*. Polity.

Townsend, P. (2019). Play and Playing. In *Creative States of Mind Psychoanalysis and the Artist's Process* (pp. 59–67). Routledge.

Washbourne. (2010). *Mediating Politics: Newspapers, Radio, Television and the Internet*. McGraw-Hill Open University Press.

Winnicott, D. W. (1968). Playing: Its Theoretical Status in the Clinical Situation. *International Journal of Psychoanalysis, 49*, 591–599.

Winnicott, D. W. (1971). *Playing and Reality*. Tavistock.

Winterson, J. (2016). We Need to Build a New Left. Labour Means Nothing Today. *The Guardian*, 24 June 2016. Retrieved from https://www.theguardian.com/politics/2016/jun/24/we-need-to-build-a-new-left-labour-means-nothing-jeanette-winterson

Yates, C. (2015). *The Play of Political Culture, Emotion and Identity*. Palgrave Macmillan.

Yates, C., & Day Sclater, S. (2000). Culture, Psychology and Transitional Space. In C. Squire (Ed.), *Culture in Psychology* (pp. 135–146). Routledge.

7

On Creative Destruction: Getting to Understand an Object Through Play

Sasha Bergstrom-Katz

I open the briefcase, which is sitting heavy on the table, and I unfasten its springy metal latches one by one (Fig. 7.1). Lifting its lid, I discover, inside, little boxes of toys, of puzzles, of blocks, of beads, of string, and little picture books (Fig. 7.2). These little things sit, dirty and used, in the little open boxes. They await tiny fingers to snatch them up and place them on the tabletop. Together, out on the surface, they begin to constitute a little scene. With my help, the green blocks become a tower, the girl doll perches on top of this, and two identical dogs watch from below. I can also enter the world of the little booklets of games. 'What's missing in this picture?' one page challenges me (Fig. 7.3). The wheelbarrow is missing a wheel. (Has it fallen off?) The rabbit is missing an ear. (Did the rabbit escape a frightening experience with a fox?) One boot in a pair is missing its shoelace. (Was this borrowed for some other household use? Or removed after a playful dog chewed at it under the table?) The teapot is missing its handle. (Did the handle get knocked off as the teapot fell off the kitchen drying rack?) The glove has only four fingers, not the usual

S. Bergstrom-Katz (✉)
Max Planck Institute for the History of Science, Berlin, Germany

G. Kinouani et al. (eds.), *Creative Disruption*, Studies in the Psychosocial,
https://doi.org/10.1007/978-3-031-63661-5_7

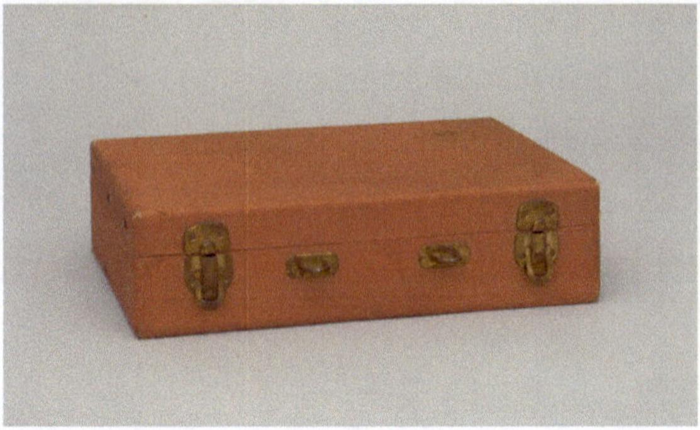

Fig. 7.1 Sasha Bergstrom-Katz, *On the Subject of Tests: Stanford-Binet Form L-M (1960)*, full, closed, 2020, digital image. (*Source:* Photos by author)

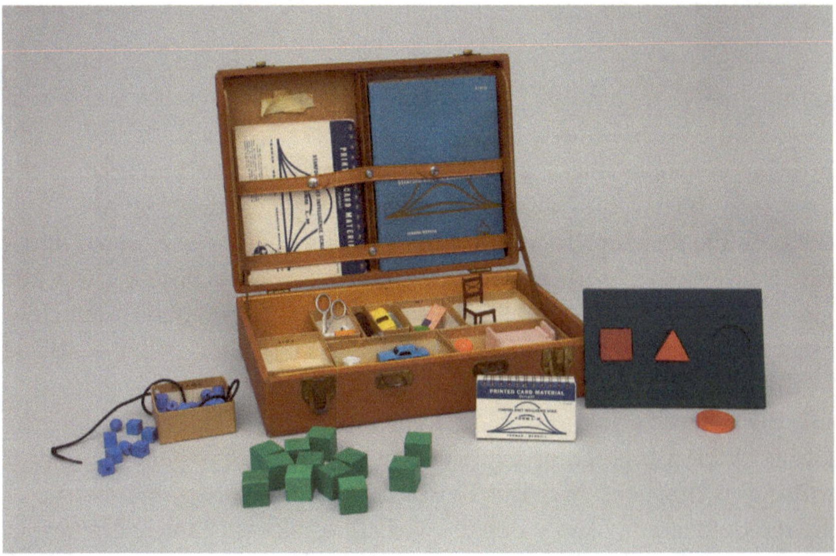

Fig. 7.2 Sasha Bergstrom-Katz, *On the Subject of Tests: Stanford-Binet Form L-M (1960)*, full, open, unpacked, 2020, digital image. (*Source:* Photos by author)

five. (Is this a bespoke glove for a person with four fingers? Or a factory error?) Back in the boxes, the shoelace paired with beads invites a new use (Is this the shoelace missing from the boot?) The beads are meant to be strung, in a particular order, onto this lace.

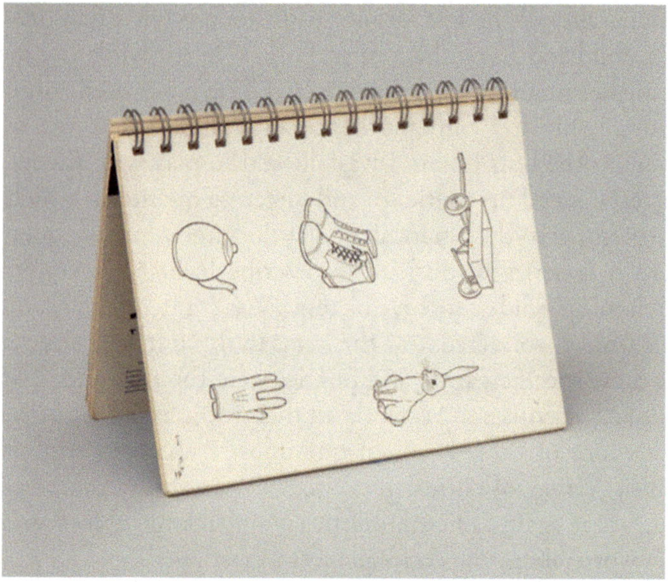

Fig. 7.3 Sasha Bergstrom-Katz, *On the Subject of Tests: Stanford-Binet, Form L-M (1960), Printed Card Material, Mutilated Pictures,* 2020, digital image. (*Source:* Photos by author)

What is this unusual selection of things? The games and puzzles are collected together in a briefcase (which is a utilitarian object most commonly associated with business) and now they are ready to be carried around, but for what purpose? This object (briefcase, toys, and booklets included) is a mid-twentieth-century intelligence test kit called the Stanford-Binet Intelligence Scale (Form L-M) (Terman & Merrill, 1960). This test plays a central role in the formation of the concept of measurable intelligence (which later developed into the Intelligence Quotient [IQ]). This test is derived from what most consider the first standardised intelligence test, the Binet-Simon test, which was created in France in 1905 by psychologist Alfred Binet and his assistant Theodore Simon (see Nicolas et al., 2013). The Stanford-Binet was the translated, revised, re-normed, and repackaged test and was first republished in 1916 after it had been under development at Stanford University by Lewis Terman, his students, and his colleagues (see Boake, 2002).

The materiality of the test kit, not its history, is what first drew me to it. I was a child and I saw this test and others like it while my mom was undergoing her training as a psychologist. I have never been administered this test or any like it, by my mother or anyone else. However, when my mom brought the tests home, I was allowed to play with them. Playing with the test opened up a series of still lingering questions, which ranged from the personal to the practical, and at the same time, the queries were connected to a series of difficult-to-describe feelings. I wondered, for example, how I would score on this test. (Was I 'intelligent'?) and, at the very same time, I wondered how the items in this test were selected. How is it that these specific games and puzzles were the *right* puzzles for psychologists and scientists to know about their subjects' intelligence? While I was conscious of these kinds of questions, I was, and still am, overwhelmed by *feelings* of curiosity, excitement, nervousness, and reticence which tug at me again as I enthusiastically unpack the objects and simultaneously worry about the consequences of testing.

Indeed, testing, and specifically intelligence testing, has been a longstanding subject of scrutiny and critique and rightfully so. Authors such as Kurt Danziger (1998), Nicholas Rose (1998), Stephen Jay Gould (1996), John Carson (2007), and Annette Mülberger (2020) have identified both the inbuilt prejudices of testing and its historical uses which materially affected the lives of people who have been tested. For example, intelligence testing is used in schools (Curtis & Glaser, 1981; Staub, 2018), in employment practices (Sokal, 1987), and in legal cases (Greenspan et al., 2015; Ilyes, 2020) and the results of group or mass testing have been used to reinforce racist stereotypes (Carson, 2007; Gould, 1996). Some scholars have attempted to rescue testing from the 'all bad' critique, emphasising the ways that, for example, social activists have used testing to advocate for equality by proving that children in lower economic and social standing have equal intellectual capacity to their peers in high-income areas (Mülberger et al., 2014). The history of the creation of tests, however, evidences a multitude of embedded ablest theories about the value of 'intelligence' and conceptions about who possesses this 'trait'. Intelligence testing's relationship with eugenics, for example, shaped the development and uses of the tests themselves and influenced both legal decision-making and cultural attitudes about heredity, procreation, and intelligence.

The history of testing is embedded not only in the test and its uses but also in the materiality of the test itself. The space of this short chapter allows for a brief telling of a creative and practice-based aspect of my wider material research into intelligence test kits, but it must be emphasised succinctly here that the ableist, racist, and sexist histories of intelligence testing are absolutely present within the tests and emerge again and again in the staged encounters I ultimately built with these tests.

Playing with Toys

My wider project on intelligence tests ties together how the objects that constitute the tests were gathered, developed, and reconstructed for use and how these objects were borrowed from interestingly disparate places, such as asylums, eugenics labs, playrooms, and popular magazines. Therein, the project ties this material history to the various historical concepts and theories of intelligence, ability, and disability as scientific objects (Daston, 2000). Further, I study the formation of the tests in relation to the growing professionalisation of the field of psychology in the United States (Sokal, 1981) and understand the test kits themselves as actors in this endeavour. However, this chapter does not have the space to delve deeper into these queries but, instead, proposes play as an especially well-matched framework for 'getting to understand' the affective dimensions of the test kits.

In the creation process of this research project, I found psychoanalyst and paediatrician Donald Winnicott's theorisations of play to be potent. In Winnicott's theory of play, play is a serious activity that engages unconscious processes and materialises them in the creative impulse to *destroy* and simultaneously to create. He describes play, first, as a "creative experience taking up space and time", and within this, he illustrates a space that exists within and between the internal psyche and the external world (2010, p. 68). Further, he is adamant that "playing is doing" such that it is a creative action that is not passive and is, in fact, *productive* (Winnicott, 2010, p. 55). In his clinical work, he sees allowing patients to play with things as providing space for self-discovery, even if they play with the most mundane things (spatulas, food cartons, string).

In Winnicott's terms, to be clear, play is not limited to a physical action or activity, but instead is a *psychic* process wherein the subject imagines the destruction of an object (frequently a person) and is thereafter faced with the reality that the object is not under the subject's omnipotent control and was not *actually* destroyed. Winnicott explicates a key aspect of object-usage; the object itself "must necessarily be real in the sense of being part of shared reality, not a bundle of projections" (Winnicott, 2010, p. 118). Therein, Winnicott differentiates object-usage from a strictly *internal* process of the mind or the psyche. Object-usage instead occurs at the convergence of internally constructed objects (the "bundle of projections") and external "real" objects that can be perceived by someone other than the subject and which also has a role due to its nature as an object.

Within Winnicott's conceptualisation of play and object-relating more generally, he insists *destruction* is necessary to create production and the appreciation of cultural objects. Destruction, however, is the step necessary to *use* objects, to take them inside psychologically, and to, at the same time, understand them as separate from the subject. As an example of this process, Winnicott describes the infant's relationship to the breast which begins with the perception that the baby is "feeding on the self, since the breast and the baby have not yet become (for the baby) separate phenomena" (Winnicott, 2010, p. 119). In the next stage, the baby is "feeding from an other-than-me source, or an object that can be given cavalier treatment without effect on the baby unless it [the breast] retaliates" (Winnicott, 2010, p. 119). It is the *transition* between the perception of self-same and self-other that Winnicott wishes to focus on, because, he says, this happens again and again throughout life. The process that occurs is sequential. After "'subject relates to object' comes 'subject destroys object' (as it becomes external); and then may come 'object survives destruction by the subject'" (Winnicott, 2010, p. 120).

Performatively, Winnicott writes the following one-sided conversation, which spells out the process again: "'Hullo object!' 'I destroyed you.' 'I love you.' 'You have value for me because of your survival of my destruction of you.' 'While I am loving you I am all the time destroying you in (unconscious) fantasy'" (Winnicott, 2010, pp. 120–121). This ongoing cyclical relationship between love and destruction is central to Winnicott's theorisation of play, which is a rehearsal of this same activity with all kinds of objects and is posited as a way of getting to understand the self in relation to the external world.

For a moment, I need to return to the test kits and the fact that they are comprised of toys. A historian of science, Jacy L. Young, directly references the makeup of the tests in the title of her article "Test or Toy" wherein she also, literally, unpacks a historical intelligence test kit, the Cattell Infant Intelligence Scale, and queries "psychologists' often-uncritical equation of childhood intelligence with appropriate play undertaken with an appropriate toy and the enactment of normative visions of selfhood" (Young, 2015, p. 103). Therein, Young contextualises historical theories of play in relation to childhood development within the work of psychologists and educationalists such as Karl Groos, G. Stanley Hall, and John Dewey (Young, 2015, p. 107) and, thereafter, makes a convincing case to question the very notion of 'appropriate play' and how it was imported into the field of psychology and, more specifically, in testing. The tests do require that children (and adults) perform tasks that might appear like play, for example, stacking blocks or putting together a puzzle, but the Stanford-Binet tests do not actually engage play as the test dictates a very tight structure during which any diversion from the prescribed task is understood as an issue. There is purposely no 'creative', 'divergent', or 'psychological' dimension to the tests, though tests like the now ubiquitous Rorschach test as well as the Guilford Test of Creativity are similarly prescriptive and are, indeed, still *tests*.

The toys inside of the intelligence tests have a *use*. They are meant to engage the test-takers, by both capturing and sustaining attention, and they are meant to be 'friendly' and familiar to the test-takers. I would also call the toys stand-ins, as they are objects which are largely interchangeable, as the purpose they serve is to be named, stacked, or identified by use (Fig. 7.4). (For example, what is this [points to cup] used for?) The actual specificity of the object is fairly inconsequential. The shape of the puzzles, as another example, must simply be at a certain threshold of recognisability for the test-taker to put them together. Specific toys, however, were chosen, and from the earliest incarnations of intelligence tests

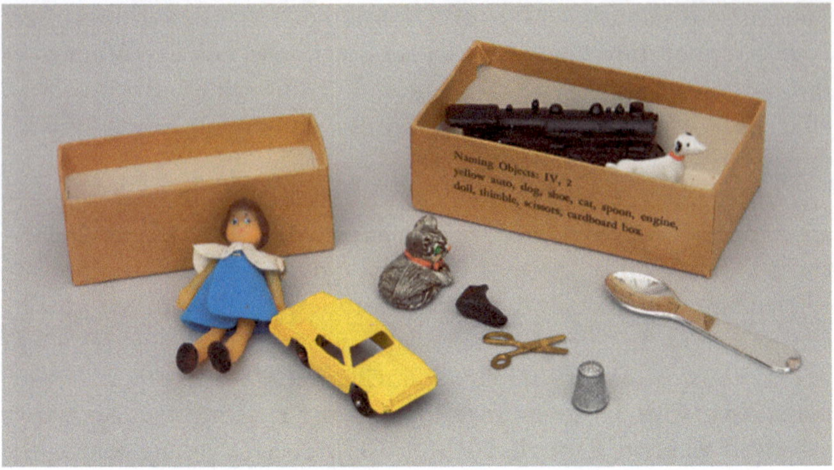
Naming Objects: IV, 2
yellow auto, dog, shoe, cat, spoon, engine,
doll, thimble, scissors, cardboard box.

Fig. 7.4 Sasha Bergstrom-Katz, *On the Subject of Tests: Stanford-Binet Form L-M (1960), Naming Objects, 2020*, digital image. (*Source:* Photos by author)

to the most recent versions, the tests are constituted of illustrative games and puzzles as well as toy figurines and objects, which are subsequently transformed into tests. At the very same time, some objects within the tests which were not originally toys (shoelaces, pennies, buttons [Fig. 7.5]) and then they are, in a sense, transformed into toys by their proximity to the other clearly toy objects and because they are meant to be used in the test in a way that is other than their original practical uses (to lace up shoes, to pay for things, to close up shirts).

What is most curious about the fact that the tests are made of toys is that the subject of the test is not allowed to play with these toys. The toys in the test are the property of the examiners, and the examiners restrict the test-taker's access to and use of the toys. As a creative method for 'opening up' the tests and 'getting to know them', I wanted to defy the very rules of testing and provide space to play with the toys, both as a transgressive act and as a method for studying the tests themselves in the intrapsychic way that Winnicott describes. As I will discuss in the next portion of this writing, I have grown ever more convinced that just by opening up and playing with the tests, I have undertaken a seemingly banal, but actually transgressive, creative, and, therein, destructive act.

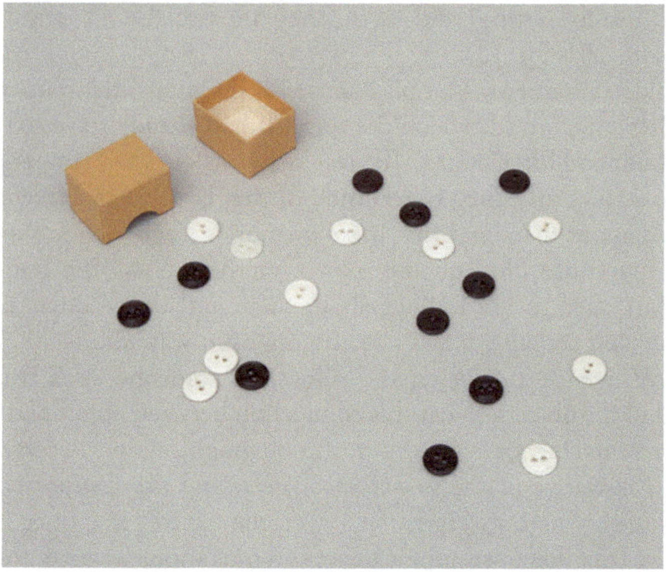

Fig. 7.5 Sasha Bergstrom-Katz, *On the Subject of Tests: Stanford-Binet Form L-M (1960), Sorting Objects by Color, 2020,* digital image. (*Source*: Photos by author)

The play, the opening of the boxes, and the getting to know the test are destructive to the function of the test, which is first off meant to test, not be tested itself through critical examination. Furthermore, by opening up and showing the test to others, the work defies the secrecy inherent in the working of the tests. If the interior is known and studied, a later conducted test cannot be considered valid. That is, this could be considered cheating or facilitating cheating, on a test. Hand in hand, the critical and functional destruction of the test happens through the playful engagement of creative exploration. Therefore, in this piece of creative research, Winnicott's conception of play becomes a space of opportunity to use objects to learn about the 'self' and to, in turn, learn about these objects *through* the self. The test kits, therefore, act as "objects to be creative into and with" (Winnicott, 2010, pp. 136–137). What Winnicott describes here, then, is the process of finding "real objects" and bringing them inside and playing with them. To use the test kits as objects, therefore, they must first go through a process of destruction, basically to test their real-ness (reality testing) and, then, they are available for creative play (Winnicott, 2010, p. 15).

Winnicott's framework of play addresses the interstitial space of interior and exterior worlds which the test kits had already traversed for me in my childhood interactions. The test kits were 'out there' impervious to my destruction, and they were inside of me, both to the extent that I fantasised about them and that these memories stuck with me such that I based my entire PhD on the subject of these tests. The test objects became attached to my feelings about them and the feelings that they stirred up, or perhaps, it worked the opposite way, the feelings I had about intelligence and being the subject of someone else's study, got attached to the objects. What this connection between object and subjectivity presents is not something autobiographical, or necessary, but instead, illustrative of the power of objects, and the distinct power of certain kinds of objects. Here, the object, the test kit, is at once: a test, a kit, a box (ripe for opening), a boxed-up operation, a suggestion of an interaction, and, notably, a collection of toys. It is also a psychic object, that is, it purports a capacity to see into the mind (for another example of a test that purports to see inside, see Galison, 2004).

Playing with Tests

The project from which this next piece of practice-based research emerged employs a multitude of modes of art and play towards getting to understand the test kits. I worked with still life and documentation, rehearsal and restaging, remixing and performing, and talking and playing (Bergstrom-Katz, 2023). Arguably, all of these methods employed play as a key aspect of *doing* research. Here, I wish to highlight one piece of the research process, which was an installation and public exhibition of two intelligence test kits and a series of related objects (Fig. 7.6). What I designed and assembled was an interactive desk where visitors could explore the interior of its drawers at leisure. The desk itself was intended to house these objects and was produced so that there were two facing sides of the structure, divided by a separating wall. Each side of the desk housed one specific test (for the purpose of time, I will only discuss the

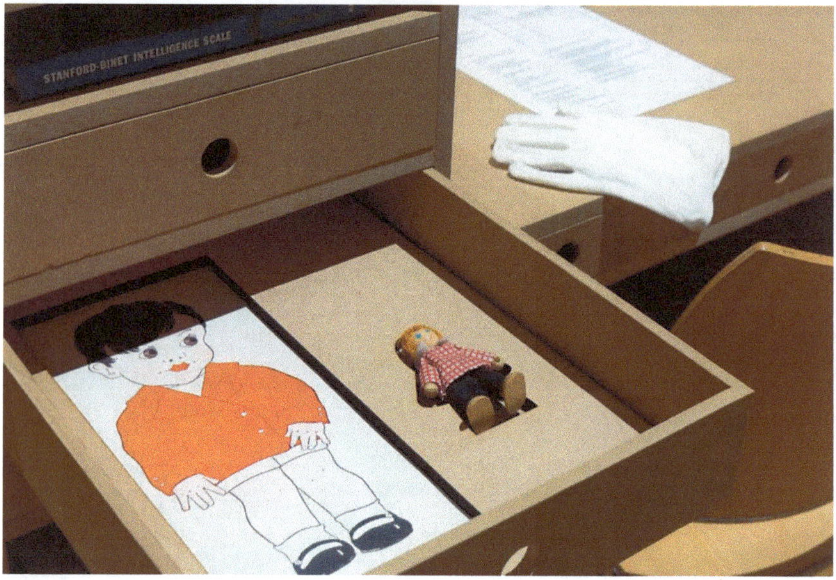

Fig. 7.6 Sasha Bergstrom-Katz, installation view of *Psychotechne* (with Tomas Percival), 2023. Peltz Gallery, Birkbeck, University of London. (*Source*: Photos by author)

Stanford-Binet test and not the Wechsler Intelligence Scales for Children-Revised [WISC-R] here), and objects I identified as related to the objects within the test. Each drawer held one object from the test and was paired with objects that were not from the test kit. The other objects in the drawers were historically, materially, or associatively related to the test object. For example, a form board puzzle was in a box with a laser-cut version of the first form board used in psychiatric hospitals in France (the Seguin form board) and was paired with a toy box top and two postcards of trained parrots playing with a version of the original test object. The objects related to both the history of this specific object (the form board) and its future incarnations outside of the test, including testing animal intelligence in relation to human intelligence (Fig. 7.7). While one main aim of the exhibition was to re-contextualise the test kits as archives of their own histories and uses (Bergstrom-Katz & Percival, 2023), it is

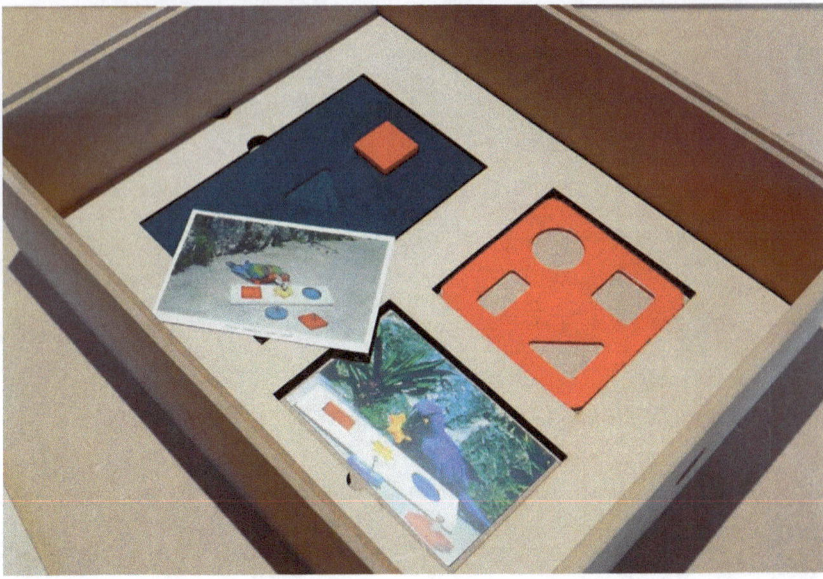

Fig. 7.7 Sasha Bergstrom-Katz, *Desk as Archive*, 2023; detail. (*Source*: Photos by author)

more important, here, to emphasise the ways in which this project employed and thereafter invited play as a process of understanding.

Visitors to the exhibition were invited to sit at one side of the desk or the other, but the playful nature of the installation was not employed to 'snare' audiences into participation or engagement. Instead, it was intended to provide the space for play, which, again, is to be understood as a creative and critical encounter. While referencing cubicles and testing spaces, the divided desks also provided privacy and open access to the tests, which is markedly different from how individuals would encounter the tests when being tested. In the scene of testing, the examiner faces the subject from across a table and provides instructions for what to do with each object, one by one. Here, in the exhibition, visitors did not have to face an examiner or even someone who could occupy the seat of the examiner. Instead, the visitor could be alone with the test. Without the examiner, then, this person is no longer exactly the subject of the test, yet the visitor's own relationship with the test might produce a different kind of subjectivity.

One purpose of this exhibition was to stage interconnected research on the histories of the testing, education, and childhood studies and, through the selection process, playing with the tests such that I could better understand my own affective relationship with the objects. Therefore, I explicitly did not methodically collect and order responses to the exhibition, beyond a guestbook and one closed workshop. Instead, I wanted to leave the space largely unobserved, and the visitors and participants unassessed, so that the power of the tests, which study their 'subjects' was reversed, and participants, including me, could study the tests and assess their own reactions to them. The invitation to play, therefore, was the key transformation in the tests, and within the process of the construction of the installation, I could observe my own playing, which happened while I selected, paired, and placed the objects together. My self-observation during and after play is, therefore, what I think is the most appropriate way to end this section, both to connect Winnicott's theory of play with my own process and to serve as an invitation to the reader of this chapter to play with the objects and ideas presented within this text and these images.

I will focus on one pairing: a small, fairly smooth, speckled rock, and a picture booklet, purposefully opened to a page that illustrates a disembodied, flexed arm (Fig. 7.8). While writing, even now, I can complicate my own reasoning for this pairing. I had, at first, paired the rock, an insistently material object, with a booklet of illustrations, to reference a pedagogical technique developed by Elizabeth and Charles Mayo called 'object lessons'. Object lessons sought to teach children about the word through an engagement with material *things*: for example, rocks (and more specifically, minerals), shells, rubber bands, and string (for more on the materiality and history of object lessons, see Ann-Sophie Lehmann, 2016). The pedagogical method was supported by a kit of a different kind than the tests. Object lesson cabinets were meant to be used by teachers in the classroom so that children could play with and learn about their material world through sensory means. Later, however, the box was replaced by text and image booklets, which belied the very purpose of the cabinets. In my pairing, I forced the image (and more specifically an

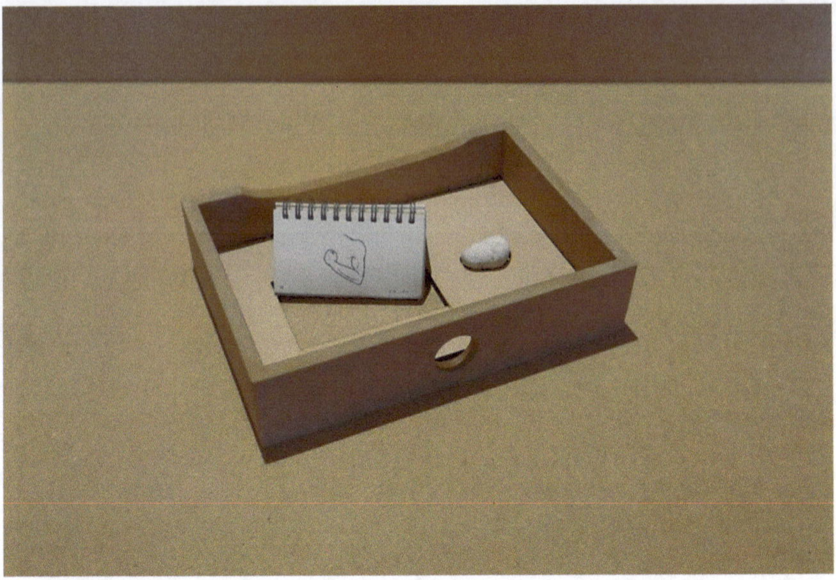

Fig. 7.8 Sasha Bergstrom-Katz, *Desk as Archive*, 2023; detail. (*Source*: Photos by author)

illustration) into potential conflict with the 'object world', both wishing to reify the booklet itself as an object and to undermine the 'reality' of the drawings inside. The very process of making this set of decisions was informative about the nature of things and their relations to representations of those same things. At the same time, I ended up, as I stated at the beginning, opening the booklet to a specific page of a flexed muscle. Later, I questioned myself: Was this pairing intentional? Was the softness of a human muscle made evident through the pairing with the rock? Or is this muscle 'rock-hard'? The play that I get to do in my mind gets at the kind of play that I wanted to provoke for others, which is sensorial, self-reflexive, associative, and historical, all wrapped together. At the same time, I realised prior to and even more evidently during the exhibition that the queer pairings had the capacity to act again as a test for visitors. What did I concretely mean by making this pairing? What is the visitor supposed to make out of them, and is there a correct answer? Finally, the page of the booklet could be changed, and throughout the exhibitions, new pairings were presented. Sometimes the booklet was flipped so that the cover was facing out, and sometimes a new pairing was on display.

Making the exhibition knowing individuals would interact with the tests also presented me with useful ethical quandaries. The tests might provoke anxiety or unpleasant memories from undergoing psychometric or educational testing. The connection between testing, ablest violence, and racism would be unwieldy to adequately address in the exhibition context. Further, offering the tests up for play might come across as flippant. At the same time, the tests' relationships to education and cultural concepts of intelligence are such that the tests belong to a public history and should thus be critiqued publicly. The second quandary was that I had already studied the tests and was presenting them without robust context. They were decontextualised further as people were meant to explore the tests without instruction by an examiner. Further still, they were deconstructed and divided into drawers. They were also removed from their original site, the United States, and the objects inside might appear foreign. Finally, the pairings I made recontextualised the test objects alongside not always apparently connected things. I had to trust that visitors would make their own sense of the test kits and their pairings and would, perhaps, begin their own research into these objects, their histories, and what they meant to them.

Over the span of the project, I was also struck by the pervasive difficulty of playing with the tests without answering the tests (that is solving the puzzles or guessing the answers to questions). The difficulty was then destroying the power of the tests and moving past the temptation to prove one's own intelligence to oneself. It took a real effort to *play* with the test, to understand it as not always already internal, that is, to remove the possibility that the test was already always testing the onlooker's intelligence by destroying its function, and reinventing it, through creative destruction and critique. To play with the test is to try to control it, to say to the test, 'You are not real, I can destroy you', and to wait to see how the test answers back. Through the simple act of trying to, for example, answer the questions differently than the test demands, the onlooker can undermine the test's logic. Is something actually really missing from this picture? Perhaps not. By removing the instructions, a box of blocks is again just blocks, without a 'correct' use, and an assortment of toys are no

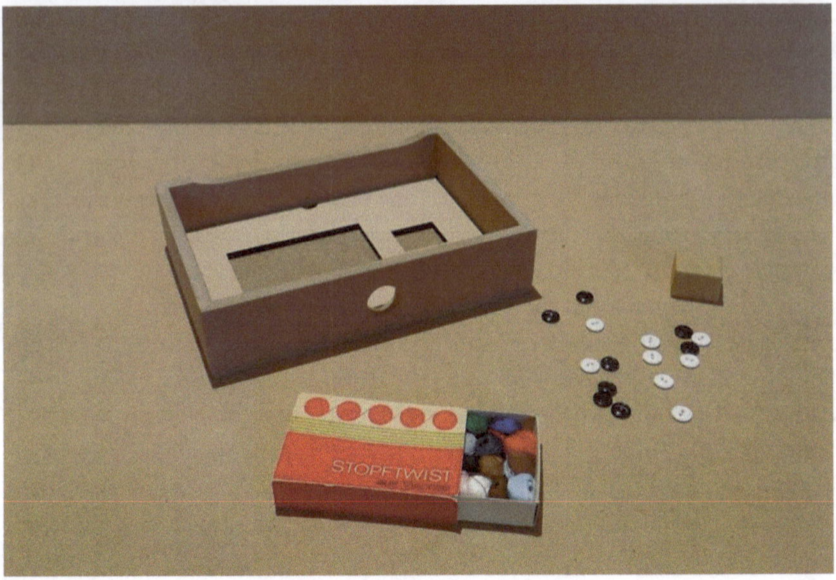

Fig. 7.9 Sasha Bergstrom-Katz, *Desk as Archive*, 2023; detail. (*Source*: Photos by author)

longer grouped just to demand that a subject identify them by use (Fig. 7.9). Instead, the person playing with the test may wish to construct a story that includes all of the objects. The test is destroyed by playing with it as long as it isn't put to correct use, and yet I found its power returning again and again. The creative destruction here, I argue, is critique, which has to be repeated each time the test resurrects. With each new creative critical engagement, observations about the materials of the test, which are not apparent within the test scenario, are revealed.

Acknowledgements This chapter builds on the methodology outlined in my PhD thesis entitled *On Intelligence Tests: Psychological Subjects and Their Objects,* thus I wish to thank my supervisory team at Birkbeck, Dr Amber Jacobs and Dr Sarah Marks for their support on this project. Further, I wish to thank Tomas Percival whose work was featured in the same exhibition, *Psychotechne*, which was on view at the Peltz Gallery in 2023. *Psychotechne* was curated by Dr Sarah Marks and was generously supported by a Wellcome Trust Institutional Support Fund. The exhibition was made possible by the Peltz Gallery and especially by Louise Owen and Angel Cohn Castle.

References

Bergstrom-Katz, S. (2023). *On Intelligence Tests: Psychological Objects and their Subjects* [PhD]. Birkbeck. [Doctoral dissertation, Birkbeck]. EThOS & Birkbeck Institutional Research Online.

Bergstrom-Katz, S., & Percival, T. (2023, March). Psychotechne: Assessment, Testing and Categorisation. *The Polyphony*. Retrieved from https://thepolyphony.org/2023/03/13/psychotechne-assessment-testing-and-categorisation/

Boake, C. (2002). From the Binet–Simon to the Wechsler–Bellevue: Tracing the History of Intelligence Testing. *Journal of Clinical and Experimental Neuropsychology, 24*(3), 383–405. https://doi.org/10.1076/jcen.24.3.383.981

Carson, J. (2007). *The Measure of Merit: Talents, Intelligence, and Inequality in the French and American Republics, 1750–1940*. Princeton University Press.

Curtis, M. E., & Glaser, R. (1981). Changing Conceptions of Intelligence. *Review of Research in Education, 9*, 111. https://doi.org/10.2307/1167184

Danziger, K. (1998). *Constructing the Subject: Historical Origins of Psychological Research* (Reprinted). Cambridge Univ. Press.

Daston, L. (Ed.). (2000). *Biographies of Scientific Objects*. University of Chicago Press.

Galison, P. (2004). Image of Self. In *Things That Talk* (pp. 257–296). Zone Books.

Gould, S. J. (1996). *The Mismeasure of Man* (Rev. and expanded). Norton.

Greenspan, S., Harris, J. C., & Woods, G. W. (2015). Intellectual Disability is "A Condition, Not a Number": Ethics of IQ Cut-Offs in Psychiatry, Human Services and Law. *Ethics, Medicine and Public Health, 1*(3), 312–324. https://doi.org/10.1016/j.jemep.2015.07.004

Ilyes, E. (2020). Psychology's Eugenic History and the Invention of Intellectual Disability. *Social and Personality Psychology Compass, 14*(7), e12537. https://doi.org/10.1111/spc3.12537

Lehmann, A.-S. (2016). *Cube of Wood. Material Literacy for Art History*. Rijksuniversiteit Groningen.

Mülberger, A. (2020). Biographies of a Scientific Subject: The Intelligence Test. In A. Mülberger (Ed.), *Oxford Research Encyclopedia of Psychology*. Oxford University Press. https://doi.org/10.1093/acrefore/9780190236557.013.694

Mülberger, A., Balltondre, M., & Graus, A. (2014). Aims of Teachers' Psychometry: Intelligence Testing in Barcelona (1920). *History of Psychology, 17*(3), 206–222. https://doi.org/10.1037/a0033339

Nicolas, S., Andrieu, B., Croizet, J.-C., Sanitioso, R. B., & Burman, J. T. (2013). Sick? Or Slow? On the Origins of Intelligence as a Psychological Object. *Intelligence, 41*(5), 699–711. https://doi.org/10.1016/j.intell.2013.08.006

Rose, N. S. (1998). *Inventing Ourselves: Psychology, Power and Personhood* (1st paperback ed.). Cambridge Univ. Press.

Sokal, M. M. (1981). The Origins of the Psychological Corporation. *Journal of the History of the Behavioral Sciences, 17*(1), 54–67. https://doi.org/10.1002/1520-6696

Sokal, M. M. (Ed.). (1987). *Psychological Testing and American Society, 1890–1930*. Rutgers University Press.

Staub, M. E. (2018). *The Mismeasure of Minds: Debating Race and Intelligence Between Brown and The Bell Curve*. The University of North Carolina Press.

Terman, L. M., & Merrill, M. A. (1960). *Stanford-Binet Intelligence Scale: Manual for the Third Revision Form L-M*. Houghton Mifflin.

Winnicott, D. W. (2010). *Playing and Reality* (Reprint). Routledge.

Young, J. L. (2015). Test or Toy? Materiality and the Measurement of Infant Intelligence. *History of Psychology, 18*(2), 103–118. https://doi.org/10.1037/a0038862

8

Long Covid and the Politics of Disablement

Robert Chapman and Micha Frazer-Carroll

Introduction

Severe acute respiratory syndrome coronavirus 2 (SARS-CoV-2) was first identified in Wuhan, China, in December 2019. Despite swift intervention from the Chinese authorities, the novel virus quickly spread nationally and then internationally. Common symptoms of the virus include continuous coughing, high temperature, shortness of breath, and sore throat. While the symptoms are often like those of other common illnesses such as cold or flu, it has a higher mortality rate. Because of this, the spread of the virus soon led to one of the deadliest pandemics in recorded history, with the World Health Organization estimating that

R. Chapman (✉)
Durham University, Durham, UK
e-mail: rjpd12@durham.ac.uk

M. Frazer-Carroll
London, UK

G. Kinouani et al. (eds.), *Creative Disruption*, Studies in the Psychosocial,
https://doi.org/10.1007/978-3-031-63661-5_8

the death toll associated with Covid-19 was approximately 14.9 million between January 2020 and December 2021 alone (WHO, 2022).

The ongoing Covid-19 pandemic—along with inadequate government responses, such as failing to adequately plan or provide protective equipment for pandemic outbreaks—has not just caused the deaths of millions. It has also led to the emergence and recognition of a new disability, under pressure from those experiencing this disability, alongside support from journalists. Many people who contract Covid, and survive, retain symptoms of what has come to be called post-Covid fatigue syndrome, or, as we prefer, "long Covid." This refers to a more prolonged disability associated with a range of physical and mental symptoms including chronic fatigue, breathlessness, brain fog, and anxiety, which persist for more than four weeks past the initial infection. According to one report, a staggering 3.1% of the UK population had long Covid as of January 2, 2023 (ONS, 2024).

The emergence of long Covid thus amounts to a mass disabling, and in our view, neurodivergifying, event. While this has been destructive for a great many—including both authors of this chapter—we also suggest current historical conditions may open up new creative possibilities for a new politics of disablement that could help ground collective efforts for material and discursive change.

Focusing primarily on the British context, to establish this, we begin by introducing long Covid at greater length. In particular, we focus on how dominant discourses around the condition reflect and reproduce a medicalised lens. We then go on to introduce an alternative analysis, from perspectives developed in disability studies. While these have mainly been useful for "bodily" rather than mental symptoms, we then suggest that long Covid, as a novel and widespread bodymind condition, may help us bridge the gap towards a societal analysis of mental illness.

Long Covid as a Medical Condition

As we just indicated, long Covid is typically understood through the lens of what is described as the "medical model" of disability (Oliver, 1990; Shakespeare, 2014). The medical model, which is the dominant model used to understand disability and illness more broadly, frames disability as a problem that lies within the individual's body. Take the example of a wheelchair user who is unable to enter a building due to there being a flight of stairs at the entrance. The medical model would frame this problem as stemming from the person's lack of mobility, rather than being connected to external architectural barriers. The medical model also often positions disability as a physiological problem to be cured, usually through individual engagement with the institution of medicine. As we will explore later in the chapter, this model fails to acknowledge the social and political barriers that construct disability.

A medical model approach is often taken for granted in public discussions around long Covid. Discussion of the experience of long Covid is often individualist in its approach—usually focusing on particular bodily symptoms. One article on living with long Covid featured in *The Guardian* in 2022 began: "Crushing fatigue. Brain fog making straightforward tasks almost impossible. Shortness of breath walking up the stairs" (Ghebreyesus, 2022). Here, symptoms are centred and used for their shock value and for an implicit commitment to a direct causal link between these symptoms and ensuing disability.

This medical model approach is also visible in discussions about long Covid and employment—for example, *The New York Times* describes long Covid as "keeping a significant number of people out of work," with those affected being "unable" to re-enter the labour market (Belluck, 2023). This medical model framing positions the bodily effects of the virus as the reason that people cannot work, in the same way that it frames wheelchair users' bodies as preventing them from entering buildings with stairs. The same article also describes employers as "feel[ing] the strains of an increasingly sick work force," positioning not only people with long Covid as victims of the virus, but also their employers. This framing may seem common-sense, but it leaves untouched the role that employers might play in making the workplace more accessible for people with long Covid. The virus and its aftereffects are framed as the beginning and end of the problem.

Public discussions around long Covid also adhere to the medical model in their centring of medical cure. A large proportion of press coverage around long Covid focuses on the prospect of discovering a cure. This pursuit is often described as a "race" (Gregory, 2021), or as part of a broader "battle" (Altmann, 2022) against the condition. Once again, long Covid is seen as a clearly defined enemy that harms otherwise healthy and functioning bodies and societies—and cure is taken for granted as an obvious, exclusive, and achievable "solution" to the problems faced by people with long Covid. As the disability activist and theorist Eli Clare points out, this approach to cure "focuses intensely on the future, [and] rarely provides resources to improve disabled and sick people's present-day lives" (Alland, 2018).

In line with the medical model, much patient advocacy has centred around the need for the development of treatments or a cure. While this is surely something that should be invested in, it is worth noting that the prospect for a magic bullet cure for long Covid seems slim. This is not just because of the limited efforts from governments to fund such research. It is also because long Covid is not one unified disease with clear-cut, core features. Rather, it is a rough cluster of symptoms that relate to a variety of organs and bodily symptoms. Furthermore, it is different in each case, since for each individual different organs and systems will have been damaged and in different ways. Because of this, it seems unlikely that any single treatment could simply and straightforwardly "cure" it. And treatment that works to at least some extent for one person may not work for another, since the underlying impairments will be different in each case. This is not to say that research into long Covid treatments is futile. On the contrary, we think that funding such research is utterly vital. Still, putting hope in some kind of cure-all would be misguided. Our point, then, is that it seems wise to consider other options for developing a politics of long Covid, bettering the lives and prospects for people with long Covid today. This might be partially analogous to what we see with other, albeit otherwise quite different, disabilities that are also heterogeneous in terms of their core traits. For instance, many people with a diagnosis of autism have fiercely critiqued the utility of searching for an autism "cure," and suggest that supporting autistic quality of life through a rights-based approach would be more helpful for autistic people (Stenson, 2019). We will return to the prospects for such an approach for long Covid below.

Another promising focus of advocacy has been prevention. In this regard, practices related to masking, sanitation, and vaccines are key. It is important to emphasise here that the core impairments associated with long Covid are themselves a socially produced form of "debilitation" (Puar, 2017), which refers to instances where political and economic factors cause bodily injury and exclusion. While much of the dominant discourse has framed Covid-19 complications as a natural matter determined by individual "vulnerability," it may be more accurate, as Shelley Tremain argues, to say that certain populations or demographics are "vulnerableised" through social policy and economic and racial inequality (Tremain, 2020). For instance, deaths in nursing homes relating to Covid infection are often explained in relation to age or underlying conditions, as if the increased mortality rate for people in nursing homes has nothing to do with how nursing homes can function as carceral systems for disabled and debilitated people. Who catches Covid-19 in the first place is significantly determined by how wealthy they are, which neighbourhood they live in, and their personal living and working conditions. Black, immigrant, and economically deprived communities have been found to catch Covid-19 at elevated rates, as are people incarcerated in institutions. For instance, a 2021 study found that people incarcerated in prisons in England and Wales were around three times more likely to die from Covid-19 than members of the general population (Braithwaite et al., 2021).

Histories of epistemic and literal violence may also influence the extent to which certain populations trust the authorities, potentially shaping their willingness to follow state guidance, for example, accepting vaccines and masking (Carson et al., 2021; Cáceres et al., 2022; Okoro et al., 2021). Overall, then, we can say that impairments associated with long Covid are themselves socially produced, since the question of who catches the virus in the first place will significantly determine who ends up developing long Covid.

While prevention is vital, this does little for those already living with long Covid, which, as earlier mentioned, is 3.1% of the UK population as of January 2023. Where it is too late for prevention and where the possibility of a magic bullet cure seems slim, even with more government investment, there seems reason to turn to other approaches to supplement existing long Covid politics. It is to such an alternative that we now turn.

Long Covid as Neurodivergent Disablement

We have just covered the standard view of long Covid, which posits it as a medical tragedy that requires funding for research. We now turn to a different perspective, viewed through the lens of disability studies and the neurodiversity movement. While disability studies is not monolithic, the overall orientation has been away from viewing disability merely as a medical issue and towards viewing it as socially and ideologically produced (Union of the Physically Impaired Against Segregation, 1976; Oliver, 1990; Shakespeare, 2014). Looked at this way, enablement is also, at least in significant part, a social matter. As such, this lens may offer different conceptual tools allowing a different politics of long Covid.

Focusing more on the psychosocial symptoms associated with the conditions, what we want to stress is that it is also possible to see the disablement associated with long Covid through a social lens. Part of this perspective comes from the social model of disability, which was developed by disabled activists and scholars as an alternative to the medical model (Oliver, 1990). As earlier mentioned, the medical model holds that disability is caused by impairment (bodily or mental dysfunction). By contrast, the social model suggests that disability is caused by the material structures and environments, norms, expectations, and practices of society. To give a simple example, wheelchair users will still have impairments even in an ideal society, but if there are ramps everywhere instead of steps, and surfaces are wide and smooth enough to ride on, they will not be excluded from participating in society. As such, whether they are *disabled* from participating in society is determined in significant part by societal organisation. Looked at this way, one of the most helpful things to do for people with impairments is to restructure the world with less disabling barriers and more enabling features.

It is important to recognise that such social approaches to disablement do not just locate neurodivergent disablement in *local* contexts such as a given individual's office or school. The point is to connect the local to systems—capitalism, white supremacy, patriarchy, and so on—to push for systemic change. In this regard, it is helpful to consider the recent work of Beatrice Adler-Bolton and Artie Vierkant (2022), who describe the overall orientation towards the "surplus" class—those unable to work in line with the standardised pace and norms of the age—within a capitalist political economy as one of *extractive abandonment*. By this, they mean that profit is systematically extracted from surplus populations through new industries of care, control, and management, while members of those populations are abandoned when this is no longer profitable. Such industries include those relating to mental health institutions, nursing homes, behavioural therapy, and so on. It is true that these industries do sometimes help disabled people, but they also often harm. Ultimately, the capacity of such industries to help is limited by the orientation towards extractive abandonment that pervades the capitalist mode of production.

Historically, the social model was initially and explicitly made to understand "bodily," but not mental, disability. A focus on removing physical barriers seems less suited to alleviating mental disablement. Yet people with cognitive and psychosocial disabilities have increasingly adopted and adapted it in recent years. Most notably, the rise of the neurodiversity movement has precisely been organised around applying the social model across an increasingly broad range of mental, psychosocial, and emotional disabilities. Beginning in autistic activist communities in the late 1990s, pioneering neurodiversity activists challenged the idea of the "normal brain," and suggested that all kinds of neurocognitive styles should be valued and supported (Blume, 1998). The framework that emerged from this movement is still mainly associated with autism and other developmental disabilities such as attention deficit hyperactivity disorder (ADHD), and emphasises how the neuronormativity of modern capitalist society has become a new form of domination that must be resisted.

However, in recent years, activists with a range of other psychiatric diagnoses, which are usually seen as mental health conditions, have also begun adopting and adapting neurodiversity frameworks to reclaim their diagnoses in order to organise and demand rights and justice. Newer applications have come from those with diagnoses such as bipolar disorder and borderline personality disorder (Prism, 2017; Johnson, 2021). While all this is still controversial, and in some instances such classifications remain contested; at least some people with each of these diagnoses—or no diagnosis at all—have found adopting a neurodiversity approach useful for politically understanding categories that have historically come under the remit of psychiatry. For instance, autistic people have found organising around the autism classification useful for making political demands, despite simultaneously rejecting the validity of this classification as a medical disease (Chapman, 2020).

Part of what we want to suggest is that a similar lens can be used to understand the psychosocial symptoms of long Covid. Consider mental fatigue. Clearly, in part, one's energy levels are determined by individual health or bodily functioning. But also, in significant part, cognitive and emotional fatigue are determined by societal pressures. The concept of "chrononormativity" (Freeman, 2010) is useful here. This regards compulsory neuronormative requirements to work to highly specific schedules, tempos, or work hours, as well as the domination of clock time. Importantly, these pressures are not natural, but rather, socially determined. In England, for instance, work hours increased, and clock time became the dominant modality of temporal orientation, in the shift from the feudal to capitalist mode of production. These have intensified further through the twentieth century and again since the crushing of a mass unionised working class during the Thatcher administration. More to the point, such practices are organised around an ideal abled worker, with no impairments, rather than being flexible in such a way that allows fatigue-prone people to be able to still participate in work. To give a further example, workplaces also often require working through bureaucracy that is also socially rather than naturally determined. While this is frustrating for everyone, it will be particularly tiring for people with cognitive processing impairments, for example, many people with long Covid. However, we shouldn't overlook the fact that work could be organised in a different way that granted these groups greater access to wage labour. In thinking about this, we should draw on the disability scholar Alison Kafer's concept of "crip time" (Kafer, 2013), which resists chrononormativity and negotiates a different disabled relationship to clock time. She says that: "rather than bend disabled bodies and minds to meet the clock, crip time bends the clock to meet disabled bodies and minds."

Sensory and attentive environments have also become more harmful in recent decades, with many expanding diagnostic constructs relating to sensory pollution. It is not just that traffic and building works in inner cities have been associated with heightened rates of depression (see, e.g. Beutel et al., 2016). It is also that workplaces often have open plan offices with intense lighting, or may require having to think in crowded, loud, and busy spaces which will be fatiguing and overwhelming for people with sensory processing impairments (Baldwin et al., 2014). Again, none of this is natural, but rather reflects the way workplace design in advanced capitalist societies tends to be built around a neurotypical norm. We speculate that this norm reinforces a range of structures and practices that likely contribute to the ongoing disablement of people living with long Covid, considering that many people with long Covid have reported that brain fog can cause difficulty with multiple sensory inputs (Callan et al., 2022).

This lens may ultimately allow individuals with long Covid to understand their experience in a new way, which reframes disablement as at least partially due to external factors. Consider how we understand the concept and experience of brain fog. One way of understanding the metaphor of brain *fog* is that the brain breaks down in such a way that makes one's perception and cognition foggy. This interpretation, implicitly, reflects the dominant medical model lens, implying that the fogginess is directly caused by neurological malfunction. But another interpretation would begin from noting that fog is always external to us. That is, literal fog is something that clouds our vision from the outside rather than from the inside, even if we are within the fog and surrounded by it. This is important because, much as with fatigue, while brain fog may be experienced as occurring from a sudden onset, its causes are likely, in significant part, social. Understood this way, we can understand brain fog as a political problem. On this view, just as changes in the weather, including literal fog, are affected by political decisions that speed up climate change, so too is the prevalence of brain fog among Covid-impaired populations affected and produced by the broader political economy, policy, and the norms and expectations of the neoliberal workplace.

Towards A New Politics of Long Covid

Given what we have covered, it is our view that while the pandemic has been an overwhelmingly destructive event, bringing about millions of deaths, contributing to inflation and economic inequality, and turning out to be a mass disabling event, there is nonetheless room for creative potentials even in the limitations set by the current historical moment.

While the social model approach, like the medical model, cannot entirely alleviate disablement, it does open a new lens for organising for people with long Covid. For instance, we can position this politics as part of a broader challenge to the way workplaces, education, and public spaces tend to be designed only for those who conform to compulsory neuronormativity in terms of their sensory, emotional, and cognitive processing. As a mass neurodivergifying event, the Covid-19 pandemic, and the resultant growing population of people with long Covid, represents a potential tipping point for this political issue. More than this, the politicisation of pathology can aid the development of community-building, mutual aid efforts, community knowledge, and so on. The emergence of long Covid has led to the creation of large online and "real-life" communities of people with/seeking the diagnosis, many of which engage in self-advocacy and information-sharing. In addition to this, the very concept of long Covid has been built by these communities as much as it has by doctors and epidemiologists—with patients finding one another on Twitter in the early months of the pandemic, and attempting to define and raise awareness of their experiences long before being picked up by media, clinical, or policy channels (Callard & Parego, 2021). Yet as we have seen, so far these have tended more towards a medical model lens than a social one (e.g. patients funding research towards medical cure), which may unduly limit the kinds of knowledge and efforts that might arise through such forms of community organising.

This certainly does not mean that developing and providing treatments should be shunned. Far from it. More pressure than ever should be put on governments to properly support people with long Covid. But the creative potentials that arise from destructive forces should be harnessed as and where we find them. The collective power of around 3% of the population is, if we organise together, not insignificant. Organising through unions and the threat of withholding labour, for those still in employment, while simultaneously drawing on traditions of protest and direct action, not to mention organising as voting blocks, would allow pressures to be placed on capital and governments to alter the organisation of work and society more generally. This should take place within a broader politics of disablement, as part of a broader coalition of workers and members of the surplus class. With this collective power, beyond pushing for the development of treatments and cures, we should be organising towards systemic and structural changes that allow us to switch disabling barriers for enabling environments.

Acknowledgements We would like to thank Hannah Reeves for invaluable editorial support and feedback that has significantly helped in the development and writing of this chapter.

Funding RC is a member of the Discovery Research Platform for Medical Humanities which is supported by Wellcome (WT226798/Z/22/Z).

References

Adler-Bolton, B., & Vierkant, A. (2022). *Health Communism: A Surplus Manifesto*. Verso.

Alland, S. (2018, May 17). Eli Clare on Our Relationship with 'Abnormal' and the Promise of Cure. *Disability Arts Online*. Retrieved from https://disability-arts.online/magazine/opinion/eli-clare-relationship-abnormal-promise-cure/

Altmann, D. (2022, August 31). There's Some Good News in the Battle Against Long Covid. *Guardian*. Retrieved from https://www.theguardian.com/commentisfree/2022/aug/31/good-news-long-covid-uk-cases-scientists

Baldwin, S., Costley, D., & Warren, A. (2014). Employment activities and experiences of adults with high-functioning autism and Asperger's Disorder. *Journal of Autism and Developmental Disorders, 44*(10), 2440–2449. https://doi.org/10.1007/s10803-014-2112-z

Belluck. (2023, January 24). Long Covid Is Keeping Significant Numbers of People Out of Work, Study Finds. *New York Times*. Retrieved from https://www.nytimes.com/2023/01/24/health/long-covid-work.html

Beutel, M. E., Jünger, C., Klein, E. M., Wild, P., Lackner, K., Blettner, M., Binder, H., et al. (2016). Noise Annoyance Is Associated with Depression and Anxiety in the General Population—The Contribution of Aircraft Noise. *PLoS One, 11*(5), e0155357. https://doi.org/10.1371/journal.pone.0155357

Blume, H. (1998, September). Neurodiversity. On the Neurological Underpinnings of Geekdom. *Atlantic*.

Braithwaite, I., Edge, C., Lewer, D., & Hard, J. (2021). High COVID-19 Death Rates in Prisons in England and Wales, and the Need for Early Vaccination. *The Lancet Respiratory Medicine, 9*(6), 569–570. https://doi.org/10.1016/S2213-2600(21)00137-5

Callan, C., Ladds, E., Husain, L., Pattinson, K., & Greenhalgh, T. (2022). 'I can't cope with multiple inputs': A qualitative study of the lived experience of 'brain fog' after COVID-19. *BMJ Open, 12*(2), e056366. https://doi.org/10.1136/bmjopen-2021-056366

Callard, F., & Perego, E. (2021). How and why patients made long COVID. *Social Science & Medicine, 268*, Article 113–426. https://doi.org/10.1016/j.socscimed.2020.113426

Carson, S. L., Casillas, A., Castellon-Lopez, Y., Mansfield, L. N., Morris, D., Barron, J., Ntekume, E., Landovitz, R., Vassar, S. D., Norris, K. C., Dubinett, S. M., Garrison, N. A., & Brown, A. F. (2021). COVID-19 Vaccine Decision-making Factors in Racial and Ethnic Minority Communities in Los Angeles, California. *JAMA Network Open, 4*(9), e2127582. https://doi.org/10.1001/jamanetworkopen.2021.27582

Chapman, R. (2020). The Reality of Autism: On the Metaphysics of Disorder and Diversity. *Philosophical Psychology, 33*(6), 799–819. https://doi.org/10.1080/09515089.2020.1751103

Ferreira Caceres, M. M., Sosa, J. P., Lawrence, J. A., Sestacovschi, C., Tidd-Johnson, A., Rasool, M. H. U., Gadamidi, V. K., Ozair, S., Pandav, K., Cuevas-Lou, C., Parrish, M., Rodriguez, I., & Fernandez, J. P. (2022). The impact of misinformation on the COVID-19 pandemic. *AIMS Public Health, 9*(2), 262–277. https://doi.org/10.3934/publichealth.2022018

Freeman, E. (2010). *Time Binds: Queer Temporalities, Queer Histories*. Duke University Press.

Ghebreyesus, T. A. (2022, October 12). The Data Is Clear: Long Covid Is Devastating People's Lives and Livelihoods. *Guardian*. Retrieved from https://www.theguardian.com/society/2022/oct/12/long-covid-who-director-general-oped-tedros-adhanom-ghebreyesus

Gregory, A. (2021, April 24). The Race to Cure Long Covid, the World's Next Health Crisis. *The Times*. Retrieved from https://www.thetimes.co.uk/article/the-race-to-cure-long-covid-the-worlds-next-health-crisis-36d7vgr8x

Johnson M. L. (2021). Neuroqueer feminism: Turning with tenderness toward borderline personality disorder. *Signs: Journal of Women in Culture and Society, 46*(3), 635–662. https://doi.org/10.1086/712081

Kafer, A. (2013). *Feminist, queer, crip*. Indiana University Press.

Office for National Statistics (ONS). (2024, February 2). ONS Website, Statistical Bulletin, Prevalence of Ongoing Symptoms Following Coronavirus (COVID-19) Infection in the UK: 2 February 2023.

Okoro, O., Kennedy, J., Simmons, G., Vosen, E., Allen, K., Singer, D., et al. (2021). Exploring the scope and dimensions of vaccine hesitancy and resistance to enhance COVID-19 vaccination in Black communities. *Journal of Racial and Ethnic Health Disparities*. https://doi.org/10.1007/s40615-021-01150-0

Oliver, M. (1990). *The Politics of Disablement*. Macmillan.

Prism, I. (2017). 'Kind of Like Being a Witch or Wizard': How I Learned to Value My Neurodivergence. *The Body Is Not an Apology*. 27 Aug. 2017. Retrieved from https://web.archive.org/web/20230929140107/https://thebodyisnotanapology.com/magazine/kind-of-like-being-awitch-or-wizard-how-i-learned-to-value-my-neurodivergence/

Puar, J. (2017). *The Right to Maim: Debility, Capacity, Disability*. Duke University Press.

Shakespeare, T. (2014). *Disability Rights and Wrongs* (2nd ed.). Routledge.

Stenson, J. (2019). Why the Focus of Autism Research Is Shifting Away from Searching for a 'Cure'. *NBC News*. Retrieved from https://www.nbcnews.com/health/kids-health/cure-autism-not-so-fast-n1055921

Tremain, S. (2020, April 1). COVID-19 and The Naturalization of Vulnerability. *Biopolitical Philosophy*. Retrieved from https://biopoliticalphilosophy.com/2020/04/01/covid-19-and-the-naturalization-of-vulnerability/

UPIAS: Fundamental Principles of Disability. (1976). *Union of the Physically Impaired Against Segregation and Disability Alliance*. London.

WHO (World Health Organization). (2022). *14.9 Million Excess Deaths Associated with the COVID-19 Pandemic in 2020 and 2021*. Retrieved from https://www.un.org/en/desa/149-million-excess-deaths-associated-covid-19-pandemic-2020-and-2021

9

Involuntary Attention as Creative Disruption: Meeting the Urban Wild with Neurodivergent Strategies

Hannah Reeves

Introduction

This chapter offers a contemplation on the implications of neurodiverse, more-than-human sociality for psychosocial studies. Drawing on my experience of doing auto/ethnographic research at Crossbones Graveyard (a burial ground and "wild" garden of remembrance in Southeast London) as a neurodivergent researcher, I consider and consolidate Judge's (2018) and Davidson and Smith's (2009) propositions that a neurodiverse sociality is already a more-than-human sociality. I offer passages of my open-field (Bloomfield, 2013; Duncan, 1973; Tarlo, 2013) approach to auto/ethnography, an accidental path to materialising a neurodivergent strategy. Discussing these experiences in relation to neurotypically

'This chapter builds on an argument first outlined in my PhD thesis (Reeves, 2024).'

H. Reeves (✉)
School of Social Sciences, Birkbeck University, London, UK
e-mail: hreeve03@mail.bbk.ac.uk

G. Kinouani et al. (eds.), *Creative Disruption*, Studies in the Psychosocial,
https://doi.org/10.1007/978-3-031-63661-5_9

humanist paradigms of social science, I reflect upon the specific responsibility of psychosocial studies towards neurodivergent people and analytics. What might taking on this responsibility—or response-ability (Haraway, 2016)—mean for how we select and delimit "subject" matter, and for the processes by which we appraise ontological and epistemological coherence and intellectual "value"?[1] Further, how can we create epistemological and institutional space for neurodiverse perspectives to multiply, including—and especially—those brought forth directly by neurodivergent people themselves? (Fig. 9.1).

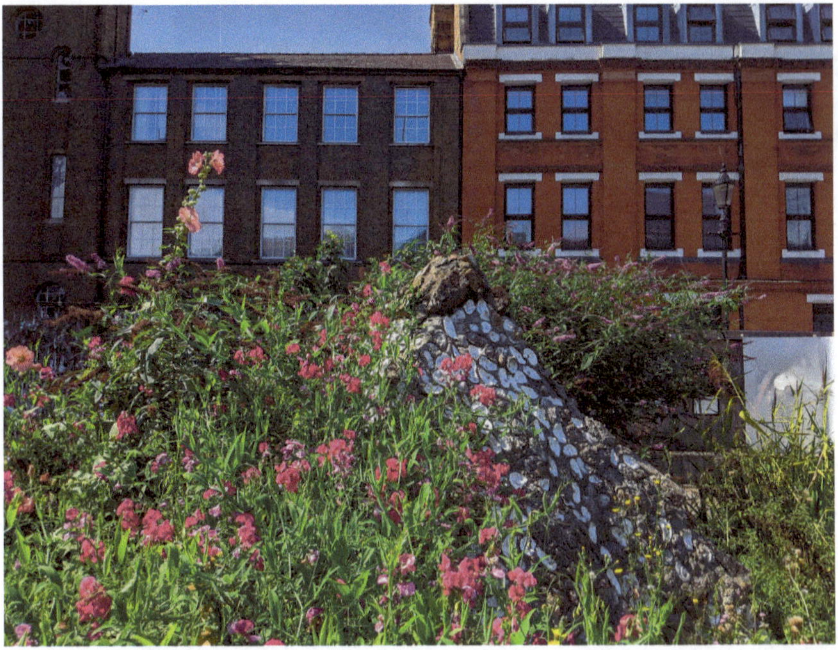

Fig. 9.1 The Pyramid at Crossbones Graveyard in summer (*Source* Photos by author)

[1] More than simple responsiveness or a distanced sense of responsibility, response-ability is about rendering each other capable of responding, of taking on the collaborative task of composing some worlds rather than others (Haraway, 2016).

Meeting the Field

I remember how nervous I felt on the way to the first interview I conducted at Crossbones. Had I selected the right questions? Would they produce the right kind of "data"? Could I perform the role of a researcher as expected: calm, knowledgeable, and in control? Could I hold my attention firmly and narrowly enough that I could seamlessly navigate this new terrain of social script? My body thought not. My heart was shuddering against whatever boundaries it could reach, and my hands were quivering ever so slightly. I was heavy with the weight of risk, chance, and my own unpredictability: the interview schedule hadn't prepared me for this. To feel such discomfort on my way to Crossbones was itself discomforting: usually my walks there are marked with familiar sights, sounds, smells, and textures; the anticipation of familiar faces; the expectation of a couple of hours of peace from the speed of life in the city. As I walk my habitual path to Crossbones on ordinary Wednesdays, I am free to daydream or lose myself in details as I please.

I remember this day with Sara Ahmed's thoughts on discomfort. Writing on the discomfort queer bodies feel when inhabiting the pervasive spaces of compulsory heterosexuality, Ahmed (2013, p. 148) describes "a feeling of disorientation: one's body feels out of place, awkward, unsettled." Even as I walked a familiar path to a familiar place in a geospatial sense, I was acutely aware of the discomforting fit between my *bodymind* (Price, 2015; Rothschild, 2000) and the path it was walking.[2] I was on my way to "the interview," a staged social encounter founded on the assumption that meanings exchanged linguistically by human subjects define the limits of what matters. The well-trodden path to the interview has been forged and consolidated by the Western humanist researcher, inevitably white, cismale, able-bodied, middle-class, neurotypical, calm, confident, and eager. He is the archetypal subject of what is most generously termed Western humanism, but which, in its historical situatedness,

---

[2] Here I follow Price's (2015, p. 27) use of *bodymind* to insist on "the imbrication (not just the combination) of the entities usually called 'body' and 'mind.'" The arguments of this chapter are based on the premise that bodies are already bodyminds. At certain points, however, I also use "bodies": to acknowledge, where appropriate, the ways in which the surfaces of bodies are shaped in *contact zones* (Haraway, 2008).

is Man's colonially enforced epistemology (Wynter, 2003). He has a habit of rendering himself invisible in social science methodological resources, but the imprints he leaves behind are all too apparent when those of us who do not align with them attempt to put abstracted methods into practice: it becomes viscerally evident that the tread of the path ahead has been smoothed by him, for him. Those of us who cannot walk this path comfortably must find a way through the bumpy surround, pushing through the friction as we go in small gestures to treading out the paths less used (feministkilljoys, 2018).

All this said, the sudden onset of this discomfort against my remembered landscape of comfortability also underscores the many ways in which normative paths through the world *have* been laid out for people with bodies like mine. I had only been free to daydream and lose myself in detail on those habitual Wednesdays because of the *comfortability* of the fit between my body and the bodies that shape it, including the organisations of matter that make up the urban landscape. I cannot forget my deviations from this normative subject position because of the discomfort that inhabiting such norms differently generates. But the extent to which I *am* at home within this position eludes me frequently. Such is the function of normativity, to make learned patterns of thought and behaviour feel completely obvious, natural, and therefore invisible.

On this remembered occasion, the discomforting fits between my bodymind and the path I thought I must tread manifested as anxiety. I locate the friction in this *contact zone* (Haraway, 2008) as produced most loudly by expressions of my neurodivergence as I attempted to inhabit what felt like firmly neurotypical terrain. There are some dimensions of this anxiety that I can, perhaps, tease out as specifically neurodivergent trouble entangled with a more "general" sense of anxiety. I was heavy with the anticipation of my baseline cognitive load (that comes with "performing" the embodied-linguistic social script) intensifying in an unfamiliar and high-stakes situation. Whereas typically at Crossbones I could allow my attention to wander with the flux of more-than-human activity in the garden, the interview would ask me to perform an intensive kind of "focus" delimited by a human-human question-answer structure.

All this said, lived experiences of neurodivergence frequently interface with a more generalised anxiety in ways that are often seamless experientially and difficult to tease out. A key potential of the *neurodiversity paradigm* (Chapman, 2020) is that such experiences can be navigated as the lived terrain of difference without obligating its *wayfarers* (Ingold, 2021, p. 181) to codify these experience as "disorders" or "disordered."[3] Neurodivergence *might* describe (but is not limited to) expressions of difference meeting diagnostic criteria for autism, bipolar disorder, schizophrenia, or ADHD, but equally, neurodivergence offers a language to describe lived experiences that traverse and trouble the boundaries of such diagnoses. As such, neurodiversity offers a mechanism of disclosure with radical potential: to reject the stigma that particular diagnoses might carry; even, perhaps to mitigate some risks attached to disclosure. The promise of neurodiversity is that difference can be understood simply *as* difference on a multidimensional, value-neutral spectrum.

While neurodivergent people might face specific challenges in such situations (which may or may not resonate with my own experiences), neurodivergence is one possible site of friction among many in the contact zones where people with bodyminds variously marked as different from Man's inhabit his shadow. A more general sense of anxiety in doing research—along with a host of other discomforting affects—may be frequently experienced, but less frequently acknowledged, by a great many researchers who diverge, in their various and often overlapping ways, from the imprints Man has left on the paths they must tread. These might include people who are BIPOC, trans, queer, disabled, or women, for example.[4] Acknowledging and honouring these discomforting affects—which can sometimes be parsed, sometimes be traced, and sometimes not—also brings forward the possibility of building allyship in the discomfort of difference.

---

[3] Following Chapman (2020, pp. 57–58), the *neurodiversity paradigm* challenges the framing of "those who fall outside neurocognitive norms" as affected by individual medical pathology, instead asserting that neurominorities are marginalised by a neuronormative society that favours neurotypical people.

[4] This is not to suggest that people whose "markers" situate them as fitting within this normative subject position cannot also experience anxiety in doing research; rather, this chapter focuses on the experiential discomfort that emerges specifically in the knowledge that one's bodymind has been marked as different.

My neurodivergence has never been incidental to my doing research: in important ways, neurodivergence pulled me into undertaking a research project at Crossbones in the first place. The monthly vigils that have been held at the gates outside the burial ground for over 15 years "honour the Outcast, both dead and alive" (Friends of Crossbones, 2019). The burial ground within holds the remains of thousands of working class and poor people buried during its intensive use during the post-medieval period; their histories stifled under layers of asphalt and concrete after the burial ground was sold on for redevelopment after its closure. The ceremony for the Outcast pushes back against the disremembering of those buried at the ground by the dominant historiography and weaves their histories through with local lore that links Crossbones—which is likely to have remained unconsecrated—to a segregated burial ground for the women who worked in medieval Southwark's brothels.[5]

The figure of the Outcast has offered a way to reclaim bodies designated "unholy" and therefore marginalised by the dominant socio-religious order of their day. Alongside foregrounding working class and sex worker histories, the Outcast has located Crossbones as a place to honour people who died by suicide, addiction, and misadventure; as well as queer, trans, and disabled people. The Outcast has done the work of gathering a fluid community of living people who recognise the Outcast in themselves. The monthly vigils emphasise that the Outcast is not simply a type of person, but also a qualitative dimension of embodiment. Honouring the Outcast is an opportunity to honour the diffuse threads of our bodily being that the dominant order implores us to cast out, or that we might otherwise wish to forget. It is this expansive quality of the Outcast that drew me to Crossbones, and which drew me to return again and again. This Outcast was present with me in the *queer failure* (Halberstam, 2011; Muñoz, 2019) of my learned attempts to present neurotypically; or otherwise, in my intermittent refusal to bother trying; the Outcast was present when my sexuality and gender expression failed to meet cisheteronormative expectations. This Outcast made me feel that

[5] Crossbones has a rich and fascinating history, but it is beyond the scope of this chapter to recount it in more depth here. For a summary of its history from the eighteenth century to the present day, refer to Berns (2016) and Reeves (2022). For further information about the grassroots campaign to protect the burial ground, refer to the Friends of Crossbones (n.d.) and Hausner (2016).

coming to Crossbones was like coming home, even as a white, middle-class, cisgendered person.[6]

Finding my place at Crossbones felt inevitable and necessary, and my deep sense of being at home there fed my yearning to study it for my doctoral research. More than simply a case study, point of comparison, or gap in the literature, exploring and sharing Crossbones' stories felt like something I had to do. Undertaking this research within a psychosocial studies department felt similarly necessary, but much less comfortable. My embodied history of fraught interactions with Western psychiatry had foregrounded a hunger to "speak back" to its formative institutions and their codifying practices. As a field founded on the critical and ethical imperative that the "individual" psyche is always steeped in, interfacing with, and coproducing the social, psychosocial studies held a particular promise as challenging assumptive notions that difference, disorder, and distress originate and reside within isolated, neatly individuated subjects. I felt a sense that developing psychosocial expertise would allow me to take a critical stance against the harm I had experienced and legitimate my claim in doing so. I hoped that I could shift my position from an *object* of the psy-disciplines to a *subject* capable of forging analyses on my own terms.

As Sara Judge (2018, p. 1102) has observed, while neurodivergent people have frequently been the object of study for neurotypical people, explicit accounts of neurodiverse experience by neurodivergent people themselves are rare in academic literature.[7] As Judge has highlighted, this is a combined consequence of the underrepresentation of neurodivergent people in academia, the potentially stigmatising risk of disclosure, as well as the often discomforting fit between traditional methodologies and

[6] All this said, it remains important to recognise that while the Outcast has done the crucial work of gathering a community who protect those buried at the ground, we cannot assume that those buried there would identify as Outcast themselves. The Outcast, like "the wild," holds a colonising potential and legacy that we at Crossbones must remain attentive to. As Lucy Coleman Talbot (2023) has highlighted, even as a bottom-up heritage site, there remains a need at Crossbones to intersectionally attend to intra-group differences.

[7] Judge (2018, p. 1102) highlights the work of neurodiverse scholars Marcia England (2016), Scott M. Robinson and Ari D. Ne'eman (2008), Temple Grandin and Catherine Johnson (2006), and Dawn Prince-Hughes (2005) as increasingly "finding room within the academy to engage with their own ways of knowing and doing."

neurodivergent perspectives. The latter presents challenges "both in terms of how the researcher works with others, and the ways in which work is communicated" (Judge, 2018, p. 1102). As an emergent field *non-innocently entangled* (Murphy, 2017) with the psy-disciplines, psychosocial studies has a specific responsibility to neurodivergent people. If ethics and reflexivity are central pillars of the field as they are often claimed to be, then a crucial part of the work psychosocial studies takes on should be for the voices of its inherited "objects" to be offered their space as subjects—and authors—of the knowledge practices that centre around them. The task is not only to make space for neurodivergent-identified people to speak within neurotypical frameworks, but also to make space for neurodiverse ontologies, epistemologies, ethics, and methods. Crucially, this also involves working towards institutional mechanisms through which such approaches can exist and be appraised, without forever being caught in the trap of assimilation to Man's epistemology (Fig. 9.2).

Finding a Way In

Despite my fascination with the disruptive potential of the psychosocial, and my fascination with the expansive possibilities of Crossbones, I had unwittingly approached my preliminary research at Crossbones using the practices of what Elizabeth Adams St. Pierre (2011, 2013, 2014, 2019) has termed *conventional humanist qualitative methodology*. I prefer to think of these practices as *neurotypically humanist qualitative methodology*: an abstracted set of methods through which Man's epistemology is frequently enacted. While psychosocial studies itself occupies a liminal space straddling the social sciences and humanities, a condition of taking up my doctoral studentship was that I undertake a year of social science methodological training. This, I was told by representatives of my funder, was to ensure my knowledge and skills were not limited to the local and specific, but would set me up for a career as a more useful researcher. With little grounding in psychosocial thinking beyond my initial interest, I began the methodological training, which was based in a politics department and designed to encompass all forms of "social research." Navigating the stabilised centres of methodological convention amidst

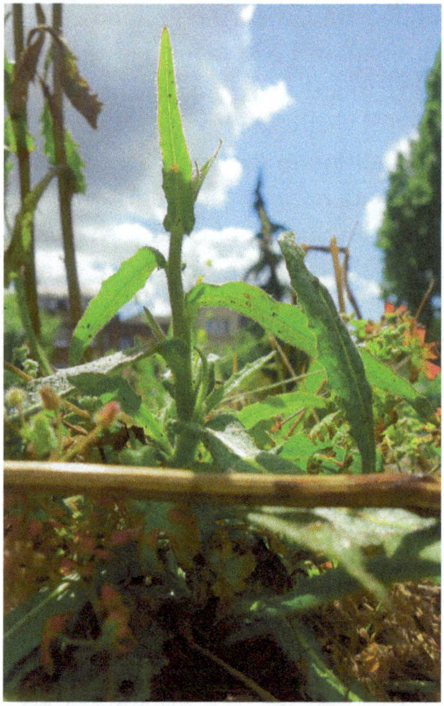

Fig. 9.2 A weedy perspective at Crossbones Graveyard (*Source* Photos by author)

my own uncertainty, inexperience, and early-doctoral-stage imposter syndrome, I had come to see neurotypically humanist qualitative methodology as the terms through which I should "prove" my capability as a social science researcher.

My discomfort around interviewing was not only around the encounter itself—although that was a significant part of it—it was also the anticipation of what would come next. As part of a set of social science research methods I was attempting to put to work (which also included using questionnaires and reviewing preexisting online data from campaigns to protect the graveyard), the interview was setting me up for the task of stepping back to see "the big picture." I worked on the fragile premise that the textual data I had gathered and transcribed would allow me to code and classify emergent themes, and from these, I would be able to infer something solid about Crossbones. Supposedly, I would be able to answer the research question I had defined at the beginning of the process. I might not have found myself so bewildered had I *stayed with the trouble* (Haraway, 2016) that came up when I had, in actuality, failed to articulate a research question in the first place. This was—and continues to be—the aspect of doing research I find most challenging. I continue to be confounded by the idea that I could know what to ask before throwing myself into the mud of the field. I queerly failed to imagine any question at all that I could reconcile with the risk of blinkering myself to the provocations that I knew Crossbones would continue to throw at me from every angle.

As I began to transcribe the interview data, it took on a flat and alien quality. The "variations in tone, intensity, and rhythm" disappeared (Scheurich, 1995, p. 240). The clang of church bells, the roar of helicopters, and the clatter of machinery disappeared; the crackling of the wind and rustling of footsteps disappeared; the soundscape of Crossbones disappeared and the words on the page felt violently excised from it. Frustrated, I began to wonder how the dynamic of the interviews might have been affected if I had tuned *in* to our surroundings rather than tuned them out and had encouraged my interviewees to do the same. Would the interview have been considered derailed? Would it be appropriate for my analysis of those encounters to focus on the fullness of their corporeality and materiality as much as the words exchanged, when my interviewees have presumably given up their time on the assumption that I am interested in their *words*? If I had verbalised the pounding in my chest or asked my interviewees how they were feeling in their bodies, would that have entailed the unwelcome crossing of an assumed boundary? If so, what does this say about the extent to which Man's neurotypical epistemology defines and delimits what counts as meaning and what counts as social? My neurodivergent trouble with the frame of the social science research interview—underpinned by the idea that language-is-representation-is-knowledge-itself—also underscores a more general problem of grappling with more-than-human materiality within the frame of neurotypically humanist qualitative methodology.

As I butted up against the task of representing something representable, I remembered how challenging I find it to respond when visitors pass by Crossbones and ask me: "so, what *is* all this?" Often these people might be rushing between work meetings, but in lieu of a concise response, I tend to insist they come inside for a quick peek at the garden. My words can't do its uncommon beauty justice, nor can I tell them what Crossbones *is* without holding them up for what would probably be an inappropriate length of time. When speaking to those accidental visitors who have enough time to hear a little more about the site, I need to feel surrounded by it—by the tenacious plants bursting from the cracks in its surface, by the mildewed ribbons fluttering from the industrial-gates-turned-shrine, by its bustling riot of critters—to put the pieces of Crossbones' story together. The site, I have so often felt, tells its own story so much better than I can. Any one of my attempts to weave its stories together feels inexpertly crude compared to what is told so seamlessly in the sedimented layers of Crossbones' more-than-human histories (Barad, 2007, p. 180).

As Elizabeth Adams St. Pierre (2019, p. 4) has argued, "the 'what is' question, Plato's question, is essentialist and not poststructural. It assumes something already exists, that something 'is,' is stable, and so can be identified and represented." The "what is" question is a central one to established practices of social science research—it is so pervasive as to be barely noticeable, given. The mesh of institutional processes within which such research takes place rests on *what is*: how could a project obtain funding without needing to answer this? "We" live in a world that has been sedimented according to Plato's question, which is precisely why accidental visitors to Crossbones ask me what it *is*: so that they can "make sense" of it in a way that is familiar, comforting, natural. When I was trying in vain to pull a coherent answer to this question out of my data, I was equally—and stubbornly—convinced that Crossbones was—objectively—simply too complex and multidimensional to be succinctly surmised, and that any attempts to draw conclusions about it would be a reductive waste of time. There is a potent extent to which I still believe this to be the case, but it is only as I revisit such moments in the writing of this chapter that I am also coming to realise that my personal neurodivergent trouble with thinking the "big picture" has also been a very significant factor in making "what is" questions about Crossbones so difficult to answer.[8] Perhaps both are true: the uncontainability of Crossbones and my own trouble with containing objects fitted comfortably together; I had found a "wild" place where my wild attention made sense.

I pick up "wild" here from Crossbones itself and let it mingle with Jack Halberstam's (2020) exploration of the term. Since being reclaimed by the local community, Crossbones has been cultivated as a "wild" garden for the Outcast dead,[9] a manifestation of the work that began at the gates outside it, in which "weeds"—nature's social Outcasts—are offered their place to thrive. For Halberstam (2020, p. 3), *wildness* names "a chaotic force of nature, the outside of categorization, unrestrained forms of embodiment, the refusal to submit to social regulation, loss of control, the unpredictable." The wild inherits its histories of having been abused, fetishised, subjected to attempted mastery and colonisation, its being defined in opposition to civilisation and those who belong to it. At the same time, the wild holds the potential for thinking across queerness, blackness, disability, animality, death, and more and offers a potential site from which those bodies marked as wild might build a more-than-human solidarity.[10]

Frustrated with the impossibility (and, it often felt, pointlessness) of the task I had unwittingly given myself—to contain Crossbones—as I

[8] Developmental psychologist Uta Frith (1989, p. 98) famously hypothesised "weak central coherence" as the key marker of autism: that is, Frith claims that while autistic people may excel at local processing, they lack a "centrally acting high-level cohesive force" that pulls such information together, resulting in "an incoherent world of fragmented experience." While fragmentation is an experience recounted by some autistic people (Davidson & Henderson, 2010, p. 467), I suggest that *equating* a preference for local over global processing with an incoherent and fragmented world is a neurotypical and deficit-oriented leap, implicitly contested in many of the beautifully coherent—but different—experiential accounts of neurodiversity highlighted by Judge (2018) and Davidson and Smith (2009).

[9] If we take "the wild" or wilderness as it is popularly conceived, that is, a place apart from or unchanged by humans, cultivating a wild garden is evidently a contradiction in terms. However, since a pure and untouched wild is little more than a fantasy, I let this apparent contradiction hang here in the hope of gesturing to a different kind of wild. What the garden of remembrance at Crossbones offers instead is an urban wild in which humans are embedded, in which humans negotiate with and learn from more-than-human others as a path of mutual flourishing (Reeves, 2022, n.d.).

[10] Judge (2018, p. 1108) similarly notes that "important threads of marginalisation and solidarity emerge between subjectivities that have been rendered less-than-human, however, creating space for empathetic common ground."

shifted into the next stage of my research, away from abstracted methods and into the grounded transdisciplinary field of the psychosocial, I took a turn. Taking the sage advice of my supervisor to "touch the earth," I found a way into the site that started instead with the thickness of auto/ethnographic detail. This immediately became the only way to grapple with the field that felt truly available to me in my neurodivergence: I could stay lost in detail and incrementally build up a picture of Crossbones through acts of noticing caught up in *polyrhythmic* (Tsing, 2013) temporalities producing incremental change. As such, I sought to address the question of what the site "is" through its dynamic fluctuations, as read through my dynamically fluctuating attention. I hoped that another kind of whole could emerge this way, without me ever having to step back far enough to be the one to define or delimit it.

Whereas basing my research on textual data had by default implored me to direct my attention to the human participants in Crossbones' community, it never occurred to me that thick description of Crossbones should begin and end with human people. Setting out to write without a plan, I took refuge in Crossbones-as-place first and foremost; I treasured writing as an opportunity to spend quiet moments surrounded by more-than-human kin. I could write immersed in company—medicinal herbs, self-sown wildflowers, bulging bodies of fungi, mischievous grey squirrels, the bones of the Crossbones dead and the rats that carry their DNA above ground—becoming-together as a post-industrial landscape rich with the kind of urban debris that would have marked Crossbones a wasteland, had it not been met with such warmth and welcome by the people that tended it and the nonhumans that enveloped it.

Without the purposeful care of a community of living humans, there would be no "Crossbones" to speak of; I cherish their work and am proud to count myself among them. Nonetheless, I am also aware that at Crossbones, living people come and go. Many of Crossbones' other participants also transgress its boundaries; but many too inhabit it for many more hours a week than living people do, not least the Crossbones dead (thanks to the sustained, collaborative efforts of humans and nonhumans). With the obvious exception of myself, as a body with a view from somewhere rather than a view from nowhere (Castro-Gómez, 2021; Haraway, 1988; Mignolo, 2009), the living human people in Crossbones' community thus move into and out of my account of it, rather than being automatically central to it.

Just as Crossbones is iteratively constituted by *more-than-human sociality* (Tsing, 2013), neurodiverse sociality is also a more-than-human sociality (Davidson & Smith, 2009; Judge, 2018). Whereas neurodivergent (and particularly, autistic[11]) people are frequently characterised as "asocial," such an interpretation neglects to account for the often profoundly social connections neurodivergent people can feel with more-than-human others: from biotic critters such as animals and plants, through rivers and winds, stones and seashells, buildings and artworks, and prominently in my case, human remains in their dissolution into the more-than-human flux (Plumwood, 2008). What is frequently neurotypically perceived as a lack or deficit might as lived neurodiversity be sensorially and affectively rich, comforting and even awe-inspiring engagements. What could appear neurotypically as "alienation," or even "disassociation," might, from a neurodivergent perspective, indicate or open up connection with something other than human conversation.[12] What might be neurotypically construed as "distraction" from an isolated and isolable object might,

[11] This chapter avoids the use of people-first language when discussing autism, following the preferred terminology of the majority of authors directly and indirectly cited in this chapter, and taking note of arguments put forward by autistic self-advocates such as Jim Sinclair (2013). Given this chapter's critical stance against the "disordering" of difference, I also avoid referring to autism as ASD (autism spectrum disorder).

[12] This may sound a counter-intuitive point to grasp. To offer an explanation based on personal experience: I recall, recently, being surrounded by florescent lighting and chattering human voices, which quickly became sensorially overwhelming to the point that I felt I was floating outside my body and unable to focus on holding conversation or basic decision-making. After leaving, I sat down at the base of a tree in the nearest green space, my sensory sensitivity still intensely heightened. The pressure of participating in human-human social interaction was removed and I could simply be in my current state without needing to "perform." The dampness of the earth was more comforting than ever, the flowers brighter, the fractured sunlight more vivid, the rustle of leaves in the trees more textured and dynamic than I had ever heard it. The same sensory sensitivity that had made it so difficult to be in the busy indoor environment actually deepened my experience of more-than-human connection.

for a neurodivergent person, be a nourishing dance of involuntary attention.[13]

That more-than-human dimensions of sociality have so frequently been ignored in social research is clearly not a product of neurotypicality alone, as many Indigenous authors and allies have attested in their critiques of Western anthropocentricism (Kimmerer, 2013; TallBear, 2015; Todd, 2015; Watts, 2013) reductive materialism (2008), and related binary constructions of living/non-living (TallBear, 2017). Rather, the historic failure of social research to attend to more-than-human sociality is a consequence of the human exceptionalism that underpins Man's epistemology. Mel Chen (2012) offers a helpful critique of the *animacy hierarchies* that situate Man at its pinnacle, with his wild human others occupying lower rungs, vying for animacy alongside other de-animated beings such as animals and plants, and at the very bottom of the pile, ostensibly inert matter such as rocks. Thinking through neurodiverse sociality as more-than-human sociality is an attempt to thicken one of many strands of knowing-in-being subjugated under Man, in the hope of joining myriad divergent threads in incrementally weaving together an otherwise.

In the following section, I share some of my burgeoning attempts to find a neurodivergent way into the "what is" question via a form of auto/ethnographic poetry, or *anthropoetry* (Kusserow, 2017). This small gesture to treading out the path less used was also the only one I felt able to take, the only path that could sustain my neurodivergent bodymind through a research project spanning several years. Rather than resigning myself to the search for a representable object, I search instead for a way to navigate the muddy middle spaces where moments and words live vividly in unexpected jolts and small details (Fig. 9.3).

[13] Psychology contrasts *involuntary attention* to *directed attention*. Directed attention requires homing concentration onto specific tasks and will eventually lead to fatigue, including in neurotypical people. Involuntary attention, on the other hand, is "resistant to fatigue" (Chung et al., 2018). People can rapidly recover from the fatigue associated with directed attention by switching to involuntary attention, which is also, pleasingly, referred to as "fascination."

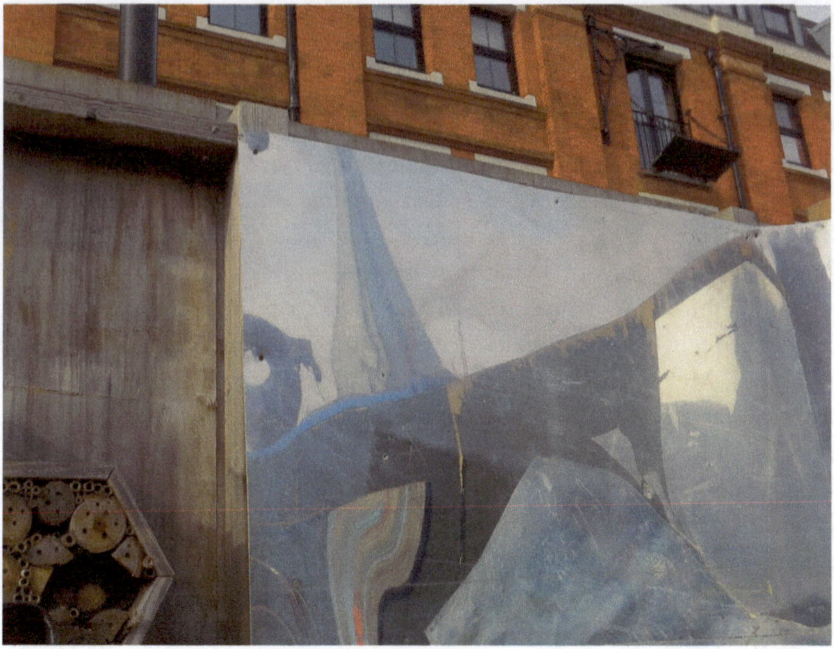

Fig. 9.3 The Shard reflected in the mirrors in the Irish Corner at Crossbones Graveyard (*Source* Photos by author)

Friday the 4th of December 2020

g a t e s   c l a n g   o p e n

and the magpie
caws disapprovingly

Time to share this place with human people for another
couple of hours.

up
up
and under
the Goose's
Wing

I prop my bike up against the wall, the one that's seen so
much over the years.
My front wheel nearly crushes a tiny solitary stem of
buddleia bursting up through the cracks.
I know the sapling can't stay here; wandering roots can't be
left to fracture the foundations in which the bones of the
dead are embedded.
But I won't be the one to enforce this, not today.

I follow a flash of colour eastwards
to something unfamiliar

the green roof of our volunteer hut,
the Clink, is finally green again

six months ago, it had
almost turned to dust

now
the disorderly textures of

euphorbia
bubbling

floundering
sedums

and dead grasses

spill over the Clink's edges

the plaque on the substation wall behind screams

1996

a wandering
buddleia grows
sideways,
solitary, from
the Clink's
wood-plated
wall, from a
crevice that was
never intended
to be this
hospitable.

I turn around

deep into winter, the salvias in the infinity beds still sing bright

crumpled brown   from that colossal London plane
leaves   over the way

nest suspended in
clusters of salvia's
foliage

this one, Hot Lips, has deep red
petals edged with white

I look closer
pause at an unexpected pocket
of mutation
a cluster of flowers

completely red   and on the   completely white
opposite side
of the plant

and wonder

how this sage came to be Hot Lips and whether I am watching them struggle to
become whatever they were before, again.

Notes: Friday the 4th December 2020

"The Clink" is named after the Liberty of the Clink—the medieval jurisdiction in which Crossbones was located—and the Clink prison, which operated nearby until the late eighteenth century.

The Goose's Wing is a sculptural shelter that envelops visitors as they enter Crossbones, built by Arthur de Mowbray in 2015. Its "goose wing" shape references the Winchester Geese, who worked in brothels locally during the medieval period.

Buddleia

close to the buddleia's centre

the drawn out, high-pitched
frequencies of passing trains

scream in
from the
northwest

rippling through the site and jolting me into a

different kind of awareness

I follow the noise to its source, towards the railway

arches that cross the northern end of Redcross Way

to the leggy

cascade of

buddleia

spouting

from the

Victorian

brickwork

introduced into cultivation in 1896

brought to Kew Gardens from China by Basque
missionary Father Armand David, who gave his name to
14 of his "discoveries," including *Buddleia Davidii*

its highly dispersible

~~lively~~ ~~wayward~~

seed

**has since escaped cultivation on multiple
occasions**

often associated with habitation

**additional dispersal can be facilitated by the air
currents generated by cars and trains**

I run my fingers over the cluster of woody protrusions at the centre of
the buddleia's trunk

they remind me of the diagrams I've seen of human
hearts, veins and arteries cut off close to the organ as
they weave in and out of it. I suppose it would be
impossible to follow them to their limits

seeing and feeling that what remains of these branches were cut at
different times

pale beige insides,
rough and moist to
touch
centres turning
hollow

deep,
dark,
earthy
browns

tender green shoots erupt amongst the
stumps

finding their way through folds of dry,
brown, leafy debris

I wonder

just how many years I am witnessing
calibrated here
compressed into this space
across this spectrum of texture and tone?

nodes
sprout
young
growth
along
exposed
above me tracts of
bare
branches

Most of the flowering heads have now gone to seed.
A few dense clusters of flowers remain, each an
explosion of tiny, purple, trumpet-shaped flowers.

I b r e a t h e in their just-lingering scent
lilac

that's what I've read
it should smell like.

A damselfly
or a dragonfly
(I never know)
stops to feed on a
flower
and another
a bee follows
and another

I squat down, following the leafy shoots that
spiral around the trunk down to its base, where
it meets the foundations
am met right away with a flush of euphorbia
and the knowledge that this buddleia is not alone
they burst from these cracks
in complex community

I remember that every one of these leaves, every strip of bark, is saturated with others too small for me to see.

Notes: Buddleia

This piece draws on direct quoted material from the Non-Native Species Secretariat (n.d.): the relevant text is rendered in bold. Where ellipses might typically be used to indicate that phrases of quoted material have been omitted, line breaks are used instead.

For All Suicides

A grey squirrel darts out
onto the stepping stones
that run alongside the
infinity pond and looks
straight at me, belly
exposed, pauses.

The squirrel looks surprised to
see me, but not remotely afraid

reminding me that for every 2
hours we human visitors spend at
Crossbones

the critters that live here
spend 22 more

breathing
digesting
touching
sleeping

with the dead

As one of two volunteers left in here as opening hours wind down, it feels they have been waiting for the (living) humans to leave so that business as usual can resume.

The squirrel holds my gaze
for a moment more before
they bound away

I walk around to greywashed,
splintered coffin resting in the Irish
Corner, bend down to read the
plaque:

Thomas Ball,
3rd Nov 1822
died by suicide after being fined for having an
altercation with his wife

a year before the Burial of Suicide
Act 1823 prohibited
the traditional crossroad burial with a stake
through the heart, replacing it with an
interment in the unconsecrated part of the
churchyard.

I pause for a moment, breathe
and attempt to commit Thomas' name to memory.

I look up, southwestwards, to
the shrine N
FOR ALL SUICIDES L O V E
and notice sticky letters spelling out V
in D I E S
green R
silver
purple
gold glitter
for the first time.

I move closer
read the names of

meet the familiar
face of the crow
painted on rusty
corrugated tin

IRVING

Marshall Leadbetter Jr.

Graeme Payne

IMOGEN GOLDIE

Jan

MONKEY Resh
DAVE

ED

inked bold and dark over the layers of names since
faded beneath

heralded by a withered
crow feather

I breathe to remember

look down to the young clump of feathery yarrow in
vibrant green unfolding from the cracks beneath the shrine

in the presence of this
involuntary gathering

of the dead we living choose to remember.

Notes: For All Suicides

Thomas' coffin was a replica built by local sculptor Adrian for an exhibition curated by Lucy Coleman Talbot (2021), *We Are Here*, held at Crossbones in October 2020 and based on Talbot's archival research. The bold-rendered text in this piece indicates direct quotations from the exhibition guide (Talbot, 2021, p. 2); as with the previous piece, line breaks are used instead of ellipses when omitting phrases from quoted material.

Discussion: Making-in-Writing as Wild Sociality

As I approached the task of transposing my chaotically scribbled field-notes—meandering the page, refusing to stay within the lines, shifting scales, doubling back on themselves—I ran into moments of tension that felt impossible to express within a neurotypical grammar. "Writing up" once again seemed to implore me to translate my notes into a tidy neurotypicality of which I felt incapable, and which felt far removed from the sensorial immediacy of the encounter with Crossbones. I hit moments of friction as I sought to translate the disorderly text of my notes into structured sentences complete with tenses, pronouns, and punctuation. The very shape of the paragraph became problematic. I found myself having to make decisions about what happened "first" for the sake of putting forward a coherent narrative, when in actuality both things had happened at once, and my attention had been split between them at the time. At other times, I read my surroundings in two or more different and sometimes conflicting ways at once; other times still, I would read my notes but another, remembered dimension of the encounter almost drowned out the words as I did so. Other times, my embodied encounter with the site—or the process of writing it up—was punctuated equally loudly with remembered conversations and fragments of information reverberating through me. Wild sociality does not obey the rules of neurotypical sociality—it is multiple, cacophonous, polyrhythmic, and nonlinear.

When I heard in passing of open-field poetics—an approach to poetry that treats the page as space, or even "a place or a landscape" (Bloomfield, 2013)—I was immediately entranced by the possibility that a page might let some of these tensions hang. I wondered if the page, as a *field of play* (Richardson, 1997), might hold the space for certain tensions: between different *intra-actions* (Barad, 2007) on the edge of being determined; between different strands of more-than-human knowledge in their co-presence; between the presumptive linearity of narrative and the *dance of attention* (Manning & Massumi, 2014) that noisy, lively, neurodiverse, more-than-human worlds necessitate. I wanted the reader to "hear" multiple voices and engage multiple, partial strands of attention at once (as I am so used to doing). As I arranged text on the page, I found that making space for these tensions made it feel less like I was writing in a foreign, neurotypical grammar. As Judge (2018, p. 1112) aptly highlights, the "continuous and actively fluid communicative spectrum" that is neurodiverse expression "requires an openness to different ways of knowing and expressing that may challenge solely verbal frameworks." The incorporation by necessity of a non-verbal component—the spatiality of the page, the white space, the tension—allowed me to approach "writing" as a material process of embodied making in a way that felt severely limited within a neurotypical grammar. The tension helped the words to feel alive, and holding this tension as resonance was deeply and sensorially satisfying to my neurodivergent brain, a moment of space from and disruption to the neurotypical grammar of language-as-representation that constantly insists that I "make sense" through a rational, linguistically bound and temporally linear narrative. Opening up the space for something other than words on the page let me call out to a world that is not delimited by language, a world in which meaning is not only present in words, and so a world that is also more-than-human.

As I played with moving text around on the page, I unexpectedly found myself reinhabiting the spatiality of the encounter with Crossbones. I was summoned back to the embodied memory of being there; it was co-present with me as I wrote up at my desk. I could navigate and express Crossbones' spatiality without being obliged to narrativise it every step of the way. I could place my more-than-human kin there without always needing to explain their presence. "I" could emerge and dissolve as placeholder or spatial location, rather than having to stay stuck within the position of stable narrator. Caught up in the perpetual struggle to sit still at my desk, I could reinhabit the embodied experience of moving around Crossbones, surrounded by the movements of more-than-human others. I could move around the page even as I stayed within it, making it easier to stay with the page and so with my work. As Davidson and Henderson (2010, p. 471) have highlighted in their readings of autistic autobiographies, for neurodivergent people, "movement is often a means of stabilizing volatile space, of reordering one's place in the environment in more manageable ways."

That my editing process has become one of making and moving has demanded I work slowly and closely—a temporal disposition that often feels undervalued or nigh impossible within *chrononormative* (Freeman, 2010) trajectories of doctoral research—but which feels deeply satisfying and necessary to me. While in certain ways, then, these neurodivergent strategies have afforded me ways to navigate my work in a way that feels more engaged, stimulating, comfortable—and crucially, possible—as I carve out the space to do this work, I run into different kinds of friction. Against the pull of the institutional demands on me—swimming upstream with diverse others who have variously found themselves "out of sync" with Man's temporality—I slow down to work in a way that allows me to express my neurodivergent encounters with Crossbones in a way that now feels unavoidable (Fig. 9.4).

Tentative Conclusions/Parting Notes

What I offer in this chapter is just one possible expression of a neurodivergent research practice among many potential others. "Potential" being key, as so far, the scope of overtly neurodiverse strategies has largely not been realised, due to the limiting factors of underrepresentation, disclosure, and epistemological and institutional support. I have found the epistemological space to share these neurodivergent strategies in the capacious spaces of psychosocial studies, and yet much work remains to be done if psychosocial studies is to sufficiently grapple with neurodiverse and more-than-human sociality. The neurodivergent strategies that have

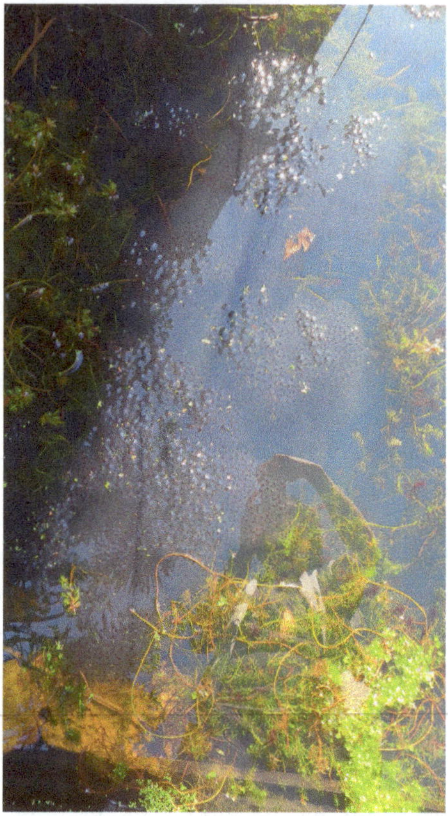

Fig. 9.4 Frogspawn in the eco-pond at Crossbones Graveyard (*Source* Photos by author)

burgeoned through my engagement with Crossbones are not solely my output; they are generated as a path of wild attention, itself demanded and produced by the lively more-than-human community within which I work. They are my co-creators of epistemic space.

A key contention of this chapter is that if psychosocial studies is to take seriously neurodiverse sociality, it should also purposefully attend to expanding its sense of sociality beyond the human. The transdisciplinarity of psychosocial studies opens up a host of pathways through which this might be realised. At the same time, it should take care that the "psycho-" in psychosocial does not crowd out more-than-human sociality.

While the psychosocial intends to disrupt the psycho/social binary, there is a risk that the "psycho-" in psychosocial implicitly insists that its analyses always come back to an ostensibly internal and somehow exclusively "human" mind, thus reiterating the binary it attempts to dismantle. As our gut bacteria will attest, no such thing exists.[14] Perhaps a more meaningful psychosocial engagement with more-than-human sociality could offer unexpected paths to thinking queerly beyond the psycho/social binary.

As I have argued here, psychosocial studies has a particular responsibility towards enacting conditions by which neurodivergent people can participate in the field *in their neurodivergence*, and not exclusively through the many ways in which they have had to learn to speak the neurotypical language. In this chapter, I have contextualised my neurodivergent strategies within a largely neurotypical grammar. This is a technique I have had to go to great effort to learn and doing so generates more than enough friction. That I have done so is also a marker of a privilege that many neurodivergent people do not have: the learned ability to traverse neurotypical modes of communication steadily enough to be able to express myself through them, however intermittently. Crucially, then, if psychosocial studies is to take seriously the work of neurodiversifying its perspectives, a neurotypical epistemology and grammar should not be regarded as the only framework through which neurodiverse strategies can become legible. This frame of legibility should not be limited to being literally understood, but rather, should also seek to recognise neurodiverse strategies as performative modes of criticality. That is, psychosocial studies should afford the space for neurodiverse strategies to *just be* rather than always to insist on their assimilation within a neurotypical frame.

Epistemic space can be an important refuge for neurodivergent people and also, therefore, a site of healing and justice. As a transdisciplinary field concerned with contemplations on critical epistemology, psychosocial studies might just afford the epistemic wriggle room within which neurodiverse perspectives can articulate themselves. As has been

[14] Recent years have seen an explosion of research around the brain-gut-microbiota axis, with profound implications for understanding human-nonhuman entanglement. Dinan and Cryan's (2017) review of key studies in the field highlights the accumulating evidence of the role of the brain-gut-microbiota axis in modulating depression, anxiety, and neurological difference.

discussed, overtly neurodivergent perspectives are rare in academia not only because of underrepresentation and inadequate mechanisms for recognising their value, but also because of legitimate concerns around disclosure. But psychosocial studies cannot wait for underrepresentation to be rectified or for the risk of stigma to be ameliorated for more overtly neurodivergent perspectives to suddenly appear. Rather, to create the space for neurodiverse perspectives to flourish, psychosocial studies should embolden its commitment to a more general diversifying of critical approaches through which all manner of wild epistemologies can come to take up space. It should be open to diverse forms of writing, and to diverse and collaborative approaches to appraising such writing. This stands to benefit not only neurodivergent people, but a great many others who tread the lived terrain of divergence from Man and his epistemology.

Further, psychosocial studies should take seriously the potential of *more-than-verbal* (Judge, 2018, p. 1102) methods to grapple with its material. While writing can, for some neurodivergent people, offer a particularly potent mode of communication (Prince-Hughes, 2002), for others, entirely non-verbal communication methods may be preferable or necessary. These methods might be actualised through mediums more often figured as creative, such as movement, performance, video, sound, painting, or sculpture, for example. The response-ability the field should take on is to build capacity to recognise the criticality already present within such forms of communication.

Acknowledgements I am very grateful to a generous handful of people who provided feedback on this chapter at various points in its life cycle: Dr Margarita Palacios, Dr Ben Gidley, Professor Heather Anne Swanson, Clau di Gianfrancesco, Dr Silvia Posocco, and Dr Annette-Carina van der Zaag. I also express my deep thanks to Guilaine Kinouani and again to Clau in their capacity as co-editors, for keeping me inspired and committed as we put together this volume. I also reiterate my thanks to Silvia for offering advice and enthusiasm at key moments during this project, in her capacity as PhD programme leader for Psychosocial Studies.

Declaration This research was supported by the Economic and Social Research Council under grant number ES/P000592/1. The author has no known conflicts of interest to declare.

References

Ahmed, S. (2013). *The Cultural Politics of Emotion*. Routledge.

Barad, K. (2007). *Meeting the Universe Halfway: Quantum Physics and the Entanglement of Matter and Meaning*. Duke University Press.

Berns, S. (2016). In Defense of the Dead: Materializing a Garden of Remembrance in South London. *Material Religion, 12*(2), 165–188.

Bloomfield, M. (2013). Landscaping the Page: British Open-Field Poetics and Environmental Aesthetics. *Green Letters, 17*(2), 121–136. https://doi.org/10.1080/14688417.2013.800338

Castro-Gómez, S. (2021). *Zero-Point Hubris: Science, Race, and Enlightenment in Eighteenth-Century Latin America*. Rowman & Littlefield.

Chapman, R. (2020). Neurodiversity, Disability, Wellbeing. In *Neurodiversity Studies*. Routledge.

Chen, M. Y. (2012). *Animacies*. Duke University Press.

Chung, K., Lee, D., & Park, J. Y. (2018). Involuntary Attention Restoration During Exposure to Mobile-Based 360° Virtual Nature in Healthy Adults With Different Levels of Restorative Experience: Event-Related Potential Study. *Journal of Medical Internet Research, 20*(11), e11152. https://doi.org/10.2196/11152

Davidson, J., & Henderson, V. L. (2010). 'Travel in Parallel with Us for a While': Sensory Geographies of Autism. *The Canadian Geographer/Le Geographe Canadien, 54*(4), 462–475.

Davidson, J., & Smith, M. (2009). Autistic Autobiographies and More-Than-Human Emotional Geographies. *Environment and Planning D: Society and Space, 27*(5), 898–916.

Dinan, T. G., & Cryan, J. F. (2017). Brain–Gut–Microbiota Axis—Mood, Metabolism and Behaviour. *Nature Reviews Gastroenterology & Hepatology, 14*(2), 2. https://doi.org/10.1038/nrgastro.2016.200

Duncan, R. E. (1973). *The Opening of the Field*. New Directions. Retrieved from https://www.proquest.com/pq1lit/publication/publications_2065371?accountid=213250

England, M. R. (2016). Being Open in Academia: A Personal Narrative of Mental Illness and Disclosure. *The Canadian Geographer/Le Géographe Canadien, 60*(2), 226–231.

feministkilljoys. (2018, November 8). Queer Use. *Feministkilljoys*. Retrieved from https://feministkilljoys.com/2018/11/08/queer-use/

Freeman, E. (2010). *Time Binds*. Duke University Press.

Friends of Crossbones. (2019). *Testimony*.

Friends of Crossbones. (n.d.). *History: Crossbones, the Strange but True Story Behind the Garden of Remembrance*. Crossbones. Retrieved April 19, 2019, from http://crossbones.org.uk/history/

Frith, U. (1989). *Autism: Explaining the Enigma*. Basil Blackwell Ltd.

Grandin, T., & Johnson, C. (2006). *Animals in Translation: Using the Mysteries of Autism to Decode Animal Behavior*. Houghton Mifflin Harcourt.

Halberstam, J. (2011). *The Queer Art of Failure*. Duke University Press.

Halberstam, J. (2020). *Wild Things*. Duke University Press.

Haraway, D. (1988). Situated Knowledges: The Science Question in Feminism and the Privilege of Partial Perspective. *Feminist Studies, 14*(3), 575. https://doi.org/10.2307/3178066

Haraway, D. (2008). *When Species Meet*. University of Minnesota Press.

Haraway, D. (2016). *Staying with the Trouble: Making Kin in the Chthulucene*. Duke University Press.

Hausner, S. L. (2016). *The Spirits of Crossbones Graveyard: Time, Ritual, and Sexual Commerce in London*. Indiana University Press.

Ingold, T. (2021). *Being Alive: Essays on Movement, Knowledge and Description*. Routledge. https://doi.org/10.4324/9781003196679

Judge, S. M. (2018). Languages of Sensing: Bringing Neurodiversity into More-Than-Human Geography. *Environment and Planning D: Society and Space, 36*(6), 1101–1119. https://doi.org/10.1177/0263775817748944

Kimmerer, R. W. (2013). *Braiding Sweetgrass: Indigenous Wisdom, Scientific Knowledge and the Teachings of Plants*. Milkweed Editions.

Kusserow, A. (2017). Anthropoetry. In A. Pandian & S. J. McLean (Eds.), *Crumpled Paper Boat: Experiments in Ethnographic Writing*. Duke University Press.

Manning, E., & Massumi, B. (2014). *Thought in the Act: Passages in the Ecology of Experience*. University of Minnesota Press.

Mignolo, W. D. (2009). Epistemic Disobedience, Independent Thought and Decolonial Freedom—Walter D. Mignolo, 2009. *Theory, Culture & Society, 26*(2–8), 159–181.

Muñoz, J. E. (2019). *Cruising Utopia*. New York University Press.

Murphy, M. (2017). Alterlife and Decolonial Chemical Relations. *Cultural Anthropology, 32*(4), 4. https://doi.org/10.14506/ca32.4.02

Non-Native Species Secretariat. (n.d.). *Buddleia, Buddleja davidii.* Retrieved September 13, 2021, from http://www.nonnativespecies.org/factsheet/factsheet.cfm?speciesId=581

Plumwood, V. (2008). Tasteless: Towards a Food-Based Approach to Death. *Environmental Values, 17*(3), 323–330.

Price, M. (2015). The Bodymind Problem and the Possibilities of Pain. *Hypatia, 30*(1), 268–284.

Prince-Hughes, D. (2002). *Aquamarine Blue 5: Personal Stories of College Students with Autism.* Ohio University Press.

Prince-Hughes, D. (2005). *Songs of the Gorilla Nation: My Journey Through Autism.* Crown.

Reeves, H. (2022). Lessons from Crossbones Graveyard: A More-Than-Individuated Ethics of Care. *Weather Matters, Fall Series.* Retrieved from https://www.weathermatters.net/lessonsfromcrossbones

Reeves, H. (2024). *Lessons from Crossbones Graveyard: A More-Than-Individuated Ethics of Care for Place, Community and Ecology* [Unpublished doctoral dissertation]. Birkbeck, University of London.

Reeves, H. (n.d.). *Buddleia. Pieces of Crossbones.* Retrieved October 27, 2022, from https://piecesofcrossbones.blog/2022/03/11/buddleia/

Richardson, L. (1997). *Fields of Play: Constructing an Academic Life.* Rutgers University Press.

Robertson, S. M., & Ne'eman, A. D. (2008). Autistic Acceptance, the College Campus, and Technology: Growth of Neurodiversity in Society and Academia. *Disability Studies Quarterly, 28*(4).

Rothschild, B. (2000). *The Body Remembers: The Psychophysiology of Trauma and Trauma Treatment* (Vol. 1). W. W. Norton & Company.

Scheurich, J. J. (1995). A Postmodernist Critique of Research Interviewing. *International Journal of Qualitative Studies in Education, 8*(3), 239–252. https://doi.org/10.1080/0951839950080303

Sinclair, J. (2013). Why I Dislike "Person First" Language. *Autonomy, the Critical Journal of Interdisciplinary Autism Studies, 1*(2).

St. Pierre, E. A. (2011). Post Qualitative Research: The Critique and the Coming After. In N. K. Denzin & Y. S. Lincoln (Eds.), *Sage Handbook of Qualitative Research* (4th ed., pp. 661–635). Sage.

St. Pierre, E. A. (2013). The Posts Continue: Becoming. *International Journal of Qualitative Studies in Education, 26*(6), 646–657.

St. Pierre, E. A. (2014). A Brief and Personal History of Post Qualitative Research: Toward "Post Inquiry". *Journal of Curriculum Theorizing, 30*(2).

St. Pierre, E. A. (2019). Post Qualitative Inquiry, the Refusal of Method, and the Risk of the New. *Qualitative Inquiry*, 1077800419863005. https://doi.org/10.1177/1077800419863005

Talbot, L. C. (2021). *'We Are Here': Crossbones Graveyard.* Unseen Histories.

Talbot, L. C. (2023). Not Their Heritage Theme Park: Honouring the Outcast at Crossbones Graveyard. In T. Biers & K. S. Clary (Eds.), *The Routledge Handbook of Museums, Heritage, and Death*. Routledge.

TallBear, K. (2015). An Indigenous Reflection on Working Beyond the Human/Not Human. *GLQ: A Journal of Lesbian and Gay Studies, 21*(2), 230–235.

TallBear, K. (2017). Beyond the Life/Not-Life Binary: A Feminist-Indigenous Reading of Cryopreservation, Interspecies Thinking, and the New Materialisms. In *Cryopolitics: Frozen Life in a Melting World* (pp. 179–202).

Tarlo, H. (2013). *Open Field: Reading Field as Place and Poetics* (pp. 113–148). Brill. https://doi.org/10.1163/9789401208857_007

Todd, Z. (2015). Indigenizing the Anthropocene. In *Art in the Anthropocene: Encounters among Aesthetics, Politics, Environments and Epistemologies* (pp. 241–254).

Tsing, A. L. (2013). More-Than-Human Sociality. In K. Hastrup (Ed.), *Anthropology and Nature* (pp. 27–42). Routledge.

Watts, V. (2013). Indigenous Place-Thought and Agency Amongst Humans and Non humans (First Woman and Sky Woman go on a European world tour!). *Decolonization: Indigeneity, Education & Society, 2*(1).

Wynter, S. (2003). Unsettling the Coloniality of Being/Power/Truth/Freedom: Towards the Human, After Man, Its Overrepresentation—An Argument. *CR: The New Centennial Review, 3*(3), 257–337. https://doi.org/10.1353/ncr.2004.0015

10

The Clinician as Killjoy (Without Killing Joy)

Rebecca Esho Greenslade

It is dinnertime. I am a participant at a symposium that meets annually to consider and critique the legacy of the work of RD Laing. A colleague begins to talk in more detail about a female client she had mentioned in her presentation that day, speaking about the challenges of working with her chaotic behaviour. Another colleague says, *sounds like a pretty severe case of BPD to me*. Others agree and begin to contribute their own BPD analysis of my colleague's client, one stating that they won't take female BPD clients as they are too difficult and manipulative. I listen for a couple minutes before speaking. *What's happening here?* I ask. *We're here because we say we're committed to extending our understanding of distress beyond psychiatric diagnosis yet everyone here has jumped at speculating this client has BPD. Is this the best we can do together?* The table falls quiet. *When you do this, are you including an understanding of how women are disproportionately given the label BPD, how neurodiversity is often misdiagnosed as BPD, or the fact that you are discussing a client at a dinner table, attributing a diagnosis to them that they have not consented to and considered*

R. E. Greenslade (✉)
Birkbeck University, The Feminist Therapy Network, London, UK

G. Kinouani et al. (eds.), *Creative Disruption*, Studies in the Psychosocial,
https://doi.org/10.1007/978-3-031-63661-5_10

it to be useful to them? Silence. Then, *I hear what you're saying Rebecca*, one participant says, *but I have an ex-partner with BPD and she sounds just like her*. I am angry. *I'm sorry too*, I say. *I'm sorry that despite all our proclamations to radical practice, here we are doing the same shit we're here to critique. This conversation is harmful to the client. Right now, we are harming someone*. I am disappointed. I am raging. People start to leave the table. Through killing joy, I have become the problem. I have also killed my joy.

Becoming a Feminist Killjoy

> Feminist killjoys are creative not *despite* being killjoys but *because* of being killjoys. And yet creativity might seem far from the life situation of the feminist killjoy whose modus operandi might appear to be rather destructive (Ahmed, 2023, p. 178).

Sara Ahmed begins her story of becoming a feminist killjoy being seated around a table. It's a story I am sure many of us resonate with. The story I began with here also took place around a table. Usually these are tables of polite conversation, tables of unspoken etiquette, tables that maintain a particular status quo. Sometimes at these tables something is said that will jar us, perhaps a racist or transphobic comment, perhaps a sexist 'joke' or, in my case, this time, a misogynistic pathologisation. A feminist killjoy chooses to speak up, to name the transgression, but our doing so meets disapproval; *we* become the transgressor because we have transgressed the politics of politeness that keeps things running smoothly at the table. We have made thing less smooth. We have killed joy. Ahmed describes, "When you expose a problem, you pose a problem. It might just then be assumed that the problem would go away if you would just stop talking about it" (2017, p. 37). For Ahmed, therefore, being a feminist killjoy means you are willing to create unhappiness. To be involved in activism or a politics of transformation is "to be involved in a struggle against happiness" (2010, p. 2).

It might seem unusual for a psychotherapist to be writing about her "struggle against happiness". Although, as an existentially trained psychotherapist, I was never taught how to make people feel better, or how to think their way into happiness. Happiness is not an existential concern. Instead, I learnt to be attentive to mechanisms of bad faith, paradoxes in living, calls to conscience and reconciling facticity.[1] I learnt how to use phenomenological inquiry and description to stay in close proximity to my clients, as a means of resisting reductive pathological language. However, it was not until I completed my training, and, freed from the limitations of its curricula (white, male, Eurocentric), that I was able to extend my understanding of bad faith to the psychotherapy profession itself. I saw that the exclusion of Beauvoir and Fanon on my existential therapy training was in bad faith, their exclusion a means to maintain a particular brand of existential thought that mirrored those that taught me, their exclusion an exclusion of the very analyses that would justify their inclusion! Beauvoir and Fanon's existential analysis of oppression began to show me how their deeply engaged political philosophies could also be applied to an emancipatory existential psychotherapeutic project, concerned with not only individual but social change (Greenslade, 2018). Enter feminism.

Feminism and feminist psychotherapies have taught me about what Ahmed describes as the "happiness myth of neoliberalism" (2023, p. 221). They have taught me just how much my profession has caused unhappiness. The psy-disciplines are the only profession I am aware of that has a survivor movement, not for having survived their unhappiness, but for having survived the unhappiness caused by people and institutions claiming to be able to alleviate it! They have taught me that, many psychotherapies, with their predominant emphasis on introspection and individual solutions, is more part of the problem than the cure, perpetuating the alienation from environment and community that pervades contemporary lives. Ahmed describes killing joy as a "world-making project" where "speaking out and speaking with … acts of spreading the word, are world-making" (2017, p. 261). She has most recently explored feminist killjoy work through the lens of cultural critic, philosopher, poet and activist; here I offer an additional lens: the feminist killjoy as

---

[1] For those unfamiliar with—yet interested in—existentialism and/or existential psychotherapy, I recommend Emmy van Deurzen's *Everyday Mysteries: A Handbook on Existential Psychotherapy* (2009) and Thomas E. Wartenberg's *Existentialism: A Beginner's Guide* (2008) as good introductory readings.

clinician. In this chapter, I am suggesting that clinicians who try to refuse and resist the normalisation of coercive and hegemonic therapeutic practices in attempt of an alternative liberatory and anti-carceral therapeutics, are actively engaging in a praxis of killing joy. Through doing so, psychotherapeutic practice widens its berth, it becomes part of a "world-making project". The clinician as killjoy undertakes, to draw upon Clare Hemming's (2012) analysis of 'affective solidarity' as a means to a feminist politics of transformation, a movement from, and between, affective dissonance to affective solidarity, or from "individual experience to collective feminist capacity" (p. 150). The killjoy clinician becomes of psychosocial interest through their undertaking of a relational praxis that is concerned with the interstices between social and psyche and their attempts to identify and attend to points and places of connection and disconnection through locating "affect, emotion and feeling into public as well as personal spaces" (Woodward, 2015, p. 4). Killing joy is a psychosocial intervention, a means of creative disruption where we unlearn and learn anew clinical "habits of being" (hooks, 2009).

Here, I focus on the role and function of collective practices and solidarity work that are so essential to sustaining the survival work that underpins a clinical killjoy practice; specifically I will discuss the ongoing praxis of monthly Feminist Therapy Supervision groups that I facilitate, reflecting on the ways these groups have engaged with cultivating a collective ethics of resistance where solidarity work creates possibilities for joy amidst the work of killing joy. Ahmed has written at length on the feminist killjoy and I cannot do justice to the nuance, clarity, playfulness, and depth of her killjoy analyses. It is a joy to read Ahmed write about killing joy. If you are unfamiliar with her writings on the feminist killjoy, I urge you read some. Please do not take this essay as fully representative of her words—it is not. I am writing my response to how I have read her words, to particular resonances and inquiries that have arisen for me. I am writing from personal story. We all have our own stories and mine will not be the same as yours. I dedicate this writing to killjoy clinicians, in loving solidarity.

This contribution to 'Creative Disruption' is inspired by a question posed by a former student, supervisee, now colleague and friend, Ruth. In one of the early Feminist Therapy Supervision groups we were reading the 'Introduction' to Ahmed's *Living a Feminist Life* (2017). Here, Ahmed introduces us to the figure of the feminist killjoy (it is not her first introduction to the feminist killjoy but it was the group's first introduction). As we began to discuss our relationship to feminist killjoy work, Ruth asked the group, *but how we can kill joy without killing our joy*? I love this question! It is a question that has refused to leave me, it is still working me, a question so alive for those of us that are trying to extend the psychotherapeutic project from, to use Gloria Anzaldúa's words: "inner work to public acts" (2002). Ruth's question has become a koan that I carry into my feminist life, a commitment to cultivating conditions of joy alongside my commitment to refuse the adaptive, status quo practices of my profession. So, thank you, Ruth. I am grateful for your question and your permission for the question to also become a title, enabling me to write into and out of it here.

Through taking up Ruth's question, I am not privileging joy as an affective aspiration. To do so would be to risk an alignment with the personal pursuits of happiness that fuel the wellbeing industries and positive psychology discourses. Happiness becomes a neo-liberal enterprise that seeks to exclude affective responses such as discontent or pessimism from our lives on grounds they are an obstacle to [economic] productivity. Joy is not always affectively available, even less so to those contending with oppression and marginalisation. I am, however, considering the generative reciprocity between joy and affective solidarity in the context of a heterogeneous group of clinicians trying to find ways to creatively disrupt and transform the status quo,[2] Ruth's 'our' reminds me of Sara Ahmed's reflection on the 'our' of feminism: "I think of that our as the promise of feminism, ours not as a possession but as an invitation to combine forces", showing up for our intersectional commitments towards each other.

[2] The group membership currently embodies different social locations across race, gender, sexuality, neurodivergence, spirituality and age. Where group members share commonality is being sufficiently financially resourced for counselling/psychotherapy training, the capacity to be present and participate in a 2.5 hour Zoom group together and similar political beliefs. However, there was less heterogeneity when the groups began. One woman of color left the first group because there were only two women of color in her group of six. In a discussion on white liberal feminism, one white, queer group member said to me, *if I hadn't known you already, Rebecca, I would never have joined a feminist supervision group set up by a white cis-woman therapist*, an important reminder of those clinicians who will choose *not* to join the group because of the positionalities I embody.

In his recent essay collection, *Inciting Joy* (2022), poet and essayist Ross Gay explores how joy can be a radical and necessary act of resistance and belonging. He considers the practices and habits that can render joy more available to us, as well as ways that cultivating joy can contribute to a more expansive sense of solidarity and care. In this chapter, I am contending that opportunity to share moments of killing joy is one such practice, one which, when we bring it into the foreground of our lives and therapeutic practices, can transform into a new habit of being. Foregrounding joy is not the same as hierarchising it. It is recognising how emotions co-exist, even when it feels like they shouldn't belong together. Similar to how Zadie Smith reminds us that joy is not the same as pleasure but present in "all that makes life intolerable" (2018, p. 334), Gay reminds us not only that pain and joy are companions, fundamentally knotted up with one another, but adds a *what if*? "What if joy is not only entangled with pain, or suffering, or sorrow, but is also what emerges from how we care for each other *through* those things?" (2022, p. 4). For Gay, we incite joy when we care for each other, joy can be strengthened in the times we must rely on each other. Joy "gets us to love, as being a practice of survival" (Gay, 2022, p. 10). For Ahmed, killing joy is also a practice of survival. Perhaps it can also get us to love.

Gay offers us a perspective of joy that is similar to Audre Lorde's perspective in her essay *Uses of the Erotic: The Erotic as Power* (1978) where she wrote: "the sharing of joy, whether physical, emotional, psychic, or intellectual, forms a bridge between the sharers which can be the basis for understanding much of what is shared between them and lessens the threat of difference" (1978, p. 46). To lessen the threat of difference is not to erase difference, but as Lorde has taught us, it is to use our differences as bridges of solidarity and care. An older member of one of the Feminist Therapy Supervision groups shared how the gender fluidity in her group is so contrasting to the gendered socialisation that she was raised with that some behaviours and preferences of other group members can feel alienating to her. She was nervous to name this difficulty but when she did, was met with love, with recognition that the group is committed to helping each other understand each other, that we *want* to understand each other. When she voiced a fear of causing offence one group member said, *even if you do cause offence I'm pretty sure we can work with that here.*

That filled me with joy! Through voicing her difference and acknowledging her positionality, the group was able to, in that moment, renew its intentions of collectively solidarity and care towards each other.

The Clinician as Killjoy

I am interested in what a feminist therapeutics needs to do to actualize its radical potential. I am interested in returning to feminist therapy's past in order to re-imagine a feminist therapy for the present.[3] Lola Olufemi (2020) "calls for a feminism that is expansive, that builds from relations of care and that recognizes that feminist work is justice work" (Ahmed, 2023, p. 284). I am interested in feminist therapy's part in this work, in how our training and experiences as both therapists and feminists can support re-imagining structures of care and ways of being in relationship with each other. This may mean transgressing and subverting some of the therapeutic orthodoxies we have been trained in. This will mean killjoy work. Lola Olufemi was one of the first feminist writers we read together in the Feminist Therapy Supervision groups. As a result, one of the group's members argued for Olufemi's inclusion on the curriculum of their psychotherapy training course, requesting it replace another text

[3] Throughout my five years as a trainee psychotherapist, I was not introduced to feminist perspectives or feminist psychotherapeutic practice. Now, as a visiting lecturer and training supervisor myself, it has become increasingly apparent that despite feminism's significant influence upon twentieth-century psychotherapeutic theories and practice, its impact and role within contemporary psychotherapy training curricula has been in decline the past decade. Feminist theory has a minimal presence within broader contemporary psychotherapeutic praxis and pedagogy (note, I am not commenting on the inclusion of feminist perspectives within psychoanalytic trainings but within integrative psychotherapy trainings, which now constitute the most popular training pathway within the psychotherapy profession). In the UK, it is not possible to train and accredit as a feminist psychotherapist, and it is my experience that trainee therapists are nowadays rarely introduced to the history and practice of feminist psychotherapies; by consequence, the relationship between feminism and psychotherapy is rarely considered as a viable, meaningful therapeutic approach to pursue. Two well-established therapist directories, www.counsellingdirectory.co.uk and www.welldoing.org, respectively, list 39 and 52 types of therapy that people searching for a therapist can choose from [last accessed 25 April 2021]. Neither directory includes feminist therapy within these listings. My own engagement with radical feminist psychotherapeutic herstories and literature has led me to both question its decline and resolve to be active in reinvigorating an interdisciplinary conversation between contemporary psychotherapeutic praxis and feminism. This was a key motivation for why I founded The Feminist Therapy Network.

selected by the course tutor that was problematic in its analysis of trans care. Now, psychotherapy students at that institution are introduced to the feminist questions and provocations Olufemi proposes. They are asked to consider these questions in relationship to their therapeutic work. This intervention was killjoy work.

What else might the killjoy clinician be intervening in? Mark Fisher utilised the term 'capitalist realism' to refer to how neo-liberalism has circumscribed our social and political possibilities to a reality entirely dominated by capitalism (2009). What Fisher termed 'post-capitalist desires' are rendered unimaginable, impossible to conceive and to actualise (2021). Neo-liberalism, has in Fisher's terms, operated a programme of 'consciousness deflation'—a squashing of the expanding collective consciousnesses of 1970's counterculture and suppression of imagining an *otherwise*. The psy-disciplines have not escaped this consciousness deflation; by contrast, they have become a site of reproduction of neoliberal capitalist ideology (see, for example, Rose, 1990, Smail, 2005, Parker, 2014, Rustin, 2015, LaMarre et al., 2019). The dominant practice model of mainstream psychotherapy is entrenched within, and operates from, notions of individualism, commodification and privatisation. We see this in the multiple crises of care that are the result of slashed public funds on care services, we see this in the increasingly manualised treatments of the NHS' IAPT (Improving Access to Psychological Therapies) service where there are long waiting lists for inflexible short-term behavioural therapies, we see this in the narrowing of our conceptions of care, we see this in the utilisation of therapists in job centres to psychologically coerce people back to work, in the pathologisation of distress and ever expanding categorisation of 'mental illness'. We see this in polypharmacy and unmonitored psychotropic prescriptions. We see this when first year students talk about social change and final year students talk about how much to charge in private practice.

In an interview with *The Morning Star* discussing the closure of London's Women's Therapy Centre (1976–2019), co-founders Susie Orbach and Luise Eichenbaum reflected how the work that still needs to be done within the psy-professions "is standing up to the neoliberal ideology that dismantles the building blocks of progressive institutions".[4] Orbach and Eichenbaum contend that whilst the women's movement has been experiencing a revival, particularly through the #MeToo movement, and that there has been progress in shifting from the personal experience to greater understanding of the social and psychological construct of patriarchal social relations, the patriarchy remains nonetheless in place and continues to fuel similar struggles that were facing women forty years ago.

Black Lives Matter has instigated a surge of trainings and workshops for therapists in anti-racism and intersectionality. I welcome these opportunities for consciousness-raising, for drawing attention to the blind spots of our privileges and the consequences of these blind spots. Yet, many of these trainings are not invested in undertaking lasting solidarity work or with building alternative practices of care. Recently, I saw a therapist claim they were a "certified anti-oppression" practitioner. I can imagine Audre Lorde writing a poem about that! I wonder how becoming "certified" in anti-oppression could also become another mechanism for the moral indifference that Lorde describes. Certificates mark the end of something, a moment of completion. Perhaps the ending becomes a gateway to something new, something more. But also, perhaps the ending forecloses further consciousness-raising and action. I am certified now, I've done the work, my certificate says so, I will collect another. And yet I also write this in grateful acknowledgement that there *are* therapists and therapeutic organisations that are undertaking critical practices of therapeutic care that are deeply committed to actualizing an anti-racist, anti-capitalist and anti-carceral therapeutics. There always have been. There always will be. You are Creative Disrupters. Thank you. Part of killjoy work is to visibilise your work, to share it, to include it in our conversations, trainings and reading lists.[5] We must persist in the otherwise. We must subvert when we can. At the same time, we must also acknowledge that creative disruption work is often self-funded, voluntary

[4] https://morningstaronline.co.uk/article/f/londons-womens-therapy-centre-1976-2019-feminist-project-committed-change [Last accessed: May 21st 2021].

[5] In acknowledgement: Maytree Suicide Respite Centre, Campaign for Psychiatric Abolition, Gaia Therapy Collective, Healing Justice Ldn, Project Lets, Recovery in the Bin and the Hearing Voices Network.

or low waged work. It is *in addition to*. It is rarely funded as it is critical, political work and it is hard to find funding for work that is critical and political and when we are sold a myth of scarcity, pitted against each other to compete for what meagre resources might be available to us, and then, under what conditions of compliance?

So, killjoy clinicians might draw attention to hegemonic and oppressive aspects of therapeutic practice, killjoy clinicians might come together in refusal of neutrality, objectivity or impartiality. Perhaps we will protest together. We might try to resist adaptive therapeutic approaches that privatise pain and accommodate people to their oppression and suffering. At times, this requires us to be the dissenting voice, the killjoy that critiques and challenges a colleagues' language or framing of distress. We might question the medicalised narratives that terms like 'trauma', 'addiction' and 'mental illness' have become so embedded within, we might draw attention to the systemic and structural conditions suffering is situated within. We might resist the weaponsiation of psychological language. Killjoy clinicians come together to try to imagine alternatives, to practice otherwise, amidst criticisms of utopian idealism or accusations that, for example, by criticising psychiatry and the mechanisms of power it upholds, we are denying emotional and psychological distress exists at all (this is a Twitter favourite!).

How might this manifest in our therapeutic work with clients? Perhaps instead of requesting a new client's GP details, or 'emergency contact' information as a matter of procedure, we will engage our clients with 'pod mapping', a transformative justice tool that originated with the Bay Area Transformative Justice Collective, which in the context of psychotherapy can help clients let us know who, in times of particularly difficulty, we can call upon *together* to support their ongoing safety and care in ways that are consensual and non-carceral. Perhaps instead of reaching into a psycho-educational 'toolbox', we commit to the critical work of 'conscientization', a pedagogical practice that places critical, reflexive dialogue in recipriocity with collective, socially engaged action.[6] When trying to understand a client's concerns, we will challenge our intra-psychic

---

[6] Community psychologist, Sue Holland's, Social Action Therapy is a good example of conscientization in therapeutic praxis (see, for example, Holland, 1991, 1992).

assumptions by also considering how systems of oppression might be showing up in these concerns. Perhaps we allow ourselves to question the monogamous imperative of therapy when it may be of service to our clients to choose to practice polyamorous psychotherapy, recognising that a weekly therapy session with us is just one relationship amongst many potential constellations of care. Perhaps, we negotiate ways of being together that align with the conditions of our client's lives, not a punitive rote therapy contract that refuses flexibility with working shifts, or chronic illness, as examples. We do not send automated email responses with a crisis line number.

Sometimes—perhaps often—killjoy clinicians won't know what to do. I am reminded of these two sentences from Gloria Anzaldúa in La Prieta: *I believe that by changing ourselves we change the world ... a going deep into our self and expanding out into the world. And yet, I am confused as to how to accomplish this* (1983, p. 208). The first time I read this, I cried in relief at Anzaldúa's uncertainty, at her not knowing how to reconcile the contradictory and challenging aspects of her life and work, yet whilst at the same time meeting this uncertainty with the vulnerability and humbleness that infuse her writings. The metaphysics of interconnectedness that is foundational to her spiritual activism does not necessitate that we always know *how* to act in the world, yet we are compelled to do so. In Zen, we will often hear the phrase: *not-knowing is most intimate* (*The Book of Equanimity*, Case 20). This statement may seem counter intuitive, yet I have come to understand that releasing our preconceptions and ideas about what's best for other people actually connects us more fully to them. It is a humble learning for a psychotherapist. We move beyond what we think we know into undiscovered, more intimate possibilities. Perhaps I am suggesting that not knowing how to act is another means to creatively disrupt, a subversion of the expertise and professionalism that so often serves to separate us from our clients.[7] This statement by Ahmed is also Zen statement!

[7] Here, I can't resist a note to academics researchers of 'mental health' with their paragraphed, peer-reviewed models of understanding and 280 characters of insight. Each time, with every client, I am trying to *live* my way to understanding them, the lives they have lived and the lives they want to live. I do this over and over, each time different questions, each time different answers. Your research methodology is not the same as mine.

> To live a feminist life is to make everything into something that is questionable. The question of how to live a feminist life is alive as a question as well as being a life question. (Ahmed, 2017, p. 2)

So, without always knowing what to do, a killjoy clinician makes living questions out of their killjoy critiques. These questions invite a radical re-imagining of psychotherapeutic cultures that have been built from and upon white, capitalist, cis-heteropatriarchial, imperialist systems of thought and praxis, a re-imagining where we move from therapeutic practices of independence towards therapeutic practices of *interdependence*. A killjoy clinician intervenes in both pedagogical and therapeutic spaces, disrupting epistemological orthodoxies, refusing the lens of capitalist realism and insisting instead on rendering 'post-capitalist desires' as *imaginable*, *possible* and *actualizable*, creating new pathways of practice: "paths we can call desire lines, created by not following the official path laid out by the disciplines" (Ahmed, 2017, p. 15). These living questions might include, how could we practice differently in order to cultivate an ethics of care that considers the collective, interdependent subject, as well as the individual? How can we centre ethics at the heart of undertaking solidarity work in psychotherapeutic practice? How do we organise our work around points of connection without erasing our differences, where do we resist the politics of politeness or the desire to smooth over discomfort? How can our collective therapeutic ethics transform the social contexts that make oppression and suffering possible? How do our practices still render carcerality possible, still refuse people and still pose possibilities for therapeutic captivity? These are all questions that have surfaced in the Feminist Therapy Supervision groups, killjoys gathering together, not always knowing what to do.

Feminist Therapy Supervision Group

I have been offering two monthly Feminist Therapy Supervision groups for about eighteen months now. Really, they are the kind of group I would like to belong to! It is a group that people have usually found their way to in response to a feeling of affective dissonance, whether experiencing a sense of isolation or alienation in their work, a lack of representation on their trainings, an incongruence between their therapeutic practice and personal values, or the absence of opportunities to consider dissident feminist ideas and their relationship to psychotherapy. We spend the first part of the group responding to a feminist text everyone has read in advance. Sometimes the text is directly on feminist psychotherapy, often it is a text by a feminist writer and we undertake the shared work of considering its ideas in relationship to psychotherapeutic practice. I am not providing a set 'feminist therapy' curriculum for the group; in fact there is no method other than offering a reading that I hope will creatively disrupt their therapeutic thinking and practice![8] (Group members are also welcome to suggest a reading they would like us to work with together.) Usually, we will use our conversation on the reading as a springboard into helping a group member think through their therapeutic work with a client they are working with. We try to bring a critical feminist lens to thinking about our therapeutic work together. We notice when this feminist lens might rub against, or enliven, the modalities we are trained in. It is not necessary to identify as a feminist therapist to be a part of the group, or to identify as a feminist, although it is necessary to be curious and open to feminist ideas and how they might be applied to, and disrupt, therapeutic practice. As is the format with many supervision groups, we spend some time initially 'checking in', letting the group know what we might need to know about ourselves that day to help us be together as fully as we can. However, another aspect of our 'check in' is the invitation to share with the group any time when we have killed joy the past month. This invitation is never a requirement or imperative. Our capacities for killing joy depend upon the bodies we inhabit, the context of our lives and how resourced we are. Nor do we create killjoy hierarchies. One type of killing joy is not elevated over another. All are valued.

At first, this was just a playful suggestion on my part; I invited killjoy sharing as a way to consolidate having read some of *Living a Feminist Life*

[8] As example, some of our readings have so far included writings by Bonnie Burstow, Sara Ahmed, Lola Olufemi, Vikki Reynolds, Laura Brown, Audre Lorde, AnaLouise Keating, Myisha Cherry, and bell hooks.

together. Yet, when we did, we noticed how much we appreciated the killjoy stories each other brought. Some have made us laugh, some have made us angry, some have required us to take a collective breath together, steadying ourselves at hearing a particular injustice or transgression. We have listened to killing the joy of a partner in a discussion about shared domestic labour, to using killjoy humour in response to a sexist 'joke', to challenging a course tutor on an absence of feminist perspectives in their classes, to speaking up to unexamined male privilege in a process group, to publically withdrawing from a conference presentation due to the inclusion of a trans-antagonistic speaker, to challenging the pathological language of a colleague, to addressing a heteronormative assumption at a GP surgery, to contacting a boiler installation company to let them know that it is not appropriate for their engineers to enter women's homes and refer to them as "love" or say "I bet you make a nice cup of tea", to challenging and ending a supervisory relationship due to a supervisor's refusal to engage with a racist remark about a client. Sometimes, group members have courageously and tenderly shared times when a client has killed *their* joy, a time when an unexamined privilege may have played out as a therapeutic transgression, a moment of harm that required a client to labour in a relational repair caused by our own infraction. Part of that repair is for us to hear and be accountable to our mistake. It is a reminder of the work it takes to be receptive to our joy being killed, when well-established defensive mechanisms are always ready to close us down if not attentive to them. Abolitionist and narrative therapist Vikki Reynolds describes the times we transgress our values as "spiritual pain" (2014). Sometimes this spiritual pain arises in response to the incongruence between our values and those of the therapeutic institutions we may work for, to "the discrepancy between what feels respectful, humane, and generative, and the contexts which call on us to violate the very beliefs that brought us to this work" (2014, p. 4). Reynolds encourages us, encourages me as a supervisor, not to try to smooth over this discomfort for my supervisees, but instead to see this spiritual pain as a potential resource for their practice. It is an ethic I try to centre at the heart of these groups, each transgression an opportunity for insight and an invitation to accountability and repair. For this is also the killjoy work of a clinician.

Some group members began to start by saying, *a few months ago I wouldn't have said this, but I imagined you all with me when I did.* Through this sharing of killing joy, we noticed that we were building our collective strength. Killing joy is strength building. It has become part of our solidarity work together, building a collective ethics that informs our therapeutic practice. Recently Ruth, whose question inspired this writing, shared how she and her wife have decided to take their mothers' premarital names as an act of feminist solidarity. Now Ruth Nanayakkara Bruce, this matronymic recovering disrupts a lineage of patriarchal namesaking. This disruption has both killed joy and created joy. Sometimes when we killjoy we are creating it at the same time. I love how Ruth is happy to share her name here, resisting the mechanism of privatisation which keeps our inner lives secret, which keeps us away from each other. Instead, by sharing her name, Ruth is disclosing her feminist commitments. In writing about feminist therapy ethics, Valli Kalei Kanuha insists that those of us who identify and practice as feminist therapists must make "public testimony" to our ethical principles (1990, p. 31). Ruth's name is public testimony to her clients that she is a therapist willing to resist and subvert patriarchy, that her therapeutic ethics are also feminist ethics.

To return to the 'our' of feminism, through killjoy work as solidarity work, we build our collective strength, we combine our force. Sometimes, we might act collectively, sometimes, we act seemingly independently, yet we are still drawing from the affective solidarity we have cultivated together. Perhaps, this is why one group member recently shared that this group has become part of her therapist survival. We have been learning how to kill joy without killing our joy.

The Feminist Killjoy Survival Kit

Feminist work is shared work. Ahmed reminds us of the importance of resourcing ourselves to continue this work, to be able to revive ourselves following another killjoy conversation or intervention. This resourcing, is for Ahmed, survival work, which refers to "not only to living on, but to keep going in the more profound sense of keeping going with one's commitments … Survival can also be about keeping one's hopes alive, holding onto the projects that are projects insofar as they have yet to be realised" (2017, p. 234).[9] The Feminist Therapy Supervision groups are one means to this survival. To sustain ourselves in this work, to enable us to imagine alternatives, Ahmed recommends we build ourselves a Feminist Killjoy Survival Kit—a place to deposit feminist things, people and practices that nourish our feminist work. Therefore, I conclude this chapter with including here some of the contents of my own Feminist Killjoy Survival Kit. These are some of the things, people and practices that support and guide me in showing up to the work being a killjoy clinician (without killing my joy). My own kit will not look like yours but I would love to hear what you would add to your own!

A well-loved item in my Killjoy Survival Kit is Nadine Miller's *Letter to her Psychiatrist*. She wrote this letter on 4 June 1970, and it was published in *The Radical Therapist* (1971), a collection of radical therapy essays edited by Jerome Agel. This collection has long been out of print; however, it has been so important to me that I own two aged, used copies, each with fragile, cracked brown pages—more pages flake and fall from the binding each time I carefully open them. The essays are angry, subversive, urgent, sometimes humorous, but Nadine Miller's letter fills me with joy. Written after a week's vacation away from her daily routine, it is essentially a *fuck you and fuck off* letter to her psychiatrist, a realisation that her sessions with him have coerced her into accepting male supremacist structures and that she is justifiably—not pathologically—hostile towards men that maintain these structures for their own benefit. Men like him. She ends by informing him that she is donating the $28.00 she owes him to the local Women's Center. I love this letter and how it kills joy, unconcealing the patriarchal mechanisms of concealment that her

[9] Ahmed's reflection on hope as survival (and elsewhere contention that hope animates struggle and working through towards otherwise futures (2017)) appears to echo Paula Freire's (2021) and bell hooks' (2003) pedagogies of hope that situate hope as a shared, critical and reflexive praxis that emerges from struggle and enlivens us to work for social justice. Similarly, eco-feminist and Buddhist Joanna Macy argues for an "active hope" that is not a passive waiting to be rescued but a practice of awakening us towards how to act in the world. However, there are also powerful critiques of hope as praxis, for example, whilst Indigenous health scholar, Chelsea Watego's essay "Fuck Hope" (2021) shares a criticism of hope as an act of complacency, she argues for a total rejection of hope as praxis, not as a means to giving up, but in order to take back joy and sovereignty.

psychiatrist disavowed. I love that she is so direct and unnuanced. Sometimes, I don't want to be nuanced either.

Like many, the first feminist I read was bell hooks. Like many, encountering her work has had a lasting and continuous impact upon me. I love that this is not an original statement, but a statement that is shared by so many feminists. Some of her books that live in my Killjoy Survival Kit are *Talking Back*, *Teaching to Transgress* and *All About Love*.[10] If, as hooks tells us, "a culture of domination is anti-love" (2006, p. 246), a liberatory feminist therapeutics must be one that leads with love. hook's revolutionary love ethic offers us a means to consider therapeutic ethics beyond institutional ethical codes and to subvert the cultural norms of 'professionalism' and 'expertise' that have come to dominate the psy-disciplines. Love is a creative disruption. At a recent Association for Women in Psychology conference, I attended a session where a number of academics, educators, activists and psychologists shared their stories of hooks' influence on their work. I have never heard the word 'love' said so much at a conference! I am adding love to my Feminist Killjoy Survival Toolkit. Recently, whilst my supervisor and I were reflecting on over a decade working together, I began to cry. I told her I loved her. *And I love you, Rebecca*, she responded. To some this might seem uncomfortable, a transgression of professionalism, an un-boundaried declaration of love inappropriate to the work of a supervisor-supervisee relationship. Yet, to me, it was a mutual acknowledgment of how we have come to matter to each other, of how we learn with and from each other, of how at times when life has challenged me, her tight hugs and deep listening enable me to continue to show up to my own supervisees, to in turn do the work of loving them. I do not know how to be a feminist without acting in love. I do not understand a feminist therapeutics that is un-loving.

Not dissimilar to a Killjoy Survival Kit, in her Supervision of Solidarity work, Vikki Reynolds (2014) poses a series of questions to help us build our solidarity team. She asks therapists to consider what shoulders us up

[10] There are many feminist writers that are in my Killjoy Survival Kit. But, books that are currently sitting next to me are of course Sara Ahmed's *Feminist Killjoy Handbook* (2023)! Also, Audre Lorde's *Your Silence Will Not Protect You* (2017), Gloria Anzaldúa and AnaLousie Keating's *this bridge we call home* (2002), Mariame Kaba's *We Do This 'Til We Free Us'* (2021), Dean Spade's *Mutual Aid* (2020) and Laura S. Brown's *Subversive Dialogues* (1994).

in the work, be it places, things or people. Essential to her own practice is a person who she can *howl at the moon with*. This is a person who understands the therapeutic work we do, understands the proximity of this work to burning out and can listen to us howl without telling us to leave the work. Usually, when we howl at the moon we are said to be to wasting our energy in doing the impossible. Yet, although it is a myth they howl at the moon, when wolves do howl, they are usually howling *to find each other*, to help a lost wolf find their way home, or calling for help in a hunt. Sometimes in therapeutic practice, we need a person who can hear us howl and help us find our way back. So, I include in my Feminist Killjoy Survival Kit a person I can howl at the moon with. They know who they are.

Lastly, as a practising Zen Buddhist the past ten years, there are many things from my Buddhist practice that I could add; the *zafu* I take my seat upon each day, the precepts I received eight years ago or the eleventh-century poetry of Izumi Shikibu. But here, I am choosing to add *robaishin* or 'grandmother's heart' to my Feminist Killjoy Survival Kit. Grandmother's heart is the old woman in early China serving tea to the passing monks by the side of the road. Always overlooked, each time she trumps their understanding of the dharma, each time killing their joy. Monastic practice was not available to women, so *roibaishin* found otherwise ways to practice Zen, cultivating wise heart and deep insight through pouring tea and serving rice cakes. If you read the stories you will see they were wonderful creative disrupters! Ahmed says that "by naming ourselves as feminist killjoys, we not only commit ourselves to the task of killing joy, we recover a feminist history" (2023, p. 2). Including 'grandmother's heart' is recovering a part of my feminist history; the lineage of killjoy Zen women that have preceded me, that continue to teach me and that paved the way for my practice life.

This piece of writing holds a deep joy and gratitude for the killjoy clinicians in my life—particularly for those of you that continue to show up to each other in the Feminist Therapy Supervision groups—as well as for those I have yet to meet. I look forward to meeting you. And, because my words are indebted to the feminist killjoy life of Sara Ahmed, the closing words must belong to her:

> We can be part of a widening when we refuse to be narrowed … We have to create room if we are to live a feminist life. When we create room, we create room for others (2017, p. 265).

Acknowledgements I thank all the feminist killjoys who have been a part of these 'funny feminist' supervision groups the past two years. Our conversations change me. And I thank my supervisor, Niki D, for your Fierce Love and accompaniment over the past thirteen years of our practice together.

Ethics Approval Informed consent was obtained for the inclusion of the full name of a group member of the discussed Feminist Therapy Supervision Group.

References

Agel, J. (1971). *The Radical Therapist*. Ballantine Books.
Ahmed, S. (2010). Feminist Killjoys (And Other Willful Subjects). *The Scholar and Feminist Online, 3*(8), 1–8. Retrieved March 30, 2023, from https://sfonline.barnard.edu/polyphonic/ahmed_01.htm
Ahmed, S. (2017). *Living A Feminist Life*. Duke University Press.
Ahmed, S. (2023). *The Feminist Killjoy Handbook*. Penguin Random House.
Anzaldúa, G. (1983). La Prieta. In Moraga, C. & Anzaldúa, G. (Ed.), *This Bridge Called My Back: Writings By Radical Women of Color* (pp. 198–209). Kitchen Table: Women of Color Press.
Anzaldúa, G. (2002). Now Let Us Shift—The Path of Conocimiento—Inner Work, Public Acts. In G. Anzaldúa & A. Keating (Eds.), *This Bridge We Call Home: Radical Visions for Transformation* (pp. 540–578). Routledge.
Fisher, M. (2009). *Capitalist Realism: Is There No Alternative?* Zero Books.
Fisher, M. (2021). In M. Coloquhon (Ed.), *Post Capitalist Desire*. Repeater Books.
Freire, P. (2021). *Pedagogy of Hope: Reliving Pedagogy of the Oppressed*. Bloomsbury Academic.
Gay, R. (2022). *Inciting Joy*. Algonquin Books.
Greenslade, R. (2018). Existential Psychotherapy and the Therapeutics of Activism. *European Journal of Psychotherapy & Counselling, 20*(2), 1–15.
Hemmings, C. (2012). Affective Solidarity: Feminist Reflexivity and Political Transformation. *Feminist Theory, 13*(2), 147–161.

Holland, S. (1991). From Private Symptom to Public Action. *Psychology and Feminism, 1*(1), 58–62.

Holland, S. (1992). From Social Abuse to Social Action: A Neighbourhood Psychotherapy and Social Action Project for Women. In J. M. Ussher & P. Nicholson (Eds.), *Gender Issues in Clinical Psychology* (pp. 68–77). Bloomsbury.

hooks, b. (2003). *Teaching Community: A Pedagogy of Hope.* Routledge.

hooks, b. (2006). *Outlaw Culture: Resisting Representations.* Routledge.

hooks, b. (2009). *Belonging: A Culture of Place.* Routledge.

House, R. (2019). London's Women's Therapy Centre (1976–2019)—A Feminist Project Committed to Change. *Morning Star.* Retrieved January 23, 2023, from https://morningstaronline.co.uk/article/f/londons-womens-therapy-centre-1976-2019-feminist-project-committed-change

LaMarre, A., Smoliak, O., Cool, C., Kinavey, H., & Hardt, L. (2019). The Normal, Improving, and Productive Self: Unpacking Neoliberal Governmentality in Therapeutic Interactions. *Journal of Constructivist Psychology, 32*(3), 236–253.

Lorde, A. (1978). Uses of the Erotic: The Erotic as Power. In Lorde, A. (2019) (Ed.), *Sister Outsider*, (pp. 43–49). Penguin Books.

Lorde, A. (2017). *Your Silence Will Not Protect You.* Silver Press.

Olufemi, L. (2020). *Feminism, Interrupted: Disrupting Power.* Pluto Press.

Parker, I. (2014). Psychotherapy under Capitalism: The Production, Circulation and Management of Value and Subjectivity. *Psychotherapy and Politics International, 12*(3), 166–175.

Reynolds, V. (2014). Centering Ethics in Therapeutic Supervision: Fostering Cultures of Critique and Structuring Safety. *The International Journal of Narrative Therapy and Community Work, 1*, 1–13.

Rose, N. (1990). *Governing the Soul: The Shaping of the Private Self.* Routledge.

Rustin, M. (2015). Psychotherapy in a Neoliberal World. *European Journal of Psychotherapy & Counselling, 17*(3), 225–239.

Smail, D. (2005). *Power, Interest and Psychology: Elements of a Social Materialist Understanding of Distress.* PCCS Books.

Smith, Z. (2018). *Feel Free.* Penguin.

Watego, C. (2021). *Another Day in the Colony.* UQP.

Woodward, K. (2015). *Psychosocial Studies: An Introduction.* Routledge.

11

Creative Disruptions With/In Psychoanalysis

Arturo Bandinelli and Iris Aleida Pinzón Arteaga

In a recently published conversation, queer theorist Jack Halberstam and Lacanian psychoanalyst Marie-Helene Brousse (2016) discuss the (missed) encounter between psychoanalysis and queer studies. Halberstam recognises the importance of psychoanalysis as a past interlocutor but adds that, given the changing dynamics of power and desire in our time, we may have reached the limits of its explanatory capabilities. To this observation, Brousse (2016) responds that she understands psychoanalysis less as an explanatory framework than a lived experience akin to an artistic performance, since it is based on "oriented improvisation, and not explanation" (p. 26). This conversation foregrounds two questions. On the one hand, we can interrogate the role of psychoanalytic knowledge when it is employed to discuss social, cultural, and political phenomena. Such a question is central to debates concerning the place of

A. Bandinelli (✉)
Centre for Freudian Analysis and Research (CFAR), London, UK

I. A. P. Arteaga
University at Albany, Albany, NY, USA
e-mail: ipinzonarteaga@albany.edu

G. Kinouani et al. (eds.), *Creative Disruption*, Studies in the Psychosocial,
https://doi.org/10.1007/978-3-031-63661-5_11

psychoanalysis in the emerging field of psychosocial studies (Frosh & Baraitser, 2008; Hook, 2008), as well as the potentials and limitations of taking concepts that emerged as part of a clinical praxis outside this setting (Frosh, 2010; Tupinambá, 2021). On the other hand, following Brousse's intervention, we can interrogate the function attributed to knowledge within psychoanalytic discourse. If the analytic relation has more to do with oriented improvisation than with explanation, on what epistemic principles is it established?

It is necessary to locate this debate against the backdrop of the convoluted relationship between psychoanalysis and queer and trans theories. As others have profusely developed, various strands of psychoanalysis contributed to the ongoing pathologisation of queer and gender non-conforming subjects (Evzonas, 2020; Meyer, 2013; Preciado, 2021). For instance, Herzog's (2017) historical account of the dissemination of psychoanalytic theories in the aftermath of World War II emphasises the permanence and transmutation of homophobic discourses, particularly in Anglo-American schools of psychoanalysis. While Meyer (2013) documents how the promotion of heteronormative discourses and clinical practices brought about immeasurable suffering for LGBTQ+ subjects. This observation echoes a more radical layer of the debate brought forward by Paul Preciado (2021), who argues that a binary epistemology of sex, gender, and sexual difference is "the inherent and immanent condition on which the whole psychoanalytic theory of sexuality is based" (p. 36), rendering psychoanalysis unable to account for the radical diversity of contemporary subjectivities without resorting to pathologisation. Although psychoanalysis needs to take responsibility for its legacy, it is also worth noting that psychoanalytic concepts have been deployed in critical analyses of the heteronormative structures that shape the social world (Farr, 2022; Elliot, 2014; Dean, 2003), and as means to depathologise mental suffering (Gherovici, 2017; Gherovici & Steinkoler, 2022; Watson & Giffney, 2017).

This twofold dimension of psychoanalytic knowledge—both reproductive and potentially subversive of the power structures within which it has emerged—calls for an analysis that addresses it as an *ambivalent object* (Frosh, 2020); i.e., as an object of study, questioning its assumptions and history, and as a tool to open up new avenues of research. A strand of recent literature has mobilised psychoanalysis as such an ambivalent object, exploring its ideological (mis)applications (Tupinambá, 2021), as well as its ties to cis-patriarchal (e.g; Bourlez, 2018; Gherovici & Steinkoler, 2022; Watson & Giffney, 2017) and colonial world orders (e.g., Burnham, 2022; Beshara, 2019; Frosh, 2013; Khanna, 2003). All these publications speak to the two questions previously mentioned, including some valuable reflections on the ways in which psychoanalytic discourse has engaged with other schools of thought. As Tupinambá (2021) notes, psychoanalysis has frequently incorporated insights from other disciplines while at times simultaneously dismissing them as worthy interlocutors, hence taking up the position of "the judge of the validity" of other fields of knowledge (p. 26). This has in turn rendered psychoanalysis far too impermeable to internal and external critique, leading to what may be defined as psychoanalytic ideologies. In light of this symptomatic relationship to other areas of knowledge, it is worth asking whether this phenomenon is caused by inbuilt epistemic principles or whether the core of the issue lies somewhere else.

Intervening at this critical juncture, this chapter intends to clarify whether the dimension of knowledge brought to the fore by the psychoanalytic experience may inform an epistemic stance that remains open to disruptions, qualifying psychoanalysis as "a procedure for not understanding" (Hook, 2008, p. 401). To approach this analytical task, we venture outside psychoanalytic literature, taking Halberstam (2011) as a privileged interlocutor. This decision is informed by three factors. Firstly, the desire to 'extend' the dialogue with Brousse beyond its actual form. Secondly, the relevance of Halberstam's (2011) work in theorising the emergence and circulation of "knowledge from below" (p. 10), a project that entails the commitment to modes of knowing that are normally excluded from academic settings. Thirdly, the conviction that Halberstam's remarks on the disruptive potentials of *forgetfulness* and *stupidity* are especially well suited to developing a nuanced consideration of psychoanalytic epistemology, highlighting points of affinity and difference that are often overlooked when psychoanalysis is popularised. It is important to clarify that our goal is not to produce a psychoanalytic critique of Halberstam's work, but to establish a dialogue in which conceptual tensions can be put to work. Our aim is twofold: to explore how psychoanalytic epistemology may be helpful in thinking creative disruptions to established systems of knowledge, *and* to trace the limits of its conceptual reach.

The first section revisits the queer praxis of radical forgetting. We contend that, while psychoanalysis does not conceive of forgetting without remainders, it may still point to the limits of remembrance. The second section dwells on the epistemic status of the encounter with a knowledge that the subject doesn't know she knows. It explores how the experience called forth by the unconscious puts into question established ways of knowing and commonsensical understandings of truth, forging epistemic principles that might contribute to an engagement with a negative dimension of knowledge. In a final reflection, we suggest that while these epistemic principles hold subversive potential, they are limited tools that need to be supplemented with ethical, aesthetical, and political considerations.

On Remembering to Forget

In the *Queer Art of Failure*, Halberstam (2011) refers to forgetfulness as a subversive way of "inhabiting structures of knowledge" (p. 11) insofar as it points to the limits of dominant modalities of knowing, focused on mastery and explanation. In line with this approach, he casts doubt on *memorialisation* because it tends to produce homogeneous narratives by obliterating contradiction and leaving no room for disruption. Against the backdrop of this thesis, Halberstam (2011) presents two modalities of forgetfulness. On the one hand, forgetting is structural to memory work: to remember something implies retaining certain aspects of what happened and letting go of others. On the other hand, forgetting can be seen as a *praxis* that seeks to interrupt modes of transmission that contribute to the consolidation of "ideas, family lines, and normativity itself" (p. 144). Drawing on Sadyia Hartman's (2008) work, Halberstam synthesises this approach under the phrase *losing one's mother*. In contrast to remembrance, defined as a way to reinstate familiar narratives, lineages, and modes of being, *losing one's mother* designates simultaneously a survival strategy derived from a violent past and "a feminist politics that issues not from a doing but from an undoing" (2011, p. 124). In this way, forgetfulness becomes a condition of possibility for subaltern knowledge to emerge, through a necessary "release from the weight of the past and the menace of the future" (Halberstam, 2011, p. 83).

As part of this elaboration, Halberstam (2011) refers to Freud's idea that the hysteric, the psychoanalytic subject par-excellence, is someone "who suffers from reminiscences" (p. 83). Insofar as the repression of unacceptable material leads to the formation of a symptom, Halberstam defines the hysteric as an "unsuccessful repressor" (ibid). In contrast to this, he is interested in "characters who are capable of radical forgetting, total forgetting, wilful forgetting" (ibid.). It is on these modalities of forgetting that the project of *losing one's mother* is premised.

In establishing a dialogue between Halberstam's work and psychoanalysis, one could at this point raise the following question: does the psychoanalytic experience testifies to such radical, total and wilful erasures of memory? In other words, can the subject of psychoanalysis forget without remainders? Paradigmatically, the psychoanalytic vocabulary comprises three modalities of defence employing negation; namely: repression, disavowal, and foreclosure (Fink, 2014a). In a schematic fashion, one could say that repression is more akin to a process of disguise or displacement than erasure; disavowal implies a splitting through which the subject acts "as if" something was not there; foreclosure constitutes a more radical form of negation whereby the material is excluded from the symbolic altogether. Even in this latter modality, however, the subject does not 'forget' without remainders as the foreclosed material returns with devastating force in the Real of the body (Lacan, 1997). Does this mean that, within the remit of psychoanalytic theory, the best we can hope for is relative rather than radical change, adaptation rather than separation, and integration rather than disruption? In a nutshell, are we doomed to never *lose our mothers?*

In what follows, we aim to show that, even though the psychoanalytic approach to memory does not conceive of forgetting without remainders, it may still contribute to the broader project of *losing one's mother*. Yet, in order to move from the *suffering of reminiscence* to the *praxis of forgetting*, a further iteration is required; this 'detour' is premised on the hypothesis that behind the subject's (conscious) *will to forget* lies an (unconscious) *desire to repeat.* This relates to Halberstam's point regarding the link between repression and symptom formation: "memory can be painful, for it actively and passively keeps alive the experiences of events that one may do better to blow out" (p. 83). However, we would resist the definition of the hysteric as an unsuccessful repressor. If that were the case, one could assume that by bolstering repression, her suffering would be relieved, something that is contradicted by clinical experience. On the contrary, the problem is precisely that the hysteric is a 'successful repressor,' which is another way of saying that repression and the return of the repressed are two sides of the same coin. This is why psychoanalysis does not encourage more radical modes of repression, but facilitates a form of memory-work aimed at loosening it.

Now, this might at first resonate with a prevailing conception of the analytic scene where the analyst demands the analysand to *speak about her mother*, reconstructing her personal history in an almost archivist quest on the origin of her being. Through a gain in knowledge enabled by a practice of remembrance, the unconscious is 'conquered' and a form of mastery reinstated. A healthier and strengthened ego, reinvigorated by a newly acquired knowledge, would then make repression redundant. We will elaborate on the relationship between knowledge and truth in psychoanalysis in more detail in the next section. For now, let us note that counter to this understanding of analytic practice, Lacan (2002) claims that what is at stake in an analysis is not the invitation to *gnothi seauton*, to 'know yourself', but rather to experience the limits of this attempt. The goal is not to unearth a missing signifier, even though this is certainly part of the process, but coming to terms with the fact that no signifier or narrative can provide the subject with a fixed and cohesive identity. Freud is certainly more ambivalent than Lacan on this matter. Although references to mastery and conquest can surely be found in Freud's writing, so are a number of radical insights, including the idea that reconstruction does not lead to integration, but precisely to its failure.

Already in his early paper on *Screen memories*, Freud (1899/1962) reflects upon the fact that, despite the importance attributed to childhood experiences in the formation of the ego, if we try to recover these past impressions, the result is "isolated recollections which are often of dubious or enigmatic importance" (p. 303). Throughout the text, he engages in the analysis of a scene from his childhood in which he appears as a three-year-old. Despite the multiplicity of actors and actions described, Freud notes that the accent is put on almost trivial details: the yellow colour of dandelions, the taste of a piece of bread; features that seem "exaggerated in an almost hallucinatory fashion" (p. 312). Why is it that the emphasis is put on these elements? Freud suspects that the scene acts as a *screen*, its value as a memory is not related to its content per se, but "to the relation existing between that content and some other, that has been suppressed" (p. 320). Interestingly, the analysis of the recollection takes off after he introduces the question of the conditions under which it initially emerged. He recalls that the scene first came to him during his teenage years, in turn producing a chain of associations between the childhood memory and his first amatory experiences as a teenager.

Again, this approach might initially resemble the archivist deployment of memory criticised by Halberstam (2011), an attempt to "make connections between bodies, lives, scattered experiences, sexual practices, and social contexts that relentlessly pull apart from each other" (p. 370). However, Freud's emphasis is on the fact that we do not have memories *from* our childhood, but memories *relating to* our childhood, (re)formed subsequently and coloured with the expectations, preoccupations, and fears of later times. A different mode of temporality is at play here: not *restoration* of the past, uncovering its force in the shaping of present experiences, but deferred action or *retroaction*, in which "future events control the meaning of past ones" (Jones, 2004 p. 1). This is a noteworthy contribution of the Freudian approach to memory, in which to remember is closer to the mechanism of dreams than to the accurate reproduction of a factual reality. A memory is a *compromise formation*, constructed through the mechanisms of displacement and condensation. In this sense, as Sprengnether (2012) notes, for Freud memory is "a kind of trickster, a canny yet unreliable narrator, a creator rather than a transcriber of reality" (p. 322). Drawing on this, Bion (2014) writes that memory is an always "misleading record of facts" (p. 15) infused with the subject's own desires and expectations, hence signalling the impossibility of accessing a linear past. A similar reading features in Freud's study on the forgetting of proper names, in which, in line with Halberstam's (2011) proposal of an epistemology of failure, forgetting does not belong to the realm of error, but constitutes a different way of inhabiting knowledge.

In *The Psychopathology of Everyday Life*, Freud (1901/1968) analyses the occasions in which words that are familiar to us fail to appear upon our attempt to remember them. Once again, a personal episode serves as the main illustration of his theoretical analysis. In a conversation with a travelling companion, he tries to recall the name of *Signorelli*, a famous painter. Instead, two other names came to him: *Botticelli* and *Boltraffio*. Why is that so? Freud does not turn to the familiarity with the name, as the forgotten one was even more familiar than its replacements. Instead, he turns to the preceding topic he was discussing and, through a chain of associations, connects his involuntary forgetting of *Signorelli* with a failed attempt to forget something else, a tragic event, the recent suicide of a patient. As we can see, the unity of the subject is put into question in this failure to forget, in which one ends up forgetting something else, precisely something that one wanted to recall.

Despite their differences, Freud (1901/1968) underscores that these two modalities of memory—childhood recollections and the forgetting of proper names—produce in the subject "an intellectual feeling of the intervention of a disturbance" (p. 45), an encounter with an internal limit that unsettles the ego's supposed mastery. These points of subjective division provide us with moments of inversion in which "thought encounters itself as something Other, runs up against itself, or blocks its own progress" (Nobus & Quinn, 2005, p. 109). This aspect seems particularly significant for an epistemology of unbecoming: on the one hand, it resonates with Halberstam's invitation to "privilege the naïve or nonsensical" (Halberstam p. 12), losing one's expected road to find something different in this course of action; on the other, it alerts us to the ambivalences that pertain to wilful forgetting, since the (conscious) intention to forget might return as an (unconscious) injunction to remember, and vice versa.

Until now, we have discussed modalities of memory that, through the experience of fragmentation, counter identity and mastery. Despite this malleability of memory, it is important to keep in mind that, contrary to certain readings of identity as utterly fractured, in everyday life selves become lodged and routinized (Plummer, 2003). And as Halberstam

(2011) remarks, memory plays an important part in these processes of homogenisation and stabilisation. To further explore the normative dimension of memory, it is illustrative to turn to another modality of remembrance that has been widely studied from a psychoanalytic perspective, that of repetition.

More than a decade after his previous elaborations on memory, Freud (1914/1964) argues that, in some cases, instead of the memory comes the act: the subject reproduces what he has forgotten, "not as a memory but as an action; he *repeats it*, without, of course knowing that he is repeating it" (p. 150). The apparent erasure of traces from the past is possible only through the repetition of an act that unconsciously reinstates what seems forgotten. This remark has been extensively stressed in the literature on trauma: for those who have gone through an experience that occurs too abruptly or violently to be grasped by consciousness, the painful event reappears in nightmares and flashbacks, haunting the subject due to a repeated failure of symbolic inscription (Caruth, 2010; Felman & Laub, 1991). Outside of this field of inquiry, Butler's (2011) performative theory of gender also engages with the notion of repetition as a particular form of memory, "gender is the repeated stylization of the body, a set of repeated acts within a highly rigid regulatory frame" (p. 25) that solidify over time, giving rise to a sense of identity through the creation of the very essence that is supposedly being embodied. At the same time, if gender norms are anxiously repeated as an "effort to install and augment their jurisdiction" (p. 237), it is because they are funded on the impossibility of fully representing what it means to be a 'man' or a 'woman'.

Now, it is important to keep in mind that, as Lacan (1998) develops in his eleventh seminar, *repetition* is not the same as *reproduction,* it does not refer to an unambiguous replication of patterns or actions. This approach would result in a form of determinism in which certain behaviours can be identified and traced back to an ideal version of the past, whereas the temporal *retroaction* at play in remembrance would be dismissed. But if repetition is not reproduction, how can it be conceptualised? In the same seminar, Lacan (1998) draws on Aristotelian vocabulary to present two modalities of repetition: the *automaton* and the *tyche*.

The *automaton* is the dimension related to the signifier and its structuring, it refers to "the coming-back, the insistence of the signs" (p. 52), a repetition that allows for the equation of otherwise heterogeneous things. After all, it is the signifier that permits the emergence of what we identify as a *series* through the deployment of substitution or "the ability to associate a term or idea with other terms or ideas, draw relations among them, and transfer affect from one to another" (Fink, 1995, p. 224). Curiously, a good illustration of this point can be found in the literary universe of Borges (1999), whose character of Funes, a young man incapable of forgetting even the smallest of details, is bothered by the fact that "the dog of three-fourteen in the afternoon, seen in profile, should be indicated by the same noun as the dog of three-fifteen, seen frontally" (p. 72). Linking experiences and objects that are phenomenologically distinct, the *automaton* amounts to a *relational* form of repetition; but this also means that, as Funes points out, all representation is essentially founded on a *mistake: some-thing* gets inevitably lost when objects are equated in this way. For the *automaton* to operate smoothly, forgetting is thus a necessary condition. As a result, Funes is incapable of abstraction and generalisation, and yet also endlessly amused: "his own face in the mirror, his own hands, surprised him every time he saw them" (Borges, 1999, p. 153).

This leads us to the second modality of repetition, the *tyche,* which Lacan relates to the dimension of chance and surprise. Interestingly, for Lacan the effect of shock or surprise, which in the most extreme cases can produce traumatic consequences, is not merely caused by the encounter with the unknown, but by the contingent (re)appearance of the impossibility that resides at the heart of all representation. As the return of *a failure,* the *tyche* signals that beneath the relational dimension of the *automaton*, what is repeated is precisely the *impossibility of repetition*: tracing back the various iterations of the signifier, we do not find an original signified but lack thereof. This is why Lacan (1998) remarks that a "missed encounter" with the Real is what causes the automaton in the first place (p. 54). To continue our reading of Borges' story, we could say that what amuses Funes in the most ordinary of repetitions, such as the daily sight of his own hands and face, is that they remind him again and again that representation always misses the mark, hence making everything 'stand out'. In order to operate within discourse, we are required to repress that this is the case; and yet, sometimes we also *forget to forget,* and that is when repetition takes us by surprise, striking us in all its oddity. Let us point out that there is a significant difference between *remembering everything*, as in Funes' case, and *forgetting to forget*: whilst the former is a totalising and immobilising state, the latter is open to dialectical movement.

If we take note of this logic, it is also easier to grasp Lacan's (1998) idea that "repetition demands the new. It is turned towards the ludic, which finds its dimension in this new" (p. 61). Going back to Butler's performative theory of gender, we could say that what returns in the heterogeneity of gendered acts and gestures is the contingent nature of gender itself. Every iteration both repeats *and* betrays the previous one, hence Butler's emphasis on un-loyal and parodistic performances as capable of exposing the absence of the essence that is supposedly being imitated, that is, the absence of an original. Similarly, memory work in psychoanalysis is not aimed at plastering over gaps and inconsistencies of the patient's speech through the recovery of past experiences, but at reminding them that every attempt to identify the origin of their problems is always a failed one and, therefore, open to refashioning and transformation.

In this respect, the 'weight of the past' can be worked through precisely by showing the subject that what is missing—"the chapter of my history that is marked by a blank or occupied by a lie" (Lacan, 2007, p. 215)—is both what they want to forget and what they cannot but repeat. Hence, as Braunstein (2008) puts it, the goal of an analysis is not to gain something but to let go of something, it is not remembrance but forgetfulness. If one is required to undergo an analysis in order to become a psychoanalyst, it is precisely to ensure that they have developed what Bion (2014) perceptively defines as a "watchful avoidance of memory" (p. 15). This is because the psychoanalytic experience bears testimony to the fact that, in order for the subject to forget what *they think they know*, they should first engage with a corpus of knowledge that resides in the unconscious: a knowledge that *they do not know they know*. This elicits a number of questions: how can we conceptualise this particular type of knowledge? What is its epistemic stance? And why may it be useful outside a clinical setting?

Knowledge and Stupidity

Discussing the dialectic between remembrance, forgetfulness, and repetition led us to questioning the epistemic status of unconscious knowledge. From the point of view of epistemology, the disruption brought about by the Freudian discovery may be summarised as follows: (a) there exists "some" knowledge in the unconscious; (b) unconscious knowledge is produced and organised following a particular logic; and (c) the unconscious is therefore amenable to rational and systematic investigation. Drawing on this, Lacan (1999) insisted that the unconscious should not be conceived as a reservoir of unsymbolised libidinal energy, irrational impulses, or inaccessible memories, but rather as a "knowledge that is not known" (p. 96). The hypothesis of the unconscious as a logical corpus also grounds Freud's (and initially Lacan's) hope that psychoanalysis could acquire "proper" scientific status (Milner, 2020; Glynos & Stavrakakis, 2018). And yet, Freud is well aware of the contradictions that this position implies. As early as 1895, in a passage that has since become a topical point of reference, he states:

> [It]still strikes me as strange that the case histories I write should read like short stories and that [...] they lack the serious stamp of science. I must console myself with the reflection that the nature of the subject is evidently responsible for this, rather than any preference of my own. (Freud, 1955/1893, p. 160)

Freud's own subjective division is at stake here, manifesting as a conflict between the ideal of the rigorous scientist and his interest in a subject that seems to undermine this very ideal. We could perhaps state that if Freud believes that the unconscious is open to scientific endeavour, through this very endeavour a crack is produced within the discourse of science.

Now, let us clarify that we do not intend to add yet another contribution to the question as to whether psychoanalysis should be considered a 'proper' science, something that has been amply discussed and to which we don't feel we would add anything new (see for instance, Lacan, 2007; Milner, 2020; Glynos & Stavrakakis, 2018). Our focus is rather on the ways in which the hypothesis of the unconscious may disrupt established systems of knowledge, including the modern episteme in which Freud was embedded. To move further along this path, let us address an objection that could be raised at this point: why should we even consider psychoanalysis as bringing to the fore a new dimension of knowledge? After all, surely the psychoanalytic experience is not the only one that is premised on an engagement with a knowledge that is not known. Leaving on the side religion and mysticism, one could for instance point out that Socrates' maieutics is premised on an engagement with *unknown knowledge*. What is more, the latter also emerges from a dialogical exchange. The parallel between psychoanalysis and maieutics has been drawn by a number of authors, including some prominent psychoanalytic theorists. Sergio Benvenuto (1991) argues that "psychoanalysis is the last modernist offspring of maieutics'" insofar as it "elicits its reflexive, hermeneutic mirror (its pupil) in the re-cognition of one's own truth through the dialectic intervention of the analyst" (p. 81). In a similar fashion, Bernard Burgoyne (2001) sheds light on how Grote's work on Socrates' mode of questioning was very influential to the young Freud. As for Lacan (2017), he famously described Socrates as a psychoanalyst *ante-litteram*. And yet, we would suggest there are at least two key differences between psychoanalysis and maieutics, differences that are helpful to illustrate the unique dimension of knowledge brought to the fore by the psychoanalytic experience.

The first difference concerns the relationship between *unknown knowledge* and the enunciative structure of the dialogue. As Nobus and Quinn (2005) point out, even though Socrates's objective is to prove that his interlocutor, paradigmatically the slave, is endowed with a knowledge they know nothing about, the latter is essentially relegated to the position of confirming Socrates' hypothesis and answering his rhetorical questions. It is Socrates who does most of the talking, whilst his interlocutor is mostly silent. Conversely, the analytic experience inverts the terms: it is the analysand who is tasked with doing the speaking whilst the analyst keeps their mouth mostly shut.

Importantly, the analyst's aim should not be to confirm their prior knowledge, to affirm their mastery over the analysand, but as previously mentioned, to forget about it. As Bion (2014) brilliantly put it, for an analyst "the only point of importance in the session is the unknown," everything that the analyst believes to know about the patient is either "false or irrelevant" (p. 15). In like manner, Halberstam (2011) argues that forms of knowing which "lie at the very edge of memory" (p. 54), including the ephemeral and elusive, shouldn't be dismissed as 'loopy stupidity', but followed through, as they may open up to new modalities of knowing and relating.

In the case of psychoanalysis, the commitment to the encounter with the unknown goes as far as to say that if the material emerging in the session merely confirms the analyst's pre-existing knowledge, then there is a good chance that it amounts to nothing more than a reactive formation, a resistance to the analytic process. A resistance that Lacan (1997) innovatively situates on the side of the analyst rather than the analyst. Excessive conformity between the analysand's discourse and the analyst's expectations may be taken as a sign that the analyst is failing to cultivate a *watchful avoidance of memory*. Drawing on the point we made previously, we could say that if the analyst is unable to forget what they think they know—i.e., to *lose their mother*—this may be interpreted as a modality of repetition calling for a work of memory, which the analyst may be able to do in supervision or going back to the couch. In a similar fashion, the social researcher using a psychoanalytic framework is invited to take distance from any attempt to simply apply concepts or categories that provide an explanation about what the interviewee really felt or what the text ultimately means. As Parker (2005) proposes, instead of focusing on what is 'known' or in the illusion of agreement, it is more productive to draw attention to "the deadlock of perspective" (p. 167), points of *impasse* in which one does not understand, and the subject or the text appear as radically Other. Yet, this requires a reflexive engagement from the researcher, a praxis that entails also a work of memory, not as the reconstruction of a linear narrative, but as the attempt to map out how the theoretical, institutional, and political positions one has taken reshape the standpoint assumed in relation to the material (Parker, 2004).

Let us now move to the second point of divergence between psychoanalysis and maieutics, which concerns the applicability of the knowledge produced. A crucial tenet of maieutics is that the *unknown knowledge* elicited in the dialogue can be readily put to 'good use', not only by the subject who produces it, but by the whole of society. However, it is hard to see how unconscious knowledge, in all its odd and enigmatic presentations, may be easily incorporated within the given socio-symbolic coordinates from which it has emerged. As Nobus and Quinn (2005) write, unconscious formations are rather "headless pieces of knowledge, disruptive eruptions of meaninglessness against the comfortable backdrop of established reason" (p. 4). Put otherwise, unconscious knowledge appears less as 'good' knowledge than as 'waste' knowledge.

Reflecting on this in *Lituraterre*, a neologism condensing the signifiers letter, litter and littoral, Lacan (2013) defines the psychoanalytic domain as concerning *knowledge-in-failure.* He then states that *knowledge-in-failure* must be differentiated from failures of knowledge. Whilst the latter would imply an inadequate rendering or application of knowledge, the former relates to the idea that all knowledge is in a state of failure, the unconscious being the domain of this failed state. This may be taken to mean that, even though unconscious formations are not as such extra-discursive, they index a structural inconsistency within the fabric of discourse, articulating a split between the established system of reason (constructive, relational) and a 'stupid' bit of knowledge (disruptive, non-relational) that pushes towards articulation. In this regard, the unconscious is not a *constructive* but a *disruptive* corpus of knowledge, meaning that the *unknown known* depletes rather than completes the domain of the *known known.*

But how can this experience of depletion be engaged with in academic research? A good illustration is provided by Margarita Palacio's (2009) work on anticommunism in Chile, which highlights how the psychoanalytic approach to the subject stays clear of over-emphasising agency or determination, defining the unconscious as "a 'radical other' which cannot be retrieved through any process of communication" (p. 19). This notion is then put to work to problematize strategic understandings of violence, pointing to the fact that not only rationality motivates it. Such an *unknown known* reveals an *excess* in violent manifestations that challenges attempts to reduce it to specific and readily identified aims. In line with what we have been discussing so far, this bit of knowledge is *disruptive* in the sense that it produces more questions than answers, situating psychoanalytic research on the side of deciphering, and yet *against understanding* (Hook, 2008; Fink, 2014b).

So far, we have engaged with the difference between psychoanalysis and maieutics to qualify in more detail the epistemic status of the unconscious, introducing the idea that unconscious knowledge may well appear as a 'stupid bit of knowledge', ready to be discarded rather than put to good use. Whilst most disciplines aim to eradicate stupidity from their ranks, Lacan (1999) states that psychoanalysis "hang[s] together (*se tient*) by basing itself on the dimension of stupidity" (p. 12). When something 'stupid' or 'nonsensical' is reported in a session, the analyst does not interpret it as an absence of knowledge or error of application, but as a "a particular kind of knowledge that exists only in, and *as*, the very form of the unconscious, its work and its formations" (Zupančič, 2017, p. 16). This does not mean that psychoanalysis elevates stupidity to the status of an ideal to be aspired to, but rather that the psychoanalytic experience "allows someone to stay stupid," insofar as it invites both analysand and analyst (and potentially the psychoanalytic researcher too) "to experience and acknowledge the non-relational character of stupidity again and again" (Nobus & Quinn, 2005, p. 5).

There are interesting resonances between the Lacanian conception of stupidity and Halberstam's (2011) idea that stupidity does not simply refer to "a lack of knowledge but to the limits of certain forms of knowing and certain ways of inhabiting structures of knowing" (p. 12). Halberstam focuses on the ways in which stupidity may offer us a compass to read the social, its power dynamics and injustices—for instance, by reflecting on the different ways in which stupidity is gendered or racialised. Drawing on Avita Ronell's (2003) major work on the topic, Halberstam's (2011) reading of different cultural products through the lens of stupidity traces "a map of male power" (p. 58) that is aimed at unlocking "other ways of knowing" (p. 66). Similarly to the psychoanalyst, Halberstam does not reduce stupidity to a failure of knowledge, but sees it as revelatory of how discourse shapes the subject. However, whilst Halberstam is interested in how stupidity is normalised, integrated, or dismissed, the psychoanalytic lens sets its focus on what remains radically *non-relational* in stupidity, in other words, on what stupidity repeats beyond the *automaton*.

To flesh this out further, let us go back to the consulting room, where an analysand might make a slip, report on a bungled action, or speak about the suffering derived from a situation they cannot stop repeating. In some instances, these formations may be perceived by the subject as painful or reactionary; in others as nonsensical or surprising; in any case, they reveal a failure of mastery on their part; such a failure might make them feel stupid. As a result, the analysand (or perhaps the analysand's partner or parents) may complain that 'they should know better.' Through a dialectical inversion, the analyst may then invite the analysand to consider the possibility that these failures hold the key to a different dimension of knowledge: the problem is not that they should know better, but that *there is something they do not know they know*. In other words, stupidity is interpreted as the index of a split that implicates the analysand qua subject. The split is between what the analysand (thinks they) know and what presents itself as an enigmatic (and often unpleasant) truth. This is a truth that the subject cannot master via conscious knowledge, and yet that has something to do with their very being.

As we can see, the status of truth in psychoanalysis is somewhat odd. Truth is not to be situated in some archaic origin nor in a mystical *beyond of discourse*. And yet, neither is truth the end product of a certain discursive regime. Instead, truth emerges precisely in the place where knowledge encounters a limit point - i.e. as *knowledge-in-failure*. As subjective creations made of signifiers, unconscious formations are the positive articulation of this limit. In this respect, they function both as cover ups *and* access points to a *non-relation* in the Other. This means that even if the unconscious is not intrinsically 'progressive' (and surely not politically correct), it nonetheless bears the potential to expose the structural incompleteness of every discursive formation, revealing its inability to 'master' the truth.

From this perspective, if established systems of knowledge aim at control over truth, it is precisely because truth is structurally missing from them. Lacan (2007) remarks that the closure of knowledge upon truth necessitates the supposition of a meta-linguistic point or Other of the Other from which the truthfulness of knowledge is guaranteed (and the subjective 'stain' erased). He relates this meta-position to the benevolent God theorised by Descartes, someone who could guarantee that reason—'good knowledge'—leads thinking towards truth. However, psychoanalysis observes that this meta-linguistic guarantor, this all-knowing subject, is in fact only ever supposed, and it is supposed precisely because it is nowhere to be found. In the place where the Other of the Other is supposed, we find a hole instead. As Lacan (1998) states, if "in the unconscious there is a corpus of knowledge (un savoir), [this] must in no way be conceived as knowledge to be completed, to be closed" (p. 134). To complete the unconscious, plugging the gap around which its formations coalesce, would imply a closure of the rift between knowledge and truth, a rift that psychoanalysis is rather invested in putting to work. An analysis is directed towards the establishment of a different relation to the incompleteness of knowledge, a relation that is singular to each subject. The end of analysis is therefore less about reaching an "ideal point" (sexual maturity, adaptation, self-understanding, dissolution of symptoms, etc.) than about the institution of an open-ended process beyond it.

Contextually, if diagnostic categories are certainly of use in clinical settings, it is only insofar as they provide a compass for the direction of the treatment, and *not* of the patient; they should not operate as ways to categorise the analysand against some supposed standard or norm; their function is not to provide explanation but to orient questioning. A crucial implication of this line of argument is that pathologising analysands whose identities or behaviours are considered aberrant within a set of historically situated cultural norms contravenes psychoanalysis' own principles. And yet, as we have mentioned earlier, pathologisation has not been infrequent in the history of psychoanalysis. If there is no doubt that great damage has been caused to the pathologised subjects and groups, our investigation suggests that this has deleterious effects on psychoanalysis as well, effectively undermining its own *raison d'etre*.

Translating this epistemic stance outside the clinic, we would contend that the deployment of psychoanalytic knowledge should not take as its final aim providing a key to *understanding* what would otherwise seem paradoxical or counter-intuitive. That does not equal saying that explanatory hypotheses may not constitute an important part of the process, but that they should not be its end. Instead, the finality of one's research would be to isolate points of impossibility, revealing how holes in discourse are covered up, narratives straightened, impasses displaced, and responsibilities obfuscated. In a nutshell, the psychoanalytically oriented researcher may therefore be able to bring about creative disruptions less by providing better explanations than by formulating better questions.

Let us conclude with a further remark. We have laid out what we believe to be the radical potentials of psychoanalysis' epistemic stance, its ability to disrupt established systems of knowledge and power. However, it is equally important to recognise that no epistemology can be taken as a guarantee against ideological (mis)applications, but at best as a partial antidote. In fact, overvaluation of one's epistemology may well function as a means to obfuscate other points of impasse, for instance, relating to processes of institutionalisation. In this respect, welcoming internal and external critique and openness to conceptual disruption are a key part of the psychoanalytic project. A project based on questioning, undoing and depleting, rather than answering, doing and completing. *Working with incomplete knowledge to create knowledge about incompleteness*, which, it seems to us, is also a good working definition of the unconscious.

Conclusion

In dialogue with Halberstam's *Queer Art of Failure*, we investigated how forgetfulness and stupidity may disrupt certain ways of knowing and being in the world. From a psychoanalytic standpoint, we contended that the disruption may be followed through to the end by mobilising forgetfulness as a motor for memory-work, and stupidity as a motor for truth. In this regard, we claimed that memory-work in analysis is not aimed at completing knowledge about one's past, but at *losing one's mother*—(i.e. being able to truly forget), and that an engagement with unconscious knowledge is not aimed at mastering truth, but at *staying stupid* (i.e. experiencing truth as *knowledge-in-failure*).

In line with our approach, this investigation surely elicits more questions than it answers. We would therefore like to conclude with two considerations that make explicit the limitations of this chapter, in turn providing some ideas for further research. We have suggested that unconscious knowledge is not readily applicable, and that the goal of an analysis is not a gain in knowledge but a shift in relation to knowledge. However, this does not imply that nothing else can be done with the unconscious besides this epistemic re-orientation. When speaking of the end of an analysis, understood both as its aim and termination, Lacan (2018) noted how a singular invention or creation is called upon precisely to transform unconscious knowledge into a know-how (savoir-fare). In this respect, the unconscious is perhaps less a creative disruption (even though creativity is certainly not missing from it), than a disruption that calls for creation. As to the status of the creation that follows, this is where psychoanalytic epistemology ends, understood this time as the encounter with an internal limit, and where a reflection on the relationship between ethics and aesthetics begins.

Another implication of our contribution is that psychoanalytic discourse cannot take as its final aim producing better understandings, whether of psychic or social phenomena, unless it is prepared to contravene its own epistemology. The role of theory is less to elucidate the world than to isolate the points where explanations and concepts fail, including psychoanalytic ones; constructions and interpretations are surely useful, but only insofar as they enable a form of questioning. Yet, psychoanalysis has sometimes operated as a normative framework, adopting a pathologising stance on colonised, gender non-conforming and homosexual subjects. The current investigation suggests that psychoanalytic epistemology is not at the origin of this phenomenon. Our sense is that further research is required with respect to the ways in which psychoanalysis has become institutionalised, and its theories and practices sedimented. In this regard, psychoanalysis may benefit from engaging with queer theorists' efforts to critically reflect on the difficulties raised by embracing certain epistemic principles, such as the suspicion towards categorisation. Difficulties that take place, not only in the research field, but also in more practical aspects such as accessing funding or getting approval from ethics committees to carry out research projects (Pascoe, 2018). Evidently, this calls into question the domain of politics, exploring how a particular set of material relations is instated and reinstated, despite or even at the expense of one's epistemic principles. Let us therefore conclude with a question: when establishing itself institutionally and thinking itself politically, has psychoanalysis been prepared to *lose its mother* (and 'father') and *stay stupid*?

References

Benvenuto, S. (1991). Psychoanalysis and Hermeneutics. *Differentia: Review of Italian Thought, 5*, 12.

Beshara, R. K. (2019). *Decolonial Psychoanalysis*. Routledge. https://doi.org/10.4324/9780429056611

Bion, W. (2014). Notes on Memory and Desire. In *Melanie Klein Today: Developments in Theory and Practice. Vol. 2, Mainly Practice*. Routledge.

Borges, J. L. (1999). *Collected Fictions* (A. Hurley, Trans.). Penguin Books.

Bourlez, F. (2018). *Queer psychanalyse: Clinique mineure et déconstructions du genre*. Hermann.

Braunstein, N. A. (2008). *La memoria, la inventora*. Siglo XXI.

Burgoyne, B. (2001). Freud's Direction. *Psychological Inquiry [Online], 12*(3), 154–156. Retrieved from https://www.jstor.org/stable/1449395

Burnham, C. (2022). Can We Decolonize Lacan? In C. Varderwees & K. Hennessy (Eds.), *Psychoanalysis, Politics, Oppression and Resistance*. Routledge.

Butler, J. (2011). *Gender Trouble: Feminism and the Subversion of Identity*. Routledge.

Caruth, C. (2010). *Unclaimed Experience: Trauma, Narrative and History*. JHU Press.

Dean, T. (2003). Lacan and Queer Theory. In J.-M. Rabaté (Ed.), *The Cambridge Companion to Lacan* (pp. 238–252). Cambridge University Press. https://doi.org/10.1017/CCOL0521807441.014

Elliot, P. (2014). Psychoanalysis. *TSQ: Transgender Studies Quarterly, 1*(1–2), 165–168. https://doi.org/10.1215/23289252-2399920

Evzonas, N. (2020). Psychoanalytic Transphobia or a Generalized Gender Trauma. *Research in Psychoanalysis, 30*(2), 103–112.

Farr, P. (2022). The Psychoanalyst and the "Transsexual": Transgender Identities as Personal-Political Subjectivities. *Psychoanalytic Social Work, 29*(2), 193–216. https://doi.org/10.1080/15228878.2022.2124525

Felman, S., & Laub, D. (1991). *Testimony: Crises of Witnessing in Literature, Psychoanalysis and History*. Routledge.

Fink, B. (1995). The Real Cause of Repetition. In R. Feldstein, M. Jaanus, & B. Fink (Eds.), *Reading Seminar XI: Lacan's Four Fundamental Concepts of Psychoanalysis: The Paris Seminars in English* (pp. 223–230). SUNY Press.

Fink, B. (2014a). *Against Understanding* (Vol. 1). Routledge.

Fink, B. (2014b). *Against Understanding* (Vol. 2). Routledge.

Freud, S. (1955). *The Standard Edition of the Complete Psychological Works of Sigmund Freud/Vol. II (1893–1895), Studies on Hysteria/by Josef Breuer and Sigmund Freud*. Vintage.

Freud, S. (1962). Screen Memories. In *The Standard Edition of the Complete Psychological Works of Sigmund Freud: (1893–1899) Early Psycho-analytic Publications* (pp. 299–322). Hogarth Press.

Freud, S. (1964). Remembering, Repeating, and Working Through. In J. Strachey, A. Freud, A. Strachey, & A. Tyson (Eds.), *The Standard Edition of the Complete Psychological Works of Sigmund Freud—Vol. XII—(1911–1913): The Case of Schreber, Papers on Technique, and Other Works* (pp. 145–156). The Hogarth Press.

Freud, S. (1968). *The Standard Edition of the Complete Psychological Works of Sigmund Freud—Vol. VI (1901): The Psychopathology of Everyday Life*. The Hogarth Press and the Institute of Psycho-Analysis.

Frosh, S. (2010). *Psychoanalysis Outside the Clinic: Interventions in Psychosocial Studies*. Macmillan International Higher Education.

Frosh, S. (2013). Psychoanalysis, Colonialism, Racism. *Journal of Theoretical and Philosophical Psychology, 33*, 141–154. https://doi.org/10.1037/a0033398

Frosh, S. (2020). *New Voices in Psychosocial Studies*. Springer International Publishing.

Frosh, S., & Baraitser, L. (2008). Psychoanalysis and Psychosocial Studies. *Psychoanalysis, Culture & Society, 13*(4), 346–365. https://doi.org/10.1057/pcs.2008.8

Gherovici, P. (2017). *Transgender Psychoanalysis: A Lacanian Perspective on Sexual Difference*. Routledge.

Gherovici, P., & Steinkoler, M. (2022). *Psychoanalysis, Gender, and Sexualities*. Taylor & Francis.

Glynos, J., & Stavrakakis, Y. (2018). *Lacan & Science*. Routledge.

Halberstam, J. (2011). *The Queer Art of Failure*. Duke University Press. https://doi.org/10.2307/j.ctv11sn283

Halberstam, J., & Brousse, M.-H. (2016). Queering Psychoanalysis: A Dialogue between Jack Halberstam and Marie-Hélène Brousse. *The Lacanian Review Sex All over the Place, 2*, 21–29.

Hartman, S. V. (2008). *Lose Your Mother: A Journey Along the Atlantic Slave Route* (1st ed.). Farrar, Straus and Giroux.

Herzog, D. (2017). *Cold War Freud: Psychoanalysis in an Age of Catastrophes* (1st ed.). Cambridge University Press.

Hook, D. (2008). Articulating Psychoanalysis and Psychosocial Studies: Limitations and Possibilities. *Psychoanalysis, Culture & Society, 13*, 397–405. https://doi.org/10.1057/pcs.2008.23

Jones, J. (2004). The Time of Interpretation: Psychoanalysis and the Past. *Postmodern Culture, 14*. https://doi.org/10.1353/pmc.2004.0019

Khanna, R. (2003). *Dark Continents: Psychoanalysis and Colonialism*. Duke University Press.

Lacan, J. (1997). *The Seminar of Jacques Lacan. Book 3, The Psychoses: 1955–1956* (R. Griggs, Trans.). W. W. Norton.

Lacan, J. (1998). *Four Fundamental Concepts of Psychoanalysis*. W. W. Norton & Company.

Lacan, J. (1999). *The Seminar of Jaques Lacan. Book 20, On Feminine Sexuality, the Limits of Love and Knowledge*. W. W. Norton.

Lacan, J. (2002). *The Seminar of Jacques Lacan XV (1967–1968): The Psychoanalytic Act* (C. Gallagher, Trans.). Karnac Books.

Lacan, J. (2007). *Écrits: The First Complete Edition in English*. W. W. Norton.

Lacan, J. (2007). Science and Truth. In *Écrits: The First Complete Edition in English* (B. Fink, Trans.). W. W. Norton.

Lacan, J. (2013). Lituraterre. *Continental Philosophy Review, 46*(2), 327–334. https://doi.org/10.1007/s11007-013-9259-8

Lacan, J. (2017). *Transference*. Polity Press.

Lacan, J. (2018). *The Sinthome: The Seminar of Jacques Lacan. Book XXIII*. Polity Press.

Meyer, W. S. (2013). Part 2: Homosexuality Uncured: Reflections of a Former Analysand. *Smith College Studies in Social Work, 83*(1), 36–44. https://doi.org/10.1080/00377317.2013.746921

Milner, J.-C. (2020). *A Search for Clarity*. Northwestern University Press.

Nobus, D., & Quinn, M. (2005). *Knowing Nothing, Staying Stupid: Elements for a Psychoanalytic Epistemology*. Routledge.

Palacios, M. (2009). *Fantasy and Political Violence: The Meaning of Anticommunism in Chile*. VS Verlag für Sozialwissenschaften.

Parker, I. (2004). *Qualitative Psychology: Introducing Radical Research* (1st ed.). Open University Press.

Parker, I. (2005). Lacanian Discourse Analysis in Psychology: Seven Theoretical Elements. *Theory & Psychology, 15*(2), 163–182. https://doi.org/10.1177/0959354305051361

Pascoe, C. J. (2018). What to Do with Actual People? Thinking Through a Queer Social Science Method. In D. R. Compton, T. Meadow, & K. Schilt (Eds.), *Other, Please Specify: Queer Methods in Sociology* (1st ed., pp. 291–303). University of California Press.

Plummer, K. (2003). Queers, Bodies and Postmodern Sexualities: A Note on Revisiting the "Sexual" in Symbolic Interactionism. *Qualitative Sociology, 26*(4), 515–530. https://doi.org/10.1023/B:QUAS.0000005055.16811.1c

Preciado, P. B. (2021). *Can the Monster Speak?: Report to an Academy of Psychoanalysts* (F. Wynne, Trans.).

Ronell, A. (2003). *Stupidity*. University of Illinois Press.

Sprengnether, M. (2012). Freud as Memoirist: A Reading of "Screen Memories". *American Imago, 69*(2), 215–240.

Tupinambá, G. (2021). *The Desire of Psychoanalysis: Exercises in Lacanian Thinking*. Northwestern University Press.

Watson, E., & Giffney, N. (Eds.). (2017). *Clinical Encounters in Sexuality: Psychoanalytic Practice and Queer Theory*. Punctum Books.

Zupančič, A. (2017). *What is Sex?* The MIT Press.

12

The Heart of Rhythm: Congolese Music as Creative Disruption

Guilaine Kinouani

Likala Moto
I put some rumba on so I can try to think.
It is one of my favourite Congolese songs.
It is called Likala Moto*. It would simply translate as hot coal.
That song always seems to pierce through the defensive walls of my mind.
So it can make my heart sing and sink.
I know it tells a tale of unrequited love.
A tie that refuses to die.
I do not understand the lyrics.
Still, the song speaks to my heart.
It has long moved my soul.
Its rhythms lead me into a place that is strangely familiar,
and yet so intimately unknown.
A thick forest guarded by a mighty night owl.
A place where spirits reside in peace, only accessible through the senses.

This chapter was written as part of the explorations first carried out during my PhD (Kinouani, 2024b) and may form part of my doctoral thesis.

G. Kinouani (✉)
School of Social Sciences, Race Reflections, Birkbeck University, London, UK

G. Kinouani et al. (eds.), *Creative Disruption*, Studies in the Psychosocial,
https://doi.org/10.1007/978-3-031-63661-5_12

Only accessible to those who have heart.
A house, a distant howl, a sorrowful yearning
Can the heart be made into a shelter for those we love?
The man in the verse sings, his has.
Motema: one of the few words I know in Lingala.
The heart.
Here, it is the refuge that continues to offer a warm home,
long after the season has come and gone.
Despite the embittered mind of that unloved man.
I have put Likala Moto on, so I can feel to think.
It is often in the background when I need to write.
And quickly it gets inside of my heart, inside my motema.
The opening melody is so beautiful it often brings a tear to my eyes.
I mourn that I may never be able to convey it in words.
Or even just simply understand the words.
Yet, the rhythm takes hold of my body in that ephemeral moment,
when I am irresistibly pulled into moving to the music, first slow.
...and this, I allow.
Whose hands are these, that I cannot see?
I faithfully follow this ancestral track.
I depart from the realm of the known.
And I depart from the realm of the now.
These too are ties that refuse to die.
Likala moto.
My mother used to say to me 'you cannot steal someone's child.'
I always knew she meant you may steal children from Africa,
but you cannot steal children of Africa.
As I dance, each breath I take replenishes my entire being,
with the essence of both my humanness and divinity.
That soothing touch that rejuvenates my weathered body …
Whose healing hands are these, that I cannot see?
As I dance, the rhythm of the Sébène shifts and accelerates and the percussions,
oh the percussions. … how they resonate within!
Heartbeats of generations who have long come and gone, are still reverberating within me.
Every one of them invigorates that river of life that runs through my veins.

My hips are awakened by the fluidity of this musical flow.

I allow this also.

This is the Congo.

Likala moto!

The magic of rumba... It primes the entire pelvic region, our very creative core,

to roll that sensual dance.

That dance of wanting.

That dance of longing.

That dance of desire.

That dance of life.

As I dance, I feel the drums vibrating and pulsating in every untouched corner of my body, corners my mind will not allow me to touch.

I have this life force deep inside me.

And I have that old Congolese song that always connects me to a different reality.

A reality one can only see with closed eyes.

A reality that as a woman I have been prohibited to feel.

A reality so many of us children of the diaspora have forcibly been displaced from.

That song sings in a language I cannot understand with my mind.

But one that my body fully comprehends.

And one within which my soul recognises the invisible hands of my ancestors.

They come to claim me and hold me in hiding, but in community.

Like the full meaning of likala moto which does not quite meet the eyes or ears.

Words that do not convey in words the intensity of the connection they speak of.

The viscerality of ancestral entanglements.

The endurance of inheritance.

The dangerousness of attempting to rupture such spiritual bonds.

Perhaps it is true. You cannot steal someone's child.

At least not when they were birthed by Africa. (Kinouani, 2024a)

Psychosocial Commentary

A proper biography of *On the Postcolony* would be impossible without a direct reference to African music. I discovered Congolese music in the late 1980s [...] The emotional sublimity of the Congolese musical imagination taught me how indispensable it was to think with the bodily senses, even to write with the musicality of one's own flesh. (Mbembe, 2001, 2015)

I am writer. I am a music lover. I have a sweet spot for African music and for Congolese music, in particular. Rumba is one of her many children, a fact known on the continent for centuries appropriated and (mis) attributed to Latin America for decades. And rumba is sensuality incarnated. It is the erotic without inhibition, perhaps even in its purest expression.

It is all about the movement of the hips.

It is all about the touch.

It is fluid.

It is emotionally charged.

It has a tenderness and a yearning at its core. Holds the duality of both pain and joy that speaks so deeply of that geopolitical region. It grabs you firmly in the way one may be held tightly yet softly, in the arms of a skilful dance partner or lover.

Instinctively, I have relied on dancing as I have negotiated the thorny waters of whiteness for my thesis and as I have attempted to survive and thrive through timeless diasporic issues, some of which I have mirrored in *Likala Moto*. Issues of displacement, injustice, cultural homelessness, subjugation, time stuckness. The afterlives of colonialism and enslavement.

Evidence of joy's capacity to exist and be sustained in the mist of suffering, Morrison might say. Evidence too that the body can seek the musical to conceptualise and theorise. Music and through music, dancing connects me to creativity in a way no other activity can. I have always associated dancing with the conceptual and with intellectual freedom.

In *White Minds* (Kinouani, 2023), I remind readers, echoing Fanon's (1952) phenomenology of epidermalisation and De Beauvoir's (1949) theorisation on women becoming flesh, that whiteness fixes the object of its gaze in time and in space and in fact constructs it as earlier expressions of past (mythical) temporalities. In doing so, it not only freezes time and movement, but it also freezes in the object of its gaze the capacity to think freely that is to say, to link objects (Bion, 1959) and to imagine itself outside of the borders it imposes. Moving the body, and by extension expanding the mind via dancing, is accordingly liberatory practice per excellence; it makes space for alternative imaginaries. To free the body is therefore to free the mind.

And so, I tend to have Congolese music in the background when I write. At times it is the same song on a loop. On low volume. This level of repetition creates both stimulation and habituation which allow me to concentrate on complex ideas while still being fed at soul level, rhythm. At certain points, I will inevitably be moved/pulled to move. This is when notes, emotions or words go from being in the background to being in the foreground of my mind, where I go from the intellectual to the embodied, to the flesh more consciously and dance freely. Other times, I may be dancing, and I will be moved to write, as an idea I might have been struggling with may become unstuck through my dancing. I will then write freely. Thinking with the body as Mbembe (2015) might say. Feeling with the mind, as I have reformulated. This commentary will attempt to expand on this conceptual background, which underscores *Likala Moto*.

Although I do not seek support in the hard sciences to 'prove' to myself that my sense, my own body or my experience of the world is valid, I am always interested in corroborating findings across disciplines since they demonstrate (1) the futility of rigid epistemic boundaries supporting my general position that all thoroughly acquired evidence will tend to move in the same direction—the direction of truth overall, regardless of its type—and (2) that the deep truths our bodies as archives hold must be taken seriously. To that end, exciting new neuroscientific research is being carried out which establishes that dancing creates neural connections, especially in regions involved in executive function, long-term memory and spatial recognition. Incredibly, dancing is now also linked to higher conceptualisation capacities (Liu, 2011; Henley, 2021).

Thinking with the Body: Feeling with the Mind

This is poetry as illumination, for it is through poetry that we give name to those ideas which are, until the poem, nameless and formless—about to be birthed, but already felt. That distillation of experience from which true poetry springs births thought as dream births concept, as feeling births idea, as knowledge births (precedes) understanding (Lorde, 1993, p. 37).

Writing this chapter for the present creative disruption collection also meant writing my first (serious) piece of poetry. Although I have previously engaged in lyrical writing, a style of writing I wish to move my writing into, I have never had the courage to write poetry, let alone make it public before then. Lorde's words shed light on the reasons why I included poetry in this undertaking. Further, they speak too of that relationship between the creative, the conceptual and the felt as mediated and by the fertility of language when imbued with the poetic.

Lyrical writing is, as I see it, poetic writing. It is writing that aspires to be evocative, pleasurable, rhythmic or in other words vibrant while scholarly, rigorous and intellectually challenging. It is therefore a genre of writing which challenges the boundaries of academic disciplines, art and science and associated dualistic assumptions. A growing body of qualitative research and scholarly work which evokes highly sensual and affective responses and usually incorporates auto-ethnography (Yoo, 2022).

I engage here with the subject-matter which formed the basis of my initial conference presentation, Congolese music and associated onto-epistemic considerations. My intervention was centred on the live use of the hips to access of the creative and as such on the use of dancing which we practised live on the day. Dancing as a way to access the erotic. Naturally, I could not convey these musical happenings, on these pages—via language. The magic, I felt, was lost.

The poem was the closest tool at my disposal to transfer something of the energy and the essence of the experience that I intended to share at the conference since we draw from the poetic to do 'soul work', to communicate the rawness of our experience and to mysteriously draw people in our being in the world or, as Yoo puts it, 'words that convey a poetic experience are ontological rather than epistemological. Ontological knowing is not transactional or to an end but forms a destination in itself' (Yoo, 2022 p. 29).

For Lorde (1993), poetry is a necessarily liberatory tool for women which provides the opportunity to fuse head and heart, to unite the Master and the slave, we may say, to access the discarded and to 'give name to the nameless so it can be thought', to reclaim the power to dream and the power to feel and to imagine freedom. It was therefore the only way for me to attempt to communicate the embodied, the visceral, the carnal dimensions of Congolese dancing and its ancestral evocations.

The Politics of the Erotic and the Policing of Women's Desires

Thus, to write this chapter necessarily required delving into the politics of the poetic and delving into the politics of the erotic, something which has forced me to confront my relationship with both and consequent feelings of vulnerability that accompany the touching of material evocative of the sensual and only implicitly, the spiritual—but also, by extension, the dark continent, in every sense of the term.

Socially sanctioned feelings of exposure were quick to arise much more than when the presentation was initially delivered. It is noteworthy that I felt notably less self-conscious about standing up and rolling my hips—or whining as it is sometimes known amongst people of African and West Indian heritage—in front of peers and strangers than I was committing words on paper for this chapter. Perhaps this speaks to that ancestral preference for the performance of the act of dancing in community as opposed to the act of thinking about the act of dancing—which here is conducted alone. Perhaps this speaks to the ephemeral nature of dancing which means that unless it is recorded, it is only archived through/in the body as opposed to textual archives, which outlive both, the body and the performance.

I shared on the day, the story of Marie a Congolese woman in the UK, a war, rape and torture survivor who I had crossed paths with within a detention centre where I headed a well-being service a few years ago. I explained that one evening, on the day of the anniversary of the bloody murder of her young son Marie came to me and started sobbing as she was re-experiencing the brutality of war. I bore witness to her memory. To her tears, for perhaps 30 minutes, she was going deeper and deeper into sorrow reliving there is no doubt atrocities, done to her body and to that of her child. I was conscious that I was losing her. That my silent presence was not appeasing her sorrowful distress and no words of comfort were in existence to hold her in her pain. So, I stood. I played some Congolese music. I watched how she instantly stood too and danced. I joined her. And little by little she joined me. I could see her eyes becoming alive again and returning into the room. I could see too that music had brought her back from the dead and connected us to life (Kinouani, 2021).

My musical intervention with Marie was purely intuitive and unplanned. Yet engaging with Congolese dancing took us to a different realm of communication in a context where words failed us, and language was not an appropriate medium to communicate or witness. Dancing took Marie out of the depth of the agony of mourning she was experiencing at that moment. I knew it was the right thing to do to alleviate her acute suffering. Still after Marie left, once the emotionality of the encounter subsided, a wave of self-doubt enveloped me. Whiteness, the Master entered the room. How would this look? Would this be ethically justifiable? What about these sacred boundaries? Perhaps here too the intervention challenged the boundaries of art and science and associated dualistic assumptions? Or they simply challenged boundaries as borders? The same logics which normalise the detention of sexually violated, tortured and grieving asylum seekers in necropolitical state apparatuses that are detention centres.

Still, although resisted, the rationalisations for not writing this chapter and then when written, not submitting came fast and they came furious. And are encapsulated by my reactions post-intervention and as the aftermath of my intuition. How could I author a poem so erotically charged? As an analyst? What might it mean for possible analysands to be exposed to such material? And imagine me dancing? In a trans-like state?

'Trans-ing'? What new or old fantasies might these rolling hips give rise to? What might Freud say? What might Fanon say?

I am not sure I can answer all these questions or that I should in fact concern myself with them at all. I do, after all, not cease to be a full-bloodied African-descended woman when I write, think or engage in scholarship. Nor I did take an oath of prudery when I became a group analyst. Moreover, I have learnt that those who hold women and Black women, in particular, in contempt or who have trouble seeing us as human will always be quick to find 'evidence' of dysfunction, pathology or perversion in our words or actions, however human they may be. And I am learning too, to let them dance with their projections. In their lack of rhythm, which often betrays a refusal to see us with their heart.

Women are still socialised to be passive objects of the sexual desire, attraction, erotic wishes, wants and needs of (cishet) men. And because we are socialised to be the objects of desire, attraction, erotic wishes, wants and needs, we as a group tend to find gratification in denying our sexual agency. And shame in claiming erotic power, though they are not one and the same. It is so socially transgressive for women to demonstrate agentic power when it comes to their own body that even the act of dancing alone, dancing only, …can become an act of transgression. Although this may not be done consciously (although it often is), we associate dancing with love making, irrespective of the genre. Both acts involve social bonding, merging often, self-other merging and, consequently, synchrony and rhythm. There already therefore is that connection to the erotic (Schutz, 1976; Tarr et al., 2014), at least to the erotic as commonly understood, through the prism of the sexual.

Lorde on the Erotic

This conflation of the sexual and the erotic and disavowing of the erotic (and of the sexual) speaks to the afterlife of Christianity-based puritanical cultures and associated valorisation of sexual innocence myths. Part of the equation is also a perversion of what constitutes the erotic. My starting point to understand the erotic remains Lorde's (1978) seminal essay 'The Uses of the Erotic: The Erotic as Power'—an essay which, in addition to disentangling erotic power from the sexual, links it to creativity, knowledge, feeling and spirituality.

Lorde defines the erotic as a form of power which 'lies in a deeply female and spiritual plane, firmly rooted in the power of our unexpressed or unrecognised feeling' …It is 'Power of the erotic which rises from our deepest and non-rational knowledge' (Lorde, 1978, p. 87).

The use of rational here is crucial. It speaks to ways dominant systems of thought have corrupted and perverted that source of knowledge and reduced it to the depraved, the debased, the pornographic so as to serve the sexual needs of dominant men/systems.

The erotic, Lorde proposes, is a source of power in that, firstly, it allows Lorde to bear witness to the totality of her own experience of oppression and translate it in a language in which she can bear witness to the experience of others. As such the erotic becomes an important epistemic tool to define ourselves and define the world for ourselves. Secondly, as energy source the erotic is life-sustaining; it provides the fuel needed to do dismantling work. Thirdly, and linking these two points, by enriching epistemic resources and the ontological tapestry of our lives, the erotic becomes dangerous to structures of power and the status quo, political action and organisation are much more likely (Caleb, 2023).

Quite innovatively Lorde proposes that the bridge which connects the political and the spiritual is formed by the erotic. It follows that connecting to the erotic is not only a spiritual act but also an act that politicises pleasure and renders engagement with the political erotically fulfilling.

As an onto-epistemic tool of resistance, and in line with psychosocial analytics, for Lorde the erotic invites us to call into question all false binaries which force us to split and compartmentalise parts of who we are, and these include the splitting of spiritual and the political. Hence, drawing from our erotic knowledge, allows epistemic bridges between apparently polarised parts of our self, to be build built.

'For the bridge which connects them is formed by the erotic—the sensual, those physical, emotional, and psychic expressions of what is deepest and strongest and richest within each of us, being shared: the passions of love, in its deepest meanings'. In summary, the erotic allows us to be guided by what we cannot see. To 'see through emotions' (Lorde, 2004, p. 32).

And this bridge building opens the possibility of living richer, fuller and more fulfilling lives, lives which are more connected to the depth of ourselves, to others and to the universe.

The Politics of Love

So clearly not all love is sexual… although our political engagements could benefit from the erotic. When I started analytic psychotherapy, a decade or so ago I shared in an early session that I loved Congolese music with my then analyst. She stared intensely at me after I spoke these words. There was a silence. Then she said she would expect I would have difficulties with structures of power and with (white) authority. I never returned to that conversation during our work together. In truth, I was too scared. Scared I knew exactly what she meant and even though I did not understand her words intellectually or at least their depth, at the time. In the silence she had already communicated to me the gravity of her assessment, and I had sensed it with my body.

Something about my affinity with these rhythms thus caused her to pause and to think. Something about my affiliation with these rhythms caused her sufficient concern for my structural welfare. Something which spoke to a mismatch, to a clash, to my dancing to different drums. When I reflected on this experience, I wondered if it evidenced an epistemic misalignment in her eyes, a rebelliousness.

A defiance. An irreverence. I remember her silence vividly till today and my waiting anxiously for what felt like hours, as she looked at me with that serious expression on her face, like a patient expecting a deadly prognosis. One of the most evocative clinical encounters of my 13 years or so analytic journey.

West (2017) teaches us that justice is what love looks like in public. And my love for Congolese music is real. And it is spiritual. But it is clear to me too that my public love for Congolese rumba is deliberate and that it is political. In a context of raging anti-blackness and anti-African hatred or contempt, so-called savage or native art is an interesting case in point in white ambivalence. Valuable enough to remain fiercely guarded within European museums where it remains since it was looted/stolen from the continent but worthless enough to forever be imprisoned in that imaginary of the primitive.

Given the coloniality of musicology and all formations of sophistication that dominate art at large, and the enduring racist tropes the region continues to attract, in the white imagination, embracing these creative productions is an act of transgression. A musical practice of ungovernability. It is fundamentally too a decolonial act. An act of love that is also, we might say, a small act of justice. A small act that aims to free such productions (and me) from that suffocating imaginary. A practice of oppositionally gazing (hooks, 1992).

Congolese Music and the Psychosocial

So, what would Fanon say and what would Freud say?

It is not certain. But we can infer something of relevance from their politics on music and on Africa based on the following two quotes.

> A proper biography With music, I am almost incapable of obtaining any pleasure. Some rationalistic, or analytic, turn of mind in me rebels against being moved by a thing without knowing why I am thus affected and what it is that affects me. (Freud, 1914, p. 257)

> I am black. I am the incarnation of a complete fusion with the world, an intuitive understanding of the earth, an abandonment of my ego in the heart of the cosmos and no white man no matter how intelligent he may be can ever understand Louis Armstrong and the music of the Congo. (Fanon, 1952, p. 31)

The aforementioned quotes capture an important tension between the two men. For Freud, music is clearly evocative of fear, danger or at the very least suspicion. Fear of losing control of the self, of the ego relating to a fear of being in the world outside of a 'rationalistic' and an 'analytic' frame of understanding the world, it would appear.

The fear of being thrown into a dark abyss, entering a realm where the self is experienced as out of bound, unknown, verbally indescribable and intellectually ungraspable. A fear of the preverbal, even perhaps of the unconscious. A fear of losing self-mastery thus mastery of the so-called primitive. Of the other that exists within, we might say.

In Fanon's words, on the other hand, we read what seems like him embracing what felt like apprehension in Freud. The appeal of intuition, of the embodied, the visceral, which he attributes to his blackness. A wish to merge and to be at one with what is both understood though 'intuitively' still perhaps also unknown, since there is still a conscious 'abandonment'. For Fanon, an appreciation for Congolese music requires a particular ontology, an ontology he believes the 'prototypical white man' embodied by Freud's words here cannot embody.

I am not sure if I am entirely convinced by either man's position. I read in Freud a convoluted attempt at distancing himself from the feminine, 'the dark continent', from the primitive, in a way that reads to me as contrived. This impression would be consistent with an anti-black reading of his oeuvre as has been widely documented and is evidenced by him, for example, referring to his patients as 'negroes', or in *Totem and Taboo,* describing 'the Negro races of Africa' as 'uncivilised'—statements widely interpreted as attempts by him to distance Jews from blackness (Tate, 1996). Attempting to 'redeem' Jewishness from antisemitism. Fanon's words are similarly imbued with a reactionary note, it seems to me. But I see in them an act of public love as proposed by West. A 'son' challenging his 'father' and his anti-black logics attempting to redeem blackness from the grip of colonial formations. Hence, Fanon is squarely punching up.

Notwithstanding the splitting of rationality and corporeality as embodied by these two (exaggerated?) positions as well as the risks of essentialising so-called racial differences, these two thinkers do put their fingers on important onto-epistemic matters which our relationship with music thus the body and movement betray. Not only does music carry essential functions for displaced groups and migrants even when parents and older generations do not consciously seek to pass on their love for music, the traditions and stories carried within the music they listen and dance to are passed on. Same with the way they move. Music consequently helps the transmission across time and space of group histories. The passing on of music is thus also the passing on of heritage, culture and, again, connection. With this transmission, collective knowledge, worldviews, healing and resistance practices are shared and can, thus, survive.

Mauss (1934) in his formulation of 'les techniques du corps' (techniques of the body) proposes the body is used as an instrument to pass on knowledge. A technique here is an embodied action which is traditional and has the effect of transmitting 'archives of being' or 'modes of life' or the habitus of a group at a particular point in time. These techniques are postulated to be passed down through various means throughout the lifespan, across generations and include imitation, observation and formal training. Although Mauss did not elaborate, he did list dancing amongst many others as an example of such techniques to explain observable corporal differences in movement, speed, gait, and occupation of space amongst diverse cultural groups in dancing practices.

Hence, musical experience transmits implicit and explicit messages such as freedom, trust and an attitude of openness to what comes the celebration of the body or of the erotic, harmonious union. Engaging with African music necessarily takes us to a different realm of communication, as my dancing with Marie demonstrates, a different world of sense making, a dimension which challenges linear and dualist engagement with the world and separatist worldviews. The opposite of Cartesian mind-body dualism. An engagement that connects rather than splits and separates thus consequently something that calls for unity, integration and interconnectedness.

The Congo and Being and Being Congolese

The ill-defined 'Congo' has featured heavily in white imaginaries as the land of savagery, barbarism and cannibalism, projective fantasies based on the atrocities inflicted on the region. An estimated 10 million Congolese people perished due to Belgian colonial extractive practices and their consequences (Johnson, 2014).

The English, the French and, in particular, the Spanish and Portuguese atrocities have arguably been erased from the global collective consciousness and from most historical accounts of the Kongo. Swallowed by the undigestibility of the Belgian colonial monstrosity. Yet, a further 6 million souls had before this been enslaved from the same region. About half the number of those extracted for the trade, with most taken to Latin America (Micheletti et al., 2020). Genocide upon genocide.

Factoring in the well-documented mortality rate of the middle passage and those otherwise killed at sea increases the figure of the murdered and stolen lives by 15–20% (Statista, 2023) conservatively. Roughly then, 11 million Kongolese people were murdered through extractive, disposessive cannibalistic capitalism. And 17 million lives altogether were stolen from one single region of the continent alone. Seventeen million... There is no doubt the 'Congo Basin' is the graveyard of Africa. The very heart of whiteness.

Rumba originates from these dark waters. Although it predates them, it is this horrific history that provides the genealogy for the duality of the pain and joy, the life and death forces, the old and new energies that characterise the genre. And that such deeply emotional and erotic imagination could originate from and be sustained in one of the worlds (if not the world's) most bloodied, exploited, brutalised regions, a region still in the grip of neocolonial conflicts and genocidal wars, again demonstrates this poignant paradox—serenity in the face of tragedy as Mbembe may summarise. This paradoxical dance cannot but call for our attention. It is in and of itself the most arresting testament of the life drive, a story of defiant survival against all odds.

While born in the Kongo Kingdom, it was brought to 'New Worlds' during the slave trade from the sixteenth to the nineteenth century (the Kikongo word—Kikongo being one of the languages of the region, being Nkumba, which means navel). The dance of the navel thus survived. It survived across the Atlantic because the enslaved sought to conserve their rhythms, their movements, their ancestry. Across the Latin world today different versions of the genres now exist which have integrated over the centuries Latin rhythms, in places with indigenous touches, while retaining the very distinctive Congolese influences recognisable to any trained or Congolese ear. It is this influence which creates a sense of home, a sense of resonance, a sense of kinship and a sense of mutual recognition through sounds, across the oceans for displaced and diasporic souls. Through these rhythms the memory of those brutally departed remains. Through these rhythms the departed remain.

According to Lorde, the erotic is a life force. Deeply held within. Ancient. It has like Rumba survived colonialism and enslavement. Brutalisation, genocide. It has even survived the internalisation of patriarchy. It speaks intuitively. Often for many of us shyly, until we make space for it to be. And if the erotic becomes, we may say, a habit of being (hooks, 1993), since it is not what we do in the world rather it is how we do it, that procures it, it is the quality of our engagement with the creative and the depth of our capacity to feel, 'the erotic is not a question only of what we do; it is a question of how acutely and fully we can feel in the doing' (p. 54) then; rumba becomes an erotic habit. Mastered over centuries. A technology of the body which has efficiently been passed on.

Beyond the intellectual gifts Rumba provides to those willing to draw from the creative to think, to those willing to dig from the sensual knowledge of the hips to theorise, for me therefore as a Congolese descended yet displaced child to discard rumba, and the fundamental erotic of Congolese music or hide what it does to the body, to my body, is to cover it with dirt. It is to collude with colonial violence and anti-black formations. It is to become complicit in the violence done to my ancestors in the name of Christ. Often for men. And most importantly here, it is to cut me from parts of my history, parts of my ancestry, and thus encourage the continued deforestation of the Congo in me.

Like many diasporans, I do not speak the language of my ancestors, but I can dance to the same drums and my heart vibrates to the same rhythms and so, somehow, we can still be at one. I find this incredibly vital to my wellness in this world. I have previously argued that one of the reasons that there appears to be so much 'psychological distress' among so-called second or third generations of African 'migrants' within the diaspora and those even further removed from the continent is because of this disconnection (Kinouani, 2021). Disconnection from ancestral lands, cultures, ways of knowing and being. And yet, there are so many of us who deprive ourselves of African art and creations; power… because they are called African. Then go on and adore genre touched by the white hand or music that has been adapted for a Western ear and fail to see whiteness at play. We see this today with the global success (a mainstream version) of afrobeats which is to be celebrated but also to be critically interrogated.

Concluding Thoughts

Despite what we have been (mis)taught, the sensual may open the gate to what is deeply conceptual. Our relationship to the musical and how we formulate its relationship with knowing therefore hold important cues about how we inhabit the world and how we relate to it. And so, we can see that sensory mastery and control of the unconscious betray a settler colonial relationship with the self, others and the environment. They reproduce capitalistic, neoliberal socio-economic configurations. Therefore, the charge of dancing 'out of rhythm', often made against whiteness, speaks powerfully to a deep truth which must be confronted. Music, particularly African rhythms, may invite us to re-connect to the natural world, to ourselves and to others in a more intimate manner, to live in harmony, that is to say, in rhythm. Asking us to feel deeply and, in doing so, disrupting that hyper-rationalist ontology which so fundamentally cuts us off from suffering, including our own, but also the suffering we are capable of inflicting on other beings and on the planet. An ontology which sustained the genocidal extraction of the Congo region and of all colonial territories at large. Congolese music and its closely related peers, the sensual, the poetic and the erotic, provide means that allow us to creatively resist these colonial ways of existing, of being and of knowing. To speak of the deeply embodied known and/or we might say in some ways to make accessible the 'unthought known'. Our connection to an inherited past which escapes rational articulation but which I have argued exists deeply within us since it so easily comes into motion in space as we dance. Music allows us to reclaim our place within the universe as we appear to be reclaimed by ancestral entities. And this invitation to merge with multiple subjectivities across time-spaces, generations and history is a rich source of life and meaning for displaced diasporans. I have found repeatedly that becoming immersed in the musical and very specifically in the familiarity of Congolese rhythms enables me to lose myself so that I can find aspects of who I am. Or rather, aspects of who I am come and find me, often despite my intellectual self. They remind me that I exist in community. They also remind me that there are other ways, contrary to what I am told as truth. There are other realities. They force me to be present in the world differently and, in turn, the world presents differently to me. I have found that I was able to lose myself as I wrote this chapter, almost in the same way that I lose myself when I lose myself in Congolese music. I cannot dance and be self-conscious and there is something about writing that calls for the nakedness of vulnerability of the erotic. And this is where all the magic happens.

Acknowledgements A warm thank you to both my eldest sister Ursula and Race Reflections member Violeta Tatu (and her mother) who helped me to grasp the depth of *Likala Moto*. Thank you to Wenge BCBG Les Anges Adorables et Blaise Bula (1998) and all the African musicians at large—for the gift of music. Thank you to the family I am estranged from due to time and space, but who I am united with through sound. I send my love to my late father; I hope to meet and dance with you, when I too enter that 'forest'. Always and forever, to the ancestors old and new, who perished in unconscionable numbers and in unconscionable suffering, but who live and do their work through me.

References

Bion, W. R. (1959). Attacks on Linking. *The International Journal of Psychoanalysis, 40*, 308–315.

Caleb, W. (2023). Audre Lorde's Erotic as Epistemic and Political Practice. *Hypatia, 38*, 896–917. https://doi.org/10.1017/hyp.2023.76

de Beauvoir, S. (1972 [1949]). *The Second Sex*. Harmondsworth: Penguin.

Fanon, F. (1952). *Black Skin, White Mask*. Grove Press.

Freud, S. (1914). *Collected Papers* (Vol. IV). Hogarth Press.

Henley, M. (2021). Thinking about Thinking: Dance Education and 4E Cognition. *Journal of Dance Education, 21*(3), 129–131.

hooks, b. (1992). *Looks: Race and Representation*. South End Press.

hooks, b. (1993). *Sisters of the Yam: Black Women and Self-Recovery*. Routledge.

Johnson, S. (2014). King Leopold II's Exploitation of the Congo From 1885 to 1908 and Its Consequences. *HIM 1990–2015*. Retrieved from https://stars.library.ucf.edu/honorstheses1990-2015/1642/?utm_source=stars.library.ucf.edu%2Fhonorstheses1990-2015%2F1642&utm_medium=PDF&utm_campaign=PDFCoverPages; https://stars.library.ucf.edu/honorstheses1990-2015/1642

Kinouani, G. (2021). *Living while Black: The Essential Guide to Overcoming Racial Trauma*. Ebury, Penguin Random House.

Kinouani, G. (2023). *White Minds: Everyday Performance, Violence, Resistance*. Policy Press; Bristol University Press.

Kinouani, G. (2024a). *Likala Moto*. Race Reflections. Retrieved from https://racereflections.co.uk/likala-moto/

Kinouani, G. (2024b). *Whiteness as Iatrogenic and Traumatogenic: An Afro-analytic Exploration and Reformulation of Racial Trauma in the Clinic and Beyond* [Unpublished Dissertation]. Birkbeck College, University of London.

Liu, Y. (2011). *OA.MG. The Cultivation of the Sense of Dancing Based on Non-intelligence Factors*. Retrieved December 8, 2023, from https://oa.mg/work/2380952498

Lorde, A. (1978). *Uses of the Erotic: The Erotic as Power*. Out & Out Books.

Lorde, A. (1993). *Poetry is Not a Luxury*. Druck- & Verlagscooperative.

Lorde, A. (2004). *Conversations with Audre Lorde, ed. Joan Wylie Hall*. University Press of Mississippi.

Mauss, M. (1934). Les techniques du corps. Article originalement publié Journal de Psychologie, XXXII, ne, 3-4, 15 mars - 15 avril 1936. Communication présentée à la Société de Psychologie le 17 mai 1934.

Mbembe, A. (2001). *On the Postcolony*. University of California Press.

Mbembe, A. (2015). *The Value of Africa's Aesthetics*. Retrieved from https://mg.co.za/article/2015-05-14-the-value-of-africas-aesthetics/

Micheletti, S. J., Bryc, K., Esselmann, S. G. A., Freyman, W. A., Moreno, M. E., Poznik, G. D., Shastri, A. J., Beleza, S., Mountain, J. L., Agee, M., Aslibekyan, S., Auton, A., Bell, R., Clark, S., Das, S., Elson, S., Fletez-Brant, K., Fontanillas, P., Gandhi, P., et al. (2020). *Genetic Consequences of the Transatlantic Slave Trade in the Americas (Version 1)*. University of Leicester. Retrieved from https://hdl.handle.net/2381/12770804.v1

Schutz, A. (1976). Making Music Together. In A. Brodersen (Ed.), *Collected Papers II. Phenomenological* (Vol. 15). Springer. https://doi.org/10.1007/978-94-010-1340-6_8

Statista. (2023). *Share of Captured Slaves Who Died during the Middle Passage, by Broad Region of Disembarkation, Between 1501 and 1866*. Retrieved from https://www.statista.com/statistics/1070565/middle-passage-death-rate-by-destination-1501-1866/

Tarr, B., Launay, J., & Dunbar, R. I. M. (2014). Music and Social Bonding: "Self-Other" Merging and Neurohormonal Mechanisms. *Frontiers in Psychology, 5*, 1096.

Tate, C. (1996). Freud and His "Negro": Psychoanalysis as Ally and Enemy of African Americans. *Psychoanalysis Culture and Society, 1*, 53–62.

Wenge BCBG Les Anges Adorables & Blaise Bula. (1998). *Likala Moto. On Titanic*. Les éditions Simon Lowe.

West, C. (2017). *Professor West Public Lecture Given at the Harvard School of Education on 24th October 2017*. Retrieved from https://www.youtube.com/watch?v=nGqP7S_WO6o

Yoo, J. (2022). *Evocative Qualitative Inquiry Writing and Research Through Embodiment and the Poetic*. Routledge.

13

Nonprofits, Black, and White Women's Power Dynamics Through an Antebellum Lens: A Critical Fabulation Exploration

Janedra Sykes

The Happening

It was hard for the three of them to peek around the corner of the door at the same time, but they all wanted to see.

It was especially tricky because one of them had Ma'am's infant in her arms, and if she cried, there would be hell to pay. Fortunately, being small, with a child's flexibility, they could arrange themselves around the door frame like stairs and watch Cassie fix Ma'am's hair.

"Cassie, my hair needs to be in the latest style for today's luncheon. I must look my best for the committee meeting." said the Mistress of the Manor as she looked into Cassie's eyes, so similar to her own in the mirror.

Cassie's expression didn't alter, nor did she utter a sound as she twisted the Mistress's hair in another direction.

"Did you make sure my day gown with the flowers on the hem is cleaned and ready to wear?"

J. Sykes (✉)
University of San Diego, San Diego, CA, USA
e-mail: janedra@arboretagroup.com

G. Kinouani et al. (eds.), *Creative Disruption*, Studies in the Psychosocial,
https://doi.org/10.1007/978-3-031-63661-5_13

Cassie paused arranging Ma'am's hair, padded silently to the armoire, chose the dress, and quietly put it on the bed. She glanced at the door, and by the look in her eyes, the three mammies knew they needed to return to the nursery.

As they walked back to the nursery, they had the same conversation they'd had a hundred times, "What do you think happened between Cassie and the Mistress that she no longer speaks?" asked the oldest mammy, who was about ten years old.

"It must have been bad," said another.

The third mammy chimed in, "It's been years since The Happening."

That's what the enslaved people on the plantation called the incident where Cassie went silent, The Happening.

Introduction

I will use critical fabulation as a tool to explore the power dynamics in the American nonprofit workplace. Critical fabulation, a term coined by Hartman (2008) in her seminal essay, *Venus in Two Acts*, is the combining of historical and archival research with critical theory and fictional narrative (Hamer, 2020). I will make the case that current-day power dynamics in American nonprofits have their roots in American slave society. These historical roots form the foundation for resistance and self-liberation efforts that are alive today. The purpose of this chapter is to use the backdrop of the movie *Imitation of Life*, the 1934 version starring Louise Beavers and Claudette Colbert, in conjunction with critical fabulation (AFI|Catalog, n.d.). I will combine historical and archival research rooted in slave narratives with fictional narratives to explore the dynamics of Black and White women as it relates to Black women's labor and White women's self-authorized entitlement to their labor.

These explorations include personal reflections, notes, social commentary, and historical archival materials. References to historically accurate reenactments from the 1800s that show the daily routines of the White plantation mistress and her enslaved lady's maid, the cinematic relationship between Black and White single mothers in the 1930s, and my lived experiences and those of my clients who are Black women combine to demonstrate that patterns of oppression still exist. Alongside this oppression, the creative disruption of self-liberation exists as well and remains effective. For thirty-plus years, I have worked in American nonprofits, a sector in which 70% of the workers are women (Urban Institute, 2021).

In general, in the United States, the majority of these women are White (Catalyst, 2023). I have held roles ranging from front-line service provider to executive director to board member. Currently, I am an Equity, Diversity, and Inclusion Organizational Development practitioner and coach who consults with nonprofits of all sizes. In addition to my organizational development work, I coach individual women of color who work in racist nonprofit cultures. I have experienced the nonprofit sector as the "White woman's house," and I have observed distinct, predictable, and repetitive patterns of behavior that reinforce the mammy-mistress psychosocial dynamic, rooted in anti-Blackness, racism, classism, and sexism; these behaviors are the basis of the Black woman/White woman workplace dynamic.

The Cultural Touchstone

The Movie's Historical Backdrop

The 1934 movie, *Imitation of Life*, was considered cutting-edge because it explored the themes of race relations, female entrepreneurship, and a mixed-race child who rejected her Blackness and passed for White (AFI|Catalog, n.d.). Fannie Hurst, the author of the book on which the screenplay was based, was a patron of the Harlem Renaissance. At the time, Harlem was a hotbed of race mixing. Blacks and Whites interacted socially, and it is considered a golden age for Black creativity, a portion fueled by White patronage.

America in the 1930s was a time of Jim Crow, Black codes, and the lynching of Black bodies while White families held picnics underneath (National Association for the Advancement of Colored People [NAACP], n.d.). The Great Migration was in full swing as Blacks escaped the brutal oppression of the South for better opportunities. In the 1920s, the United

Daughters of the Confederacy, a respected mainstream White supremacy organization, proposed a statue of Mammy, a fantasy version of slavery in which the Black woman loved her role of servitude. The proposal was seen as a whitewashed revision of history by Black activists at the time (Shorpy, 2020).

In the movie, a Black woman and a White woman had a "partnership" while holding onto the social hierarchy. Their partnership represented the unspoken racial and gender hierarchy in American culture that is alive today. The film was wildly successful and was remade in the 1950s. Its role as a cultural touchpoint remains. It is rumored that popstar Beyoncé and actress Zendaya are considering a remake (Court, 2022).

A Personal, Social, and Historical Commentary

I was born in Los Angeles, California, to parents who were from the southern and midwestern American states. They participated in the final wave of the Great Migration of 1910–1970 (The U.S. National Archives and Records Administration, n.d.), when approximately six million Black people migrated to northern, midwestern, and western states to escape the brutal oppression of the Jim Crow South (Wilkerson, 2010).

My mother was born in St. Louis, Missouri, and my father in Columbus, Mississippi. My childhood was split between Southern California and Northeast Mississippi. My lived experiences reflect knowledge of the societal norms of overt (Mississippi) and covert (California) anti-Black racism that is rooted in American culture.

Being Black in America requires the ability to intuitively, if not consciously, recognize and navigate the power dynamics of American culture born in White supremacy. Sharpe (2016) describes anti-Blackness as the climate we live in. Living in a social environment that, as the saying goes, "loves Black culture, but not Black people," creates a cumulative amount of stress that racks the nervous system. This chronic stress, much of which happens in the workplace, contributes to poor mental and physical health outcomes. This is particularly true for Black women. Yet there are ways in which Black women, and those who truly support them, can disrupt this dynamic and create a window for healing.

The Movie and Its Present-Day Applications

The primary plot in *Imitation of Life* is that a Black woman's daughter hates her Blackness and passes for White (AFI|Catalog, n.d.). The subplot is the basis for this chapter and involves the business relationship and the division of labor of the main characters. The Black woman provides her creative product, maintains the household, and raises the children, while the White woman interacts with White males using her beauty and cleverness to build the business. Here the social hierarchy is arranged in a unique yet unimaginative manner. A Black woman as the helpmate who enables a White woman to reach her goals in exchange for financial support hints at internalized patriarchy.

In the movie, there is a scene when the White woman offers 20% of the business to the Black woman (Stahl, 1934). She declines while saying she's happy that the White woman allowed her to live with her and serve her and her daughter. She tells the White woman that she can keep the money and just use her share to give her a nice funeral. The White woman decides to put the 20% in the bank for her and does not press the issue.

The successful string of breakfast restaurants was based on the Black woman's secret pancake recipe. The racial privilege of the White woman, and the racial hierarchy, determines how each woman receives the fruits of their collective labor. In the nonprofit workplace, Black women's work is often discounted and later, with minor adjustments, co-opted by their White colleagues and supervisors (Thompson, 2021); this is especially prevalent with nonprofits that serve marginalized communities. White-led nonprofits receive the lion's share of the funding and offer their Black sub-contractors, primarily Black women, a fraction of the grant amount for community outreach and case management. If employed by White-led nonprofits, Black women are often limited to front-line worker positions with limited opportunities for upward mobility.

The process of subjugation that discounts and devalues Black women's creative labor is a social construct fueled by Whiteness and reinforced by the spoken and unspoken societal expectations that Black women are overly generous, humble, and happy to serve the needs of White women in the workplace. The current term "from pet to threat" (Donahue et al.,

2021) aptly describes the dynamic. Competing with White women by advancing their own careers is considered threatening by White women. A self-authorized Black woman who advocates and makes decisions in her own best interests is considered transgressive.

The theme that runs throughout the movie is that the Black mammy character is an eager and willing servant, which is the linchpin of the psychosocial mistress-mammy dynamic (Black Feminisms, 2021). The Black woman is fulfilled in her role as a servant. She has no personal ambitions, and therefore she is not a threat to the White woman. This fantasy has a historical throughline to the psychosocial atmosphere in American nonprofits. The movie illuminates the role and tasks of the mammy within the nonprofit sector and their echoes of enslavement.

From *William Faulkner quotes* (n.d.), the quote, "The past is not dead, it's not even past" (para. 1), remains true. In their short video, an antebellum historical reenactment, NotYourMommasHistory (2021) portrays the power dynamic that is present in many nonprofit organizations. The knowledgeable older Black woman guides the younger White woman while remaining hypervigilant about the power dynamics and the need to be subservient and agreeable. Often my clients and colleagues tell me about the gyrations they put themselves through to avoid White women's tears and being labeled as uppity while being expected to provide emotional comfort and reassurance on demand. The assumption is that Black women are happy in their roles, and any show of displeasure can be labeled as having "an attitude," "difficult to work with," and "not being a team player." This assumption serves to create and reinforce an organizational culture that keeps the social order intact.

Wilkerson (2020) argues that America has a caste system with Black women at the lowest rung; this dynamic is expressed by inequities in pay, lack of upward mobility, and few available leadership positions. Nonprofits are iatrogenic organizations for Black women because we work in organizations that limit and harm us, like the mammy in the White woman's house.

While White women could not own land, in the antebellum South, they could own Black bodies—their slaves were often part of their dowry to landed White men (Jones-Rogers, 2019); this included George Washington's wife Martha. Noted self-liberated person Ona Judge, who was Martha Washington's maidservant, escaped during Martha's practice of moving the enslaved persons back to the South to avoid freeing them according to the local laws of the Capital (The Mount Vernon Ladies' Association, n.d.). This mindset continued after emancipation in 1863, expressed by a proposed 1918 city ordinance in Greenville, South Carolina, that required Black women to work in the homes of White women under the threat of jail (The Greenville News, 1918).

Southern Roots

As a child, I had two homes. When school was let out for summer on a Friday, my younger brother and I were on the way to Mississippi the next day. Our grandparents wanted all the time they could get with us, and we wanted it as well. Although Jim Crow was outlawed, it was still present to a lesser degree, quietly operating in the background.

It was unspoken that the town's fancy swimming pool was for White children. The pool for the Black children was across town in a substandard facility. My browned-skinned mother exposed my younger brother and me, both light-skinned Black children, to this modified version of Jim Crow by taking us to the pool, sitting on the side, and waiting for us to call her mommy. She and I watched the White children swim away from us, and as the White adults started to look alarmed, she said, "Let's go."

The segregated community afforded me the luxury of being surrounded by Blackness. The locus of Black life was Catfish Alley, one long street three blocks off Main Street that contained most of the things we needed: restaurants, dentists, hairdressers, insurance agencies, and a liquor store. It was the center of everything Black. It was alive and vibrant, and it policed itself. In some ways, I was freer in a small Mississippi city than I was in Southern California.

My family was affluent and was considered one of the leading Black families. We owned a restaurant, a cab service, a funeral home, and a "by the hour" hotel. My most cherished childhood memories are of my grandmother's restaurant, named *Paradise Cafe*. This is where I learned about the power dynamics at play when interacting with White or Black people. My family behaved distinctly different, as described by Du Bois' (1903) concept of double consciousness and authenticity.

Through the eyes of a child, my college-educated grandmother embodied power. She was born in Mississippi, loved it, and had no desire to leave. Occasionally, she went to the larger cities of Birmingham, Alabama, or Memphis, Tennessee, for medical appointments because she "didn't trust these cracker doctors" in her town. She chose to exercise her authority within the boundaries of the social hierarchy.

When a fight broke out in the cafe, she did not call the police. She waded into the fracas with a kitchen knife to settle the situation. The next day, when the White police officer came to the cafe asking why the restaurant's front window was busted out, my grandmother shrank and played dumb. "You're sure there wasn't a fight?," the officer would ask, "Naw sir, I'm not sure what happened. When I came in this morning, it was like that." As a child, I knew that my grandmother was playing a game. She would look at me and laugh after they left.

When I was about ten years old, my family debated whether I should attend college in Mississippi. My grandmother wanted me to attend Mississippi State College for Women or Ole Miss. I remember my mother distinctly telling my grandmother, "She can't go there. With her mouth, she would be swinging from a tree within three months." My grandmother stared at me for a few moments, laughed, and said, "Yeah, you're right." Southern social mores required performative submission, sweetness, and docility of Black women in relation to Whiteness.

The Mammy, the Mistress, and Nonprofits (Fig. 13.1)

> "This is simply ridiculous. Grandmother Cassie was a mammy, and she sure wasn't happy about all those White children hanging about her." Maude commented as she looked at the photo in the morning edition of the New York Times. "Grandpa Thurston told me that she hated that lady and could have done without those children."

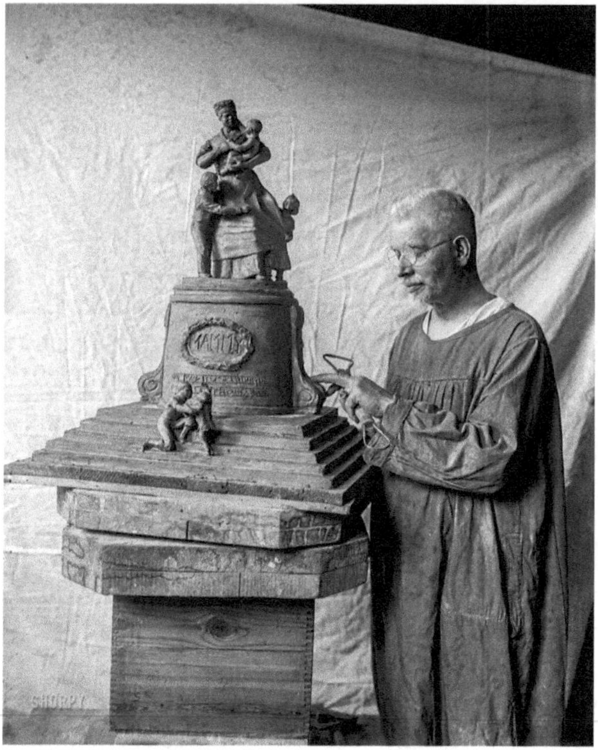

Fig. 13.1 U.S.J. Dunbar, 6/27/23 (1923)

This White fantasy was created and promoted by southern White women. In the 1920s, a White supremacist group, the United Daughters of the Confederacy, organized and proposed to Congress to erect a statue of the mammy in Washington, DC, next to the Lincoln Monument (Horwitz, 2013). It presented Black women as the beloved caregivers of Whiteness. It represented the preferred social order.

Black people protested loudly because they knew this representation was a myth. The White-fueled symbol of the Black mammy was considered an insult and historically inaccurate. Black women rarely lived into old age, and the typical mammy was usually a child herself. Her ward was an infant for whom she was responsible. The mammy portrayed by the statue was despised by Black activists of the time because it symbolized identification with the White oppressor (Rabelo et al., 2021).

In the late 1960s, I remember when the Black maids came to town to shop for their employers and came into the Paradise Cafe during the break between breakfast and the lunch rush when the cafe was quiet. These maids worked for White households. Some lived in White homes and went home to their families on the weekend; others worked in these households from 5 am to 6 pm and then went home to their families. Over coffee and lemon meringue pie, they would share their frustrations with my grandmother. I remember them saying, "Mama Evelyn, she (the mistress of the White household) thinks I love her children more than my own." My grandmother would comment sympathetically, "That's how they are."

As a young girl, I sat on a stool at the counter with my feet not touching the bottom, quietly listening to their stories. They worked the same long hours that my grandmother did, getting up at 4 am and working until the early evening. But my grandmother had the option of taking a nap in her chair located adjacent to the cash register and next to the industrial-sized coffee urn. My grandmother only had to pretend with White people during a limited portion of her day, and then she returned to Catfish Alley, where she held court. I felt so sad that these women had to pretend all day. That simple comment from that maid over 50 years ago resonates today.

The expectation that Black women's proper role is to center the needs of White women permeates the nonprofit workplace. To take the metaphor further, taking care of White women's actual children or their creative babies (i.e., ambitions, projects, and ideas) before nurturing their own is oppressive and exploitative. I often think about the chronic stress of Black women: the cumulative effects of the small, relentless insults and the micro-expressions of power leveled against us in the workplace. For example, when they ask Black women to do the tasks, they can easily do themselves. Or when they are late or come unprepared to a meeting led by Black women, demonstrating their disrespect. Or when … the list feels endless.

There is a thin continuous stream of insults that Black women swallow to survive. A thin stream that wraps around Black women's throats, cutting off our ability to advocate for ourselves and ultimately to breathe. When I have sought support from other Black women within the nonprofit sector, I get the same response that my grandmother gave those southern Black maids, "That's how they are."

Racialized Gender Roles

I have observed these dynamics in nonprofits based in Southern California. I have co-facilitated online workshops on disrupting White supremacy culture in nonprofits, and workshop participants across the country have confirmed that these dynamics are common social exchanges in their workplaces.

In current Black American parlance, going from "pet to threat" (Donahue et al., 2021) expresses the professional discrimination Black women face, often tokenized, supported by their White mentors in public yet undermined in private. There's often a paternal air. Black women are seen as subordinates rather than as peers, despite their ranking on the organizational chart.

There is a historical throughline from the American South. It was not uncommon for the White mistress of the house to refer to her Black adult female as their "girl, who is like a member of our family," who puts in long hours being the primary caretaker for their family while neglecting her own. Black women are tasked with excessive caregiving. The Sojourner Syndrome (Mullings, 2006) and the Superwoman Schema (Woods-Giscombé, 2010) outline excessive caregiving as a survival mechanism.

The concepts of Black women as laborers and White women as recipients of their care and of Black women as workers and White women as supervisors harken back to the antebellum era. This delays or omits self-care, which creates a tremendous chronic cumulative level of stress (Nisbeth, 2022). Nonprofits in America are White-led, called "snow-capped." They are primarily staffed by White women in the roles of nurses, teachers, executive directors, senior-level managers, and philanthropic program managers.

Patterns of Contemporary Enactments

The following patterns of behavior resonate with my equity, diversity, and inclusion clients, coaching clients, and my personal experiences. The elements of perfectionism, defensiveness, and fear of open conflict outlined in Okun's work on White supremacy culture are threaded throughout the dynamics between Black and White women (Jones & Okun, 2001).

"There Is Something Not Quite Right"

This dynamic is what I call the "White glove," and it has a distinct "Mistress of the House" feel to it. It's the ambiguous, undefined criticism that comes in late to the project. Often just before the deadline (thereby undermining the work of the Black woman), the White woman in self-authorized (legitimate and illegitimate) authority comes in and reviews the work where she usually finds something that's just "not quite right."

This requires further conversation, additional work, or the insertion of an idea that should have been shared earlier in the project. This behavior can undermine the confidence of the Black woman by constantly changing standards that are based upon the preferences of the White woman. In addition, it results in derailing the project.

"But That's What We Need"

One of the most exploitive exchanges that I witnessed as a consultant was between a White female-led organization and a Black female-led organization. The White female-led organization was based in a university that was funded to do health disparity work in the minority community. They had contracted with a Black-led organization to do some outreach work and had a written contract for a pre-determined amount of time and money.

As the program progressed, the Black-led organization fulfilled its contract, and other needs arose, as happens in most community-based work. The White-led organization wanted the Black-led organization to fulfill those needs without compensation but with the hope that the White-led group would include them in future grant-writing efforts. What remains unstated is that White-led groups often black-ball the Black-led groups that don't cooperate. They are labeled "difficult" to work with.

Thirty minutes passed with the Black women saying, "That's not in our contract," as the White organizations re-phrased the statement, "But this is what we need." The call ended in a stalemate. After the call, while debriefing with my Black client, at first, there was a heavy silence, and I broke it by saying, "That was exhausting." Immediately, there was group recognition and agreement. There was also confusion about what happened and the purpose of the call.

A key element that the White women never asked was: "Can you do this for us?" or, "This is what we need you to do. Can we adjust the contract?" There was just a simple statement of need with the assumption that the Black women would volunteer to do it. The tones of voices remained measured and friendly, with no hint of annoyance on the part of Black women, to avoid being labeled "difficult." The White women's tone reminded me of a tone a teacher would use with a recalcitrant student or of a nurse with a patient. The dynamic of White women simply stating their unmet needs with the expectation that Black women would voluntarily fill them is the mistress/mammy psychosocial dynamic that dominates workplace relationships between Black and White women.

Primary Deflections of White Women

In the nonprofit sector, there are two primary deflections. The enemy is patriarchy, and it is sexism, not racism. These deflections act as bulwarks against being perceived as a racist institution. What I often hear is, "We can't be racist because we do good work," as if the organization's mission is the antidote to sexism and racism.

These deflections contribute to continuous gaslighting and prevent the issues from being raised. The enemy is men, and the acceptance of sisterhood, built on this assumption, is a condition of being assimilated into the female-dominated nonprofit culture. To question the validity of patriarchy as the operating oppressor is processed as an attack on White women's individual goodness and those in her professional circle.

Tanya looked her executive director in the eye and was at a loss for words. She was concentrating on keeping her facial expression neutral and her tone without a hint of strong emotion.

Nancy, a middle-aged, affluent White woman who led an organization that provided services to domestic violence victims, continued explaining why it was okay to accept funding from sources that promoted the separation of families, arrest, and incarceration as the mandatory remedies for domestic violence.

"I know that the justice system, in general, can be a problem. They are part of the patriarchy after all, and women of color may be hesitant to seek out services if they believe they will be required to press charges against their partner. I'm very aware of the statistics that show Black and Latino men are treated very differently by the justice system, but I know the District Attorney personally. I'm working with him, and I believe his heart is in the right place."

Tanya continued to look at Nancy while thinking about her mortgage payment until she found the professionally safe response, "I see your point."

I have observed that racism operationalized by White women cannot be named without the risk of tears, clutched pearls, being deemed "angry," or not understanding that, as a liberal White female executive director (who was also my boss) told me once, "When sexism is abolished racism will be too." Racism in the form of candy-coated control via gaslighting was the basis of the culture in her organization.

In my experience, the preponderance of White female executive directors who are trained therapists and licensed clinical social workers explains the toxic nonprofit organization cultures. The misuse of the "supervision" model, adapted from the clinical training, sets up an unspoken power dynamic of the "the well and the unwell." The constant insult of being treated as less psychologically developed, plus the role of confusion of mixing the therapist/client relationship with the supervisor/subordinate relationship, creates stress.

According to the Workplace Bullying Institute, 80% of workplace bullying is between women. Research indicates that women-to-women bullying in the workplace is commonplace (Kurter, 2020). Adding a racial hierarchy to this mix sets up the mammy dynamic. A mammy is excessively caregiving and never angry. Therefore, she is a target for bullying.

Whiteness, Extraction, and Boundaries

LaDonna was as quiet as possible when she entered the office. She silently told herself she needed to invest in an insulated lunch box, so she didn't need to return from the field to get her lunch out of the refrigerator. She'd had a long morning and just wanted to grab her lunch, head out to the park and sit under a tree and eat.

As she was heading for the door, a group of her co-workers, all White women middle managers, a few rungs up on the organizational chart, were in the breakroom eating lunch. Susie, LaDonna's manager's supervisor, called out, "Hey LaDonna, sit down and eat with us. We want to pick your brain about a problem we are working on."

LaDonna hesitated. She really wasn't in the mood for this. The last time her "brain was picked," her ideas ended up being presented in the staff meeting with no acknowledgment of her contribution.

Yet she felt blessed to have a job that allowed her to help women of color manage their diabetes since she lost her grandmother last year to the disease. LaDonna, struggling with her own pre-diabetic condition, started to think about all the comfort food she could eat to reward herself for surviving this meeting without losing it.

Kinouani (2023) explains that when White women "invite" Black women into their spaces, although this may be under the guise of appreciating their capabilities, this can quickly turn into the expectation of extraction for the benefit of whiteness, often White innocence. A Black woman who resists this script and uses her expertise, creative problem-solving skills, that is to say, a Black woman who retains her agency and autonomy to challenge White patriarchy or, as Kinouani (2023) puts it, the "direction of the gaze," without performativity and fake smiles, can rarely do so without repercussions, varying in severity: from mockery, exclusion, and marginalization to more serious envy-based sadistic violence (Kinouani, 2023).

When viewed under the colonial mindset that Black creative materials are "raw," "primitive," or "missing a key element," the White woman can take ownership of the Black woman's creative product. Her processing of the "raw" and "primitive" materials makes it useable, and it becomes the means for her career advancement. Kinouani (2023) uses the term micro-colonialism to aptly capture this dynamic. Anger is a normal healthy human reaction to boundary violations that enables human beings to set healthy boundaries. Since Black women are not allowed healthy anger in the workplace, the formation of boundaries is prohibited. They are often forced into appeasement, learned helplessness, and covert acts of resistance to survive the workplace dynamics.

Creative Disruptions

> *Cassie looked at her and Ma'am's reflection in the mirror as she styled her hair, careful not to look into her eyes. She wondered how often Ma'am thought about The Happening and their current situation. Cassie knew she had a flair for fashion, make-up, and hairstyling. And that Ma'am was the first stare of fashion due to her efforts. Ma'am expressed her frustration with Cassie's silence often. She wanted the amiable companionship that the other lady's maids gave to their mistresses, jokes, gossip, and happy servitude. That stopped the day Cassie asked to tend to her dying child rather than fix Ma'am's hair. Because she asked twice, Ma'am gave her a week with the bit. After it was removed, she chose not to speak another word. Four years later, Cassie could still taste the iron on her tongue.* (Wikipedia, 2023)

Critical fabulation, historical knowledge, and psychoeducational tools are the elements of creative disruption, arguably also known as liberation. When Black women can piece together historical facts with an imagination embedded with the spirit of liberation and consciously use psychological support systems, they can begin to free themselves from the mundane, oppressive workplace cultures that entrapped them.

Disrupting Using Narcissistic Abuse as a Pathway to Resistance and Healing

William Edward Burghardt Du Bois wrote about the narcissism of White supremacy (Collins, 2019). One of the ways this is played out is by the centering of White women's needs. She is entitled to Black labor and its fruits. It's an extractive dynamic because Black women are used as suppliers for the narcissism of White women within the organization. Becoming her "pet negro" and "mammy/maid" is the unspoken purpose of the relationship; the goal is to meet the emotional and material needs of the White woman.

Accessible capacity-building, self-care, and community care strategies can help navigate this embedded narcissism. I have referred clients to the work of mental health professionals and found it to be an effective approach to coaching clients and training supervisors (Durvasula, 2024).

Disrupting Using the Nervous System/Somatic Lens Flight, Fight, Freeze, and Fawn

Viewing the mammy/mistress psychosocial dynamic through the nervous system/somatic lens has helped my clients understand and address their high levels of chronic stress (Geronimus et al., 2006). The quotes I hear most from my clients are "They're on my last nerve" and "They're line steppers," which reflect boundary violations. Accessible psychoeducation and psychological safety plans can help navigate and create support systems and opportunities for healing.

I have helped my clients find circles of support within and without their organizations. Clients who find side hustle/nurturing spaces for their creative products derive the most benefit. They can nurture a realistic self-concept outside of the mammy/mistress psychodynamic. In addition, advocating for or taking advantage of remote or hybrid workspaces reduces stress.

Disrupting by Awareness

As leaders of nonprofits, White women remain the mistresses of the house. Often, they are licensed clinical social workers and marriage and family therapists. They have infused the clinical supervision model into their management style, which creates role confusion. Toggling between acting as a therapist and acting as a boss is an unpredictable and, therefore, stressful power dynamic. Healing can happen when we name the authentic power dynamic or reject the false one, hold it in silence, or overtly state it. Using silence by refusing to pick up the call for subjugation and distancing when possible has proved effective.

Healing also happens when we claim actual power by reframing the conversation to the task at hand. For example, simply stating, "While I recognize that my feelings are important, what I'm concerned about in this moment is how to address the issue at hand"; this can align the behavior with the overt actual power dynamic, not the unspoken one. I encourage my clients to get actual therapy, if warranted, with someone who has a knowledge of racialized trauma.

Damage, Healing, and Creative Disruption: Expectation of Excessive Caregiving

Healing can happen when Black women prioritize themselves whenever possible and recognize that the care and feeding of White women is not their responsibility. Creative disruption can look like limiting caregiving while expressing your own needs; this disrupts the assumption that only White women have valid needs and challenges the call to inhabit the mammy role—test for reciprocity. Black women need to ask themselves if it is a genuine friendship they want to pursue or if they are being compelled to participate in a faux friendship or to fulfill the mammy role.

Relentless Boundary Infringement and the Healthy Clapback

Healing can happen by using the Healthy Clapback Method (Stevenson et al., n.d.). Stevenson et al. (n.d.) suggest acknowledging the harm with a safe person—rank the specific harm on a scale of 1 to 10. Fully feel your anger, shame, or embarrassment with a safe person. Express to the safe person what you really want to do and say. Then, have a brainstorming session with the safe person about the things you can do and say that address the situation but cause no unmanageable harm. Then, go back and address the situation or be prepared for the next incident.

Michelle sat across from her at the small table in her soon-to-be former office. This was her exit interview. Michelle was being laid off due to an organizational restructuring. A restructuring that prohibited her from applying for the new position, which merged her department into another.

Her supervisor, the primary architect of the restructuring, expressed her concern for Michelle's emotional state and the state of Michelle's soon-to-be-former direct reports, who, to varying degrees, were upset and dismayed by the changes in the agency.

"How are you?" she asked, looking deep into Michelle's eyes. Her voice was husky with concern. "I'm coping," Michelle simply responded.

"Have you thought about what you're going to do? You're so talented. I don't think it will be a problem for you to find another position!" she probed again. "Actually, I don't have anything lined up," Michelle responded.

A few heartbeats of silence while they gazed into each other's eyes.

She began to cry, "I feel so bad that you're leaving. This is so hard." Michelle continued to look at her and heard the voice in her head tell her, "Take your apron off. You're not here to meet her emotional needs." Michelle listened and felt free.

Conclusion

The pain that Black women feel is the product of the asymmetrical relationships they must navigate in a society whose very foundation was built upon labor done by enslaved people. Reverberations of this history flow through American society; it lives in its politics, popular culture, workplaces, family history, and lived experiences. Often, Black women experience the dynamics of their relationships with White women as narcissistic exchanges, covert and harmful power dynamics, and unspoken hierarchical roles in which Black women sit on the lowest rung.

As readers observe these interrupted patterns, they may experience discomfort. This discomfort evokes the limitations the writer must navigate when attempting to puzzle meaning out of these ongoing encounters. Invariably, the lenses of our lived experiences shape the types of data we are able to collect and the narratives we build from them. Using incomplete historical archives and memories resulting from racialized and gendered workplace happenings can thus create fragmented stories and scattered imaginaries which may limit our ability to connect with the realities, past and present, of the dynamics uncovered.

Disconnections speak to the ways trauma affects our ability not only to remember and to link events; they also highlight White supremacy's consistent violent erasure of its own presence. Finding meaning through this fragmentation, attempting to fill in the absence with what may feel like disconnected notes for many racialized trauma survivors in the nonprofit sector, is a way to reclaim agency and power in an ongoing effort to use creativity to resist. For the reader, bearing witness to that fragmentation is both disruptive and lucid solidarity.

There are ways in which Black women and those who truly support them can create a window for healing—by having an awareness of the damaging dynamics at play through observation supported by a commitment to disrupt these enduring gendered and racialized patterns. To achieve this level of acceptance requires the ability to acknowledge the mental and physical damage of such repetition, perpetration, and complicity, as well as a willingness to collectively confront the past. Hence, an understanding of American history. Not the fan fiction of the founding fathers, but the histories that are shared in slave narratives, and in our individual family histories. The use of critical fabulation can help fill in the gaps of our generational experiences, thereby bringing to people a greater understanding of how a traumatic past, rooted in antebellum America, may inform their difficult present and offer an opportunity for liberation and transformation of the self and of our communities. As

Morrison (1987) poignantly states, "Freeing yourself was one thing, claiming ownership of that freed self was another" (p. 111).

Acknowledgments I want to thank Guilaine Kinouani for her steadfast support and for introducing me to the method of critical fabulation. It opened a new world and freed me as a person and writer. I want to thank my mother, Dr. Juliet Harris Sykes, and my grandmother, Evelyn G. Sykes, who taught me how to work in a culture built to discount and devalue me while maintaining my self-worth. I felt their spirits as I wrote this chapter.

References

AFI|Catalog. (n.d.). Retrieved from https://catalog.afi.com/Film/1130-IMITATION-OFLIFE?sid=bbd0c1b9-9985-4ab2-be43-d0f09f899f4c&sr=12.167134&cp=1&pos=1

Black Feminisms.com. (2021). 5 Controlling Images that Affect Black Women. *Blackfeminisms.com*. Retrieved from https://blackfeminisms.com/controlling-images/

Catalyst. (2023, February 1). *Women of Color in the United States (Quick Take) | Catalyst*. Retrieved from https://www.catalyst.org/research/women-of-color-in-the-united-states/

Collins, D. E. (2019). Racism and Narcissism: America's Original Sin. August 18, 2019. *Al Jazeera*. Retrieved from https://www.aljazeera.com/opinions/2019/8/10/racism-and-narcissism-americas-original-sin

Court, A. (2022, February 18). Beyoncé and Zendaya to remake 1959 classic "Imitation of Life": Source. *New York Post*. Retrieved from https://nypost.com/2022/02/18/beyonce-and-zendaya-in-talks-to-remake-imitation-of-life/

Donahue, K., Gilbert, T., Halpert, M., & Migas, P. R. (2021, June 29). *The infuriating journey from pet to threat: How bias undermines Black women at work*. Forbes. https://www.forbes.com/sites/forbeseq/2021/06/29/the-infuriating-journey-from-pet-to-threat-how-bias-undermines-black-women-at-work/?sh=32e92af64903

DuBois, W. E. B. (1903). *The Souls of Black Folk*. A.C. McClurg & Co..

Durvasula, R. (2024). *It's Not You: Identifying and healing from narcissistic people*. Penguin.

George Washington's Mount Vernon. (n.d.). *Ona Judge*. Retrieved from https://www.mountvernon.org/library/digitalhistory/digital-encyclopedia/article/ona-judge

Geronimus, A. T., et al. (2006). 'Weathering' and Age Patterns of Allostatic Load Scores Among Blacks and Whites in the United States. *American Journal of Public Health*. May, 2006. American Public Health Association. Retrieved from https://scholar.google.com/citations?user=yhbccFcAAAAJ&view_op=view_citation&citation_for_view=yhbccFcAAAAJ:ZfRJV9d4-WMC

Hartman, S. (2008). Venus in two acts. *Small Axe, 12*(2), 1–14. https://doi.org/10.1215/-12-2-1

Hamer, C. (2020, July 28). *Saidiya Hartman's Critical Fabulation Can Help Inspire Today's Activists*. Study Breaks. Retrieved from https://studybreaks.com/thoughts/critical-fabulation/

Horwitz, T. (2013, May 31). *The Mammy Washington almost had. The Atlantic*. https://www.theatlantic.com/national/archive/2013/05/the-mammy-washington-almost-had/276431/

Jones, K., & Okun, T. (2001). *Dismantling Racism: A Workbook for Social Change Groups*. Minnesota Historical Society. Retrieved from https://www.thc.texas.gov/public/upload/preserve/museums/files/White_Supremacy_Culture.pdf

Jones-Rogers, S. E. (2019). They Were Her Property. https://doi.org/10.2307/j.ctvbnm3fz

Kinouani, G. (2023). *White minds*. Policy Press.

Kurter, H. L. (2020). Women Bullied at Work: Here's Why Your Female Boss Doesn't Support You. *Forbes*. Retrieved from https://www.forbes.com/sites/alyssawright/2020/04/27/a-look-to-the-nonprofit-sector-the-importance-of-women-leaders-during-the-pandemic/?sh=40e4084a47d5

Morrison, T. (1987). *Beloved*. Random House.

Mullings, L. (2006). Resistance and Resilience: The Sojourner Syndrome and the Social Context of Reproduction in Central Harlem. In A. J. Schulz & L. Mullings (Eds.), *Gender, Race, Class, & Health: Intersectional Approaches* (pp. 345–370). Jossey-Bass/Wiley.

National Association for the Advancement of Colored People. (n.d.). *History of lynching in America*. NAACP. https://naacp.org/find-resources/history-explained/history-lynching-america#How%20NAACP%20Fought%20Lynching

Nisbeth, K. (2022). *An Exploration of Motherhood: Testing Pathways of the Environmental Affordances Model on Depressive Symptoms and Allostatic Load*. [Abstract]. Retrieved from https://www.researchgate.net/publication/363334614_An_Exploration_of_Motherhood_Testing_Pathways_of_ the_Environmental_Affordances_Model_on_Depressive_Symptoms_and_Allostatic_Load

Nonprofit Trends and Impacts. (2021). Urban Institute. urban.org. Retrieved from https://www.urban.org/sites/default/files/publication/104889/nonprofit-trends-and-impacts-2021_1_0.pdf

NotYourMommasHistory. (2021, May 25). *A Day in the Life of an Enslaved Lady's Maid | These Roots Episode 1*[Video]. YouTube. Retrieved from https://www.youtube.com/watch?v=Zg94KjclLJo

Rabelo, V. C., Robotham, K. J., & McCluney, C. L. (2021). "Against a Sharp White Background": How Black Women Experience the White Gaze at Work. *Gender, Work and Organization, 28*(5), 1840–1858. https://doi.org/10.1111/gwao.12564

Sharpe, C. (2016). *In the Wake: On Blackness and Being*. Duke University Press.

Shorpy. (2020). *The Mammy Memorial: 1923*. Retrieved from https://www.shorpy.com/node/25367

Stahl, J. M. (Director). (1934). *The Imitation of Life* [Film]. Universal Pictures.

Stevenson, H., et al. (n.d.). *Racial Confrontations, Systemic Racism, and Vicarious Trauma: How to Help Clients Navigate Them* [Workshop]. National Institution for the Clinical Application of Behavioral Medicine (NICABM) [Host]. Retrieved from https://www.nicabm.com/program/trauma-racism/?itl=store

The Greenville News. (1918, October 2). Negro Women To Be Put To Work. *Newspapers.com*. Retrieved August 23, 2023, from https://www.newspapers.com/article/the-greenville-news-negro-women-to-be-pu/38314573/

The U.S. National Archives and Records Administration. (n.d.). *The Great Migration (1910–1970)*. National Archives. https://www.archives.gov/research/african-americans/migrations/great-migration

Thompson, R. (2021, October 29). #BlackWomenAtWork hashtag uncovers the everyday racism black women face at work. *Mashable*. Retrieved from https://mashable.com/article/black-women-at-work-hashtag

U.S.J. Dunbar, 6/27/23. (1923). [Photograph]. Retrieved from the Library of Congress https://www.loc.gov/item/2016847717/

Wikipedia Contributors. (2023). Slave Iron Bit. *Wikipedia*. Retrieved from https://en.wikipedia.org/wiki/Slave_iron_bit

Wilkerson, I. (2010). *The Warmth of Other Suns*. Random House.

Wilkerson, I. (2020). *Caste: The Origins of Our Discontents*. Random House.

Woods-Giscombé, C. (2010). Superwoman Schema: African American Women's Views on Stress, Strength, and Health. *Qualitative Health Research, 20*(5), 668–683.

14

Waking Up from Whiteness

Halina Pytlasinska, Nancy Blair, Els van Ooijen, Jennifer Ramsay, and Jane Ribbens McCarthy

Social dreaming is a way of 'thinking from the heart' that draws on earth wisdom: knowledge that is held between people and all species. If dreams hail from the interconnected fabric of the universe, sharing them can reveal knowledge beyond the bounds of the socially constructed ego and the White[1] European emphasis on intellect, analysis and theory. Social dreaming therefore has the potential to provide a decolonised view of life and society. The purpose of Western dream analysis tends to be the gaining of insights into the individual psyche. Shared dreaming, on the other hand, considers the greater societal and global picture and draws on intuition where knowledge lies in the relationship between people and all

[1] We have used 'black' and 'white' and 'whiteness' and 'black feminism' in lower case to be consistent in relation to social justice.

H. Pytlasinska (✉)
Buckinghamshire, UK
e-mail: halina@clipzonk.com

N. Blair
Dartmouth, Nova Scotia, Canada

G. Kinouani et al. (eds.), *Creative Disruption*, Studies in the Psychosocial,
https://doi.org/10.1007/978-3-031-63661-5_14

species. Thus, dreams may reveal systemic issues reflected in the individual and point to social injustice and environmental damage.

Concerned about climate crisis, loss of biodiversity and ecological emergency, the five of us are also aware of our privileges, in being white and having homes, food, water, education and loved ones around us. We have met weekly since February 2022. In this chapter we reflect on the work from our weekly social dreaming sessions and share what our dreams have taught us about the enmeshed issues of ecological crisis and racism.

We feel strongly that colonialism and racism lie at the heart of the climate crisis and ecological breakdown. Colonialism and racism are both rooted in an 'othering' of categories of people and non-human life that leads to profound and continuing destructive exploitation. When we heard about the proposed book on creative disruption, we agreed that sharing dreams collectively seems creatively disruptive. We wondered how social dreaming might develop our understanding of our inherent racism. Could this collective sharing of dreams, with the memories and associations inspired by them, help us to illuminate our whiteness and our white supremacy that may lie, hidden to us, in our psyches and very being-in-the-world? Could this dream work disrupt the cisheteropatriarchal system in which we live? Our desire is to 'wake up' to creative ways of being in the world to move us beyond the destructiveness of the white systems that continue to harm people of colour and the planet, our home. Inspired by our dreams we have developed a keen interest in a kinship worldview that aligns with indigenous perspectives. Can dream work help

---

E. van Ooijen
Bristol, UK
e-mail: els@nepenthe.org.uk

J. Ramsay
Madrid, Spain
e-mail: info@storyarte.com

J. R. McCarthy
The Open University, Aylesbury, UK

University of Bath, Bath, UK
e-mail: Jane.McCarthy@open.ac.uk

to enhance kinship values and enhance our ability to respect and interact with our planet and all other species as kin? We agreed to embark on this writing venture, although looking through the lens of creatively disrupting whiteness had not been our original purpose in coming together.

The process of writing a chapter with others is challenging. We struggle, at times, to find a collective voice. There are conflicts and differing points of view to be represented here. We wonder how far the trust and kinship bonds formed in the dream work will carry us through this process of writing collectively. In our co-created dream space, all differing perspectives naturally have sufficient room to intermingle, in ways that written words struggle to do.

Social Dreaming

In his development of Mpondo theory, Ka Canham discusses dreams as a significant part of *ukwakumkanya*, a central concept that drives Mpondo theorisation: 'Dreams link us to futures and pasts' (2023: 10). Nwoye explicitly contrasts the Eurocentric individualistic perspective on dreaming with the 'African dream perspective [that] recognizes … also the intriguing and interesting phenomenon of triangulation of the other in the context of dreaming and dream interpretation' (2017: 4).

As a group of white European women, however, without explicit thought we began from the methodology of social dreaming put forward by white male therapists familiar to us. Drawing from these ideas, our group uses social dreaming methodology where dreams are not about an individual dreamer, as in psychotherapy and counselling, but rather seen as wisdom from and about the collective. In social dreaming, the imaginative space co-created by the gathered dreamers is called a matrix. The matrix acts as a crucible for emerging dreams, and memories ignited by them. Once a dream is offered within the matrix, it no longer belongs to the dreamer but forms part of a dreamscape. A bricolage of dreams, memories, images and metaphors emerges. The fabric of the matrix morphs and grows, and acts like a window at times, or even a bird's eye view into society. The collective shenanigans of humankind and the impact of the Global North on the earth and all other species are revealed in the matrix. The dreams are not interpreted; the themes and knowledge need no interpretation (Lawrence, 2005). In social dreaming the focus is on the process of the matrix and where it will continue to lead.

The five of us take the bones of the social dreaming method and add our own ingredients. Into the mix we pour poetry, drawings, storytelling techniques and active imagination. At times we become dream symbols and dialogue in their voices. Through working together, the dream canvas that we co-create offers up fresh insights into the world we inhabit during the day. In the matrix, past and present comingle. Sometimes whiteness shows up, unobliterated by shame. We sit with powerlessness, hate and grief without being overwhelmed by feelings.

At times, we wonder where dreams come from. Is there perhaps a social unconscious, a space within which all of humanity is connected in a dreamscape, or parallel universe?[2] We wonder about this transpersonal space where humans may be one, connected to all of nature, including other species, the earth, the cosmos. Does the dreamworld connect us through a mycelium network? Dreams bloom from the rhizome to create the world; perhaps dreams form the roots of all creation. Previous researchers have experimented with social dreaming to address social and ecological problems that were too complex and overwhelming to be understood by individual minds (Manley & Crociani-Windland, 2018). Following this tradition, we wonder how aspects of social dreaming may help us to wake up to our whiteness.

Through freely associating to dreams, we sense a deep connection to earth, nature and each other. In one dream a white woman's head is slowly gliding along a librarian's desk, her face painted over with sticky pink nail varnish. Lacking energy, she dies. Curious, we explore the library through creative imaginings and speak with the head. How can a head survive without a body? Does this dream reflect a dissociation from the wisdom of the body and our animal being?

Through dreams, animals and plants call out. Their messages cut through habitual thinking. We ponder on the discomforts, the possibilities and limitations of this work.

[2] This differs from Jung's 'collective unconscious,' where Jung perceived a commonality of archetypal forces.

Introductions

We briefly introduce ourselves here before the dreamworld takes us beyond individuality to a collective.

Halina: I was motivated to begin a new dream group when my friend Jane shared a dream with me. I have paid attention to my dreams since childhood. Brought up in the city of Cambridge, in a Polish Irish household, the daughter of immigrants, I always felt an outlier. As therapist and trainer for thirty-two years I have facilitated many dream groups.

I learnt about racism in the playground of my primary school, where I saw a white boy being mean to a girl because her skin was black. As a teenager my father told me about the cruelty of the labour camps during the Second World War. In my late teens and twenties, I focused on radical politics, and feminism, marching in protest for CND, for social justice, and the release of Nelson Mandela. As a student in Bristol, I saw refugee artists from South Africa perform. While my peers immersed themselves in punk, I listened to jazz, blues, reggae and African music. Sam Cooke, Nina Simone, Bob Marley, Miriam Makeba, among others, these black musicians raised my awareness of my white conditioning.

Joining a social dreaming group during COVID-19 lockdown I 'woke up' to the urgency of climate crisis. It's as though white patriarchy has humankind under a spell. I want to recover from being spellbound. Will sharing dreams help?

Jane: My white English heritage is deeply rooted, across centuries, in the lives of rural labourers in Southern and West England, moving into the East End of London in the late nineteenth century. Class and gender shaped my early life. My childhood was spent in an affluent, and very white, commuter village in the Home Counties, but my own family were 'not out of the top drawer.' Somewhere along the way, I became dissatisfied with the world I lived in, and very curious about ways of life beyond my own, reading authors such as James Baldwin, Ralph Ellison and Elizabeth Gaskell. At university I was overwhelmed by the courage of a black South African man, shaking with nervousness in front of an audience of students, but determined to describe the inhuman apartheid systems in which he lived. As an adult, my experience expanded. I lived near

London, and worked through various professional roles, but remained largely unaware of the impact of racism and homophobia on a family friend of colour. I have lived through three marriages and have three children.

Over decades, I've become aware of how, both personally and professionally as an academic sociologist, my life has been shaped by the profoundly embedded English notion of 'the individual.' I have become increasingly aware of how this isolating rhetoric (fantasy?) obscures humanity's (and my own) experience of connectedness, and have explored differing approaches to understanding and experiencing our relationality. Climate activism in recent years has added a major urgency to understand the connectedness of all life, along with the imperative to understand the ways in which colonialism and racism are central to the crises we face, and the need to uncover my own whiteness.

In my late thirties, I discovered dream workshops, through a friend. These opened new windows into my soul, very different from the supremely rational, restrictive, disconnected world of English whiteness that I knew (Golding et al., in press). But in that earlier experience of dream work, held in loving group support, dreams were regarded as a window into the personal unconscious, a route into 'my own' 'individual interior.' Now in my 70s, the idea that dreaming could become a shared collective and emergent experience has been entirely novel, outside the ken of my narrow individualised white heritage.

Nancy: From my home in Halifax Harbour, I see the ocean, as an everyday part of my life. Now 70, I have worked in social justice, environment and therapy. I expect to spend the rest of my life working with others who want to build a world where all kin, human and other-than-human have their rightful place. Having experienced many years of Jungian dream analysis, listening to dreams has been a regular part of my life.

Over the past years, in Nova Scotia, I have experienced Hurricane Fiona, wildfires and floods. Living and working with two retired greyhound racers, Tyson and Taurus, inspired me to found the Animal Assisted Therapist in Counselling Chapter of the CCPA. Through working as a Pet Loss and Bereavement Counsellor I have seen how humans are shocked by their grief for the loss of a beloved pet. In my work as a

Climate Therapist, individuals express the same terrible feelings around the loss of our other-than-human kin.

Being in a social dreaming matrix is very comfortable for me, even when there are challenging and difficult issues. The dream matrix is not quite what I expected it to be, it is a unique place. The idea that all the dreams shared belong to all in the circle, took some getting used to. I became more myself in the dream circle as time went by. After sharing dreams, I feel grounded, and much more able to do the work I am called to do.

Els: Growing up during the 1940s and 1950s in post-war Nederland I had a ragdoll made from old black nursing stockings, yet my childhood was very white. Despite having been a nurse, therapist and trainer for many years, with a relational, embodied and meditative approach to therapy, for much of my life I fitted into Helms' (1990) 'Contact' state of white racialisation, regarding myself as colourblind.

George Floyd's shocking murder in 2020 tumbled me into a state of cognitive dissonance, or what Helms might call 'Disintegration' (Helms, 2019). The casual way in which the young white policeman kept his knee on Floyd's neck, ignoring the gasps 'I can't breathe' is still imprinted on my brain. I asked myself, 'Did I really not get that it truly is this bad?' Now I am running to catch up with what I should have realised decades ago: that as a white European woman I am part of the problem because, until recently, I had avoided the conscious knowledge of having swallowed a worldview of white superiority.

Always fascinated by dreams, I learnt much from a weekly Jungian dream group attended for two years. I greatly value the communal space of our current Social Dreaming group where whatever comes up is accepted and valued. It allows me to let go of defenses and let in truths that were previously unwelcome.

Jennifer: I was born in Scotland. The circumstances of my childhood led me to take refuge in the wonderful world of books.

After studying Biological Sciences, I travelled the world, where I became influenced by Rock Art in Australia and world mythology. Finally, I settled in Spain and had two sons with my partner. As our sons grew, so too did my desire to paint the ancient narratives from myths. This desire led me to become a professional storyteller. Twenty years on, stories are still at the centre of my personal and professional life. I truly believe that these ancestral tales are treasures, a legacy from the ancestors, encoded with wisdom.

As well as Gestalt Eco therapy and Art therapy, I studied Symbolic Psychodrama of Fairy Tales and dreams. I believe that both fairy tales and dreams are part of the same symbolic language, a language forgotten by many. In this social dreaming circle, many of the dreams are like stories I have been working on. I feel often that Nature is calling out to me in dreams, asking for help and support. I carry forward these dream messages through storytelling.

I grew up in Glasgow, where the names of 62 streets are linked to the slave trade. The city prospered from the import of goods the slaves produced, like sugar and tobacco. But my memories talk of the division between Catholics and Protestants in the city. Local newspapers were always full of the conflict between Celtic and Rangers football supporters and the loud Orange Walks deafened out issues around racism for me. My first real personal awakening to racism was when my mum refused to meet my Sri Lankan boyfriend and would not have him in the house. I could never have imagined that my mum was racist.

We seek to acknowledge the pain white supremacy and racism cause people of colour. Being immersed in the shared activity of social dreaming we stop being limited as individual thinkers, to sometimes more clearly see the destructive patterns and structures that white systems create. Below we share specific dreams that illustrate aspects of this experience. The relationships between the dream symbols and how they are represented in drawing reveal the racism we carry from the society we have lived.

Invitation to Reader

We invite you to read our dreams slowly, with attention, and notice what comes up in you as you read.

Dreaming Ourselves Awake to Unacknowledged Racism

'We have forgotten that we have forgotten who we are.'
Jennifer Ramsay

1st Dream

I am living in a large house with a male partner and other visitors, doing workshops together. My partner and I have conversations about being separate or together in the house. We can carry on sharing things, or we can buy things like milk and yogurt separately. Can we live more separate? All the people go for a walk together. I can see them through the windows walking up a hill outside. There are many stairs in the house, large banisters and my bra hangs on this. Upstairs there is a kitchen area and downstairs in the basement there are rooms, not currently used.

There is another even grander house, up the hill.

2nd Dream

I am a Japanese woman on a train, my breasts are bare, I wear flowing robes, and have a small penis. A black woman decides to share my bed. I think no, there is no room. The bed is beautiful, but extremely narrow. There is no room for her but she comes in anyway, I feel invaded and push her out.

There are mannequins created to take the place of people. Each couple is given a mannequin. People do not have sex with partners, only with the allocated mannequin.

Invitation

What was going on for you as you read these dreams? What thoughts, memories, ideas, reactions came up for you?

Our Responses

'The mannequins replacing people reminds me of a really painful conversation I had at the time with a black friend about the historical connotations of gollywogs—the dangerous baddies in childhood Noddy books.'

'Remember the racist plantation minstrel or gollywog symbol on marmalade jars?' (Bale, 2017; Guy, 2021).

'I really missed the little man when it was discontinued—I had no idea about anything derogatory growing up. As a child I had no idea that it was racist.'

'The pain that symbol caused black people. The pain of enslaved lives.'

'The large house in the dream reminds me of Upstairs Downstairs?'

'I loved that programme.'

'I wonder what life would have been really like in those households?'

'Pretty dire I should think. You needed to know your place.'

'Perhaps boundaries were needed, to tolerate the intimate proximity between servants and family member?'

'It also reminds me of the young, unwed Irish girls who were sent to convents to work in laundries if they fell pregnant. Also, the bodies of eight hundred children, found in the basement of one convent.'

As we share, one woman draws a picture of the dreams and associations (Fig. 14.1).

'You've left out the black woman and the Japanese woman.'

'I don't know how to draw them. Oh, hang on, I did draw the white woman.'

'In the drawing, our white group excludes the women of colour.'

'That reminds me. I had a dream where my mother did not want two black women inside, she pushed them out!'

'The drawing shows what is revealed and what is hidden.'

'The gaps between the dreamer's experience of the dream and its partial representation in the drawing reveal racism.'

'The dreams cut through our sense of shame about our hidden racism so that it can acknowledged openly between us.'

'There's a sense of verticality in the first dream. Is that perhaps symbolic of status, power over others?'

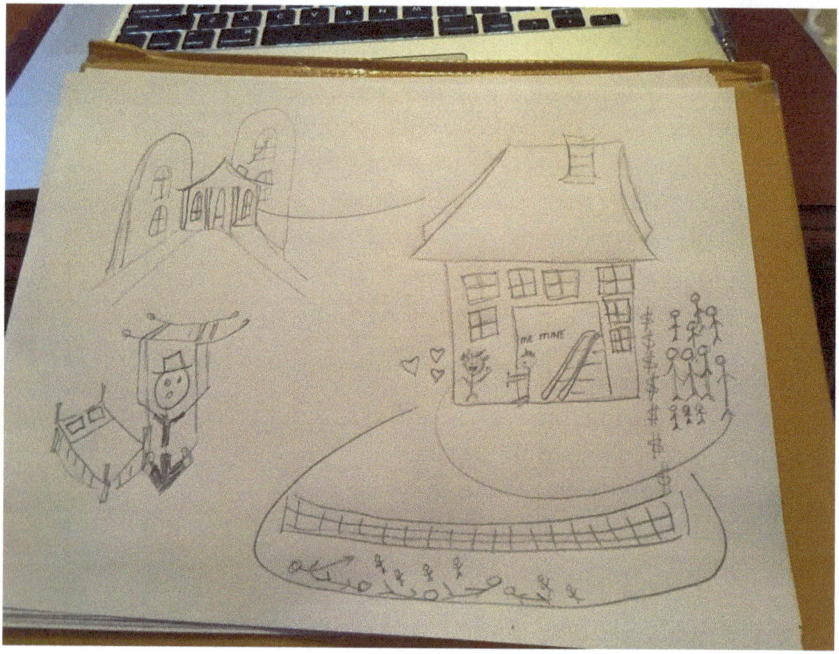

Fig. 14.1 As we share, one woman draws a picture of the dreams and associations

'And what about the small penis, that was not drawn either.'

'Are we denying our inner masculine?'

'Another hidden thread.'

'Are we avoiding our inner white patriarchal aspect?'

'What about the bra? Is it perhaps a symbol of feminine power?'

'The way the dreams and associations are captured on the page. The boundary drawn as a barrier of dollar signs appears to indicate a rift between the few people in the house and the crowd left outside. There is a lone mannequin on the bed, but the women are absent. It has taken the place of real women.'

'The words "me and mine" have been drawn between the couple.'

'A theme of ownership.'

'Control and ownership are core to the white colonial mindset.'

'The stairs looks like a slide.'

'Who is sliding out of responsibility, or out of sight?'

'The house with the white people has many windows.'

'The white privileged surveying the landscape.'

'Eerily, it looks like the house is built upon the dead babies.'

'Colonial Britain built on the backs of slavery. The white people have the space to consider their purchasing power.'

'The words "me and mine" and how ownership can impede relationship, as couples squabble over finances and status.'

'A line connects the woman in the picture to the crowd of people outside.'

'This line slices through the dollars.'

'Status, division, racism, sexism, and classism, the false separation that is at the heart of colonialism.'

'In the centre of the picture are three beating hearts.'

'Children were killed, historically, when the mother was unmarried.'

'The narrow bed from the dream becomes a double bed in the picture, perhaps reflecting white privilege.'

'White children play with dolls called gollywogs that denigrate black people. Women become sex objects with mannequin status. The theme of sex addiction—unvalidated feelings give rise to addiction.'

'Are we addicted to whiteness?'

'At times, as white women, we can "forget" about racism.'

'The presence of the bed reminds me of the fetishisation of black women.'

'At the 2014 Edinburgh Festival Brett Bailey's Exhibit B showed black performers in a glass cabinet, chained to a bed and standing stock-still while the audience walked around them, to recreate the colonial exploitation and exhibiting of black bodies including a grotesque display of Saartjie Baartman, known as the "Hottentot Venus." The show received excellent reviews in spite of recreating the denigrating circumstances of a human zoo and fetishisation of black women'. 'Objectification is how white people understand their relationship to black people'.

'I knew I had a train dream to share but couldn't remember it. After the group I found the dream in my journal and am struck by the similarities. Another case of buried racism and leaving out a woman from a different culture.'

The dream is emailed to the rest of the group in the morning.

Indian Hotel and Station

> I travel to India. The train station is derelict, British colonial, red brick like a university building. The passengers and I can't work out how to use the station, how do we catch the train, which platform do we need? Eventually, we figure out which platform to go to and gain access to a Raj hotel that is semi-disorganised but luxurious. We are given glass box rooms. I worry about room privacy then notice they have curtains. My young Indian female friend and I are offered luxurious spa treatments, where we lie-down on our hotel bed, a double bed that we share, our heads float in water. The water is scented and adorned with petals. I am excited about the opportunity of the waterbed spa. It feels such a beautiful custom.
>
> We are going to travel together but tarry awhile in the spa. We have to go to the same platform each day to continue our journey. There is always a loop of travellers searching through the dereliction for the platform and the journey forward. I hold key information on the platform. A wealthy white male entrepreneur is keen on acquiring my knowledge.

'An Indian woman, and a whole culture is left out of the matrix.'

'The glass box in this dream reminds us of the glass ceiling, separating men and women's pay.'

'The glass box could expose white privilege, and yet there are flimsy curtains, obscuring privilege still.'

'White gaze, the unacknowledged racism to simply not see people of colour.'

'When face recognition software was first invented, there were issues with the software because it was invented by white people and only recognised the features of white faces.'

'Our dreams are full of white people, contrasting with the reality of the term 'global majority.''

'At school, because of the way history is taught, I believed that most of the people in the world are white, with people of colour as the exception when in fact, white people are the global minority.'

'The proportions of classroom world maps were distorted in the 1960s, shrinking the continents of Africa and Asia and falsely enlarging the UK.'

'Dream sharing has lessened my white fragility and sense of embarrassment, so I can more clearly perceive and work with my racism.'

'Robin DiAngelo states how shame can overwhelm and motivate white people to further collude with systems of oppression' (DiAngelo, 2019).

'Guilt is sometimes a healthy response, that supports collective respect.'

'I wonder if shame on the other hand is unhealthy, arising from a notion of self that is conditioned by colonial thinking.'

'From a Gestalt perspective, it is part of the top-dog/underdog splitting that prevents authenticity.'

'An aspect of control and domination?'

'I feel guilt, as well as shame about racism.'

'Following that social dreaming matrix, in a client session I was able to honestly declare my previously denied racism without hiding it or feeling too ashamed to own up to it. It was as if the matrix dug this stuff out of me and placed it on the table for all to see.'

'Focusing on my own guilt and shame does not help anyone. Like Dabiri writes, it's what I or we do now that is important.'

During one session we decide to use active imagination to investigate our colonial binds.

'Metal bands inside and around me that dig into my body, restricting movement.'

'I see a giant cement block precariously hovering above me, while feeling boulders and stones in my belly.'

'A metal framework inside me that looks like an oil rig.'

Experienced in using imagery to work with trauma, we seek now to escape from these colonial images of prison. We are aware that black activists rightfully criticise white people for focusing on their own inner work instead of taking action. We discuss how this inner work is the first step towards taking action but not the end result.

'I use a wrench to undo the bolts, then I beam the metal cage out of my body.'

We share books by indigenous academics and black authors. Reading authors like Emma Dabiri and Kehinde Andrews we are more aware of the continual denial of the racism that exists in the UK. Sharing dreams and reflections strengthens our political views and sense of power. As white women dream-sharing enhances a desire to speak out against racism, listen to indigenous peoples and build coalition with people of colour. Together we nurture caring values from black feminism.

Different Worldviews: Kinship Versus Colonial

Invitation

We invite you to be involved with our dreams, to read them slowly, with attention, and notice what comes up in you as you read.

The Grass Dream

Asleep, aware that I am dreaming. On a road that runs along the top of the hill, near Gros Morne in Newfoundland. A narrow road leads towards cabins, there are no people. The grass on the hill is beautiful, very green. Sunny and perfect weather, so still. At the bottom of the hill, there is a wide stretch of water. On the other side of the bay, there are more hills. I am filled with gratitude for the gift of being. I give thanks to whoever called me here. And wake.

A little later this was followed by a waking dream.

I am standing on the hill and looking at the grass. Seven or eight figures are rising from the grass, people shaped, but not human. No eyes or ears or mouths but they are clearly communicating with each other. Three come towards me. They are grass; in and of the grass, not separate but wading through it. Three come towards me. They are beautiful and I am very much at peace. They touch me and I am being drawn down into the grass. I am with them but still myself, a human. For a moment I wonder if I am dying because I am being taken into the ground. But I am not dying. It is very relaxing and calming. I trust them completely. Then I wonder if the bugs will crawl into me and maybe bite me and eat me. It seems not; anyway, I am not bothered by that. I feel very cared for.

A sense of wonder pervades the group on this evening. The dream inspires an outpouring from all. We share moments of connection with trees that had felt magical. A time being filled with light in a forest. The emotion of meeting a First Nation woman in Canada, who beat a drum and sang to the trees in gratitude before taking the dreamer into the forest. A memory is shared of hearing the trees sing.

A dream is shared where fungus is eaten allowing the dreamer to understand other languages. Another dream is about the Amazon Forest and the river.

'The grass dream is saying that if we listen to plants carefully then we would be able to more fully understand each other.'

The Robin Dream

> 'Eco therapists work together in a bright room with large windows and countryside views. An old friend spills water. The clumsiness seems unforgiveable, although the lack of forgiveness threatens the friendship. A dog is presented for adoption. Then it splits in half, I retract my love for the creature. A robin flies into the room. The robin is on fire. I want to help the bird but don't know how to catch it without burning my hands.'

'Was the fire that burnt the robin caused by humans?'

We share memories of burnout.

'Fire that is warming and life affirming when contained, but lethal when out of control.'

'The bird might have been saved if the water hadn't been spilt.'

'Is the dream a caution not to waste water, or perhaps a lesson in compassion?'

'Perhaps the dream foreshadows the fires and floods across the world caused by Anthropocene climate change?'

'Animals often visit the dreaming matrix to warn of ecological damage, social injustice and racism.'

'The room in the dream is Yasmin Kapadia's, who writes about kinship' (Holding the Hope, 2023, p. 155). 'We discuss the theme of becoming ill when burnt out.' 'We explore how racism causes damage to human bodies through the tyranny of hierarchical working systems.'

'White patriarchy creates powerful distinctions based on features of human bodies.'

'Categories like racism and shadism, bend everyone out of shape.'

Thinking with the Heart to Decolonise the Mind

The grass dream motivates us to read indigenous writers like Robin Wall Kimmerer (Kimmerer, 2015), who speak about a sense of kinship with the earth and mutual reciprocity. We feel drawn to the kinship view that humankind, animals, plants, rocks, indeed the entire world is in relationship (Topa & Narvaez, 2022). Social dreaming allows room for expansion, complexity and uncertainty; an infinite field of possibility instead of the often too rigid, rational and deductive way of white colonial thinking. The liminal space of the social dreaming matrix is inclusive, welcoming diversity and contradictions.

Tiokason Ghosthorse, a member of the Lakota people in North America, writes that indigenous people think from the heart. The white patriarchal view, however, sees the human intellect as king and humans as superior to other species (Hausdoerffer et al., 2021). We realise that colonial thinking produces hierarchical systems. When the spirit of the land is no longer recognised, it becomes a thing for extractivism to feed a monstrous consumerism (Ward, 2020).

Shawanda and Manitowabi (2023) recommend that indigenous dreaming methodologies provide a decolonial perspective and can make the unknown known. Indigenous dream work furnishes a gateway to sacred knowledge from the ancestors, to be shared with elders to reveal the ethereal or spirit world that is an interconnected web with all life. Such indigenous dream methodologies can provide a glimpse into the future, offer guidance towards paths that have been lost and deepen understanding of psychological disharmony.

'Race' or 'whiteness' are manufactured constructs, with powerful consequences even while they don't actually exist. Through dreams we realise the interconnection of everything: climate change, racism, capitalism, ethics, grief and mortality. We want to shed our white individuality and become part of the shared collectivity of all life and living beings. During and after the social dreaming group members feel more awake, at peace in the body, a sense that impacts held beliefs and identities. Perhaps this is what Tiokasin Ghosthorse calls 'knowing through the earth' (Ghosthorse, 2023).

Inspired by research and writings from indigenous academics we respect their profound customs and wisdom with an awareness of the dangers of misappropriation. We wonder about our own indigenous roots. In the Middle Ages, people listened to and shared dreams readily (Wellesley, 2018). Perhaps the 'Enlightenment' caused European indigenous worldviews to be banished to the margins? Could we find continuing resonances through dreams? Jennifer studies Druid teachings, Jane attends the 'gathering' of silent Quaker meetings, Els practises Zen meditation and shamanic journeying, Halina practices yoga and chi gong. Nancy honours the original inhabitants of her homeland, Mi'kma'ki, the ancestral and unceded territory of the Mi'kmaq People. We feel the need for a new narrative not based on colonialism, extraction, competition and the acquisition of stuff. We ask, 'Where is our origin? Are the ancestors speaking through the dreams?'

We often ask our dreams for help, but sometimes receive nightmares that illuminate truths buried in the daylight hours. We remember the vision of the head in the library or dreaming being bitten by a snake. When nightmares wake us in shock, they show us what we do not notice in waking life. Damage that we ignore shows up in dreams. Animals call out warnings. We listen to the cries of the wild and strengthen our kinship bonds with other species.

The wisdom gleaned from dreams is shown through the relationships between dream symbols and the emotions evoked when shared in the matrix. A tapestry emerges between dreams and the emotions and associations they evoke. An everchanging ecosystem is created. We experience how all knowledge is unearthed through relationships. The matrix reminds us of the larger network that connects all of life.

'I am because we are' (African proverb expressing Ubuntu.)

Connectedness with All Species, and the Elements

Dream Fragment

'First we were larvae, then we were a body, then we get feathers.'

This poetic and mysterious dream fragment seems to suggest a new story of evolution. The wording is precise. The dream suggests that humanity is merely a phase, not an ultimate goal. We may be reborn as birds.

'We believe in the Global North that we are at the top of the hierarchy.'

'How would we interact with other species if we didn't feel entitled and superior?'

'The pollution of the seas. Anthropocene damage. How it might change if we view all species as equal, as kin.'

'The animal kingdom features strongly in our dreams.'

'Perhaps the animals are sending dream messages, demanding the people of the Global North wake up to Anthropocene damage.'

'This concept that animals are calling to them turned their human-centric views inside-out.'

'In a dream, humans are performing, dogs and a polar bear come to watch. The humans begin to panic but the dreamer says, "there's no need, the animals are simply curious and will not harm you."'

'Another dream features a horse that is stuck in a hedge; trapped on a boundary. In a different dream an elephant dressed ceremonially, becomes a bed. The dreamer climbs up with her husband to drink poison from a vial, she has to transmute the poison, her husband follows suit. Families appear in another dream where an ape is adopted, the dreamer and ape say they love each other.'

'As we expand our worldview to recognise a kinship with other species, through these dreams, white supremacy is duly challenged.'

'The absolute secret of the universe that I heard speaking to me in a dream'—'it's the spaces in between that count.'

'Does the dreamworld illuminate a different identity for us?'

'Instead of seeing ourselves as individuals, are we the space between everything? The background rather than the individual organisms?'

'Other cultures see animals as human ancestors.'

Penelope, from Ancient Greek mythology, believed her husband would return from the Trojan wars and her heart remained faithful to him. When pressed to choose a new partner, she promised that she would once she had completed a tapestry burial shroud for Odysseus' father Laertes. During the day she wove, but at night she unpicked her stiches to ensure the tapestry shroud would never be completed. She managed to sustain this deception for three years until a slave, Melantho, reported it to the suitors.

Like Penelope, the dream matrix seems to unpick the whiteness woven throughout our lives. By night, dreams loosen the threads of our colonial views and weave long-lost indigenous values of kinship. Mutual respect sews fresh tapestries; egalitarian principles thread new beliefs that do not need unpicking!

'A voice from a dream advises, "Maybe we can all take meds."'

'Big Pharma is embedded in this white colonial system.'

'Medicating ourselves against feeling the pain that colonialism inflicts?'

These powerful dream words creatively dampen the voice of white patriarchy that subtly and inevitably dominates us still. We have an inspired discussion around the topics of control and domination that lie at the heart of a colonial mindset. People in the Global North are often medicated or inebriated to deal with the stresses and exhaustion from the workplace. The neo-liberal managerialism of recent decades regards control and measurement of the individual as core for contemporary business practices and organisational management. If the unconscious is like the warp and weft that holds thoughts together, the warp may be the wild heart or indigenous worldview of a person in the Global north, the weft their social conditioning or patriarchal worldview that sustained whiteness.

Our dreams constantly challenge the notion of individuality. First Nations' people's way of being does not separate a person from the earth or other species. Connectedness is embraced. Similarly, the South African concept of 'ubuntu,' loosely translated to mean, 'I am because we are,' illustrates the importance of mutuality and being bound up with others. The Hindu story of Indra's Jewel Net where humans are all jewels, their facets reflecting all others, also describes connectedness. From a different context altogether, quantum physicist Karen Barad theorises about relationality in the social sciences in ways that recognise all categorisation as contingent, with the discursive and the material performing the world into being through their intra-actions (discussed by Ribbens McCarthy et al., 2023).

In indigenous worldviews, being-ness is experienced relationally. Personhood is not based in a separated embodied individuality, but in collective relationships—which in affluent Anglophone countries may be primarily experienced in domestic life and expressed through the language of 'family' (Ribbens McCarthy, 2012). From an indigenous perspective this relationality is experienced not only with human brothers and sisters but also in kinship with other species, in mutual reciprocity with the elements, with the sun, rivers, wind, in being earth.

Dream Sharing Generates Trust

Meeting regularly builds our trust. We share dreams of disrupted voyages and of communal spaces: public houses, trains, swimming pools, hotels, walled cities and castles. Over time, we grow fond of each other's gifts and talents. The space between us remains flexible, stretched now and then, to allow room for each voice to be heard.

We become liberated from the burden of carrying knowledge alone. Through sharing dreams, we bear witness to what is denied and avoided. Unspoken fears, designated to 'the back of the attic,' find a voice. We open our hearts to each other and share overwhelming and traumatic stories from the Lebanon; fears about ecological crisis; deep-seated grief; the loss of loved ones; the pain of living with cancer.

Social dreaming unveils white confidence to reveal vulnerability. We move towards kincentricism (Topa & Narvaez, 2022, p. 3), an earth-based consciousness, appreciating each other, different communities and the more-than-human world as kin. Three of us join a black feminist reading group. Els notices how she feels in relationship with her house-plants, not just seeing them as something pretty to have around. We often wonder how our dream-sharing impacts other humans, although there is no real way of measuring this.

Being Earth

Dream-sharing induces an intense sense of belonging.

'We simply know for a moment that all belongs to us because we belong to all' (D.H. Lawrence).

Dream fragments highlight the group's intimate connection with the more-than-human world:

'Ancient creatures are stirring in the bowels of the earth. Powerful and scary. Maybe they are the saviours, and they need to do away with us.'

'I have rich green earth under my feet, and I am almost stepping on sleeping baby hares with my big human feet, not even realizing they were in the same "room" as me all the time.'

'My house plant calls out, the earth between us is not solid, (I realise she needs help when I wake up and repot her).'

'A forest of baby elephants sits in the sea, they are under water and their trunks are straight up breathing the air. Nearby a tiny dinosaur falls off the shelf into the sea.'

'*Dreams featuring plants and animals centre the us in their bodies and help us to connect with our instincts and animal being*' (Abram, 2011).

In the poem, 'To learn from Animal Being,' John O' Donohue prays that Europeans learn to be in touch with their animal senses, so that we can,

> 'Feel the earth
> Breathing with us.'
> John O'Donohue (2008)

Recognising other species as kin, we share:
'I sing with the blackbird in the garden.'

'And I sing a response to the robins.'

'Instead of asking my dreams for help I begin to wonder how we can serve the natural world. I ask other species, 'what can I give you?' Instead of 'what can I get from you?'

Through receiving a dream gift, collectively we can explore how we can use it wisely for the common good of all species, perhaps taking us towards a coalition beyond allyship towards being accomplices' (Dabiri, 2021).

'The elements have featured strongly in our dreams, appearing as flood, fire, earthquake, storm across hills, rivers and seas. Dreams connect us to the sacredness of the land, to the aliveness, power and soul of it. It is not a dead thing to be dug and exploited.'

Synchronicity Leads the Way to a New Language

White European languages (Kimmerer, 2015; Jullien, 2008/2014) create a world of objects that become a basis for division, othering and ruthless exploitation. Indigenous languages are relational, using verbs that animate the world rather than nouns that categorise it (Topa & Narvaez, 2022). Dreams speak through pictures, bizarre stories, metaphor, intense emotions, evocative sensory imagery. Dream language is actively relational. Immersing ourselves in the language of dreams transforms our everyday thinking patterns and disrupts the rationality of whiteness.

'I like the sessions where we focus on movement and action in the dreams.'

'Yes, transported by car, train, or even a plane.'

'This mirrors the way we are moving in waking life, or how society is moving or stuck, like flying too high or moving in unison on public transport.'

'Remember the dream about a bicycle deeply stuck in mud?'

'Yes, shows society's entrenched values, perhaps reflecting colonial thinking that is stuck, trapping the wheels of sustainability and inhibiting momentum.'

'Through dream sharing, we have become more aware of synchronicities. When animals appear in dreams and in waking life, we pay attention. Remember the time we shared dreams of bees online, Jennifer's room is invaded by a giant hornet!'

'And the day after the dream about a green comet appeared in the matrix, I read about a green asteroid circling.'

'As people of colour inhabit our dreams more freely, opportunities appear, unexpectedly and repeatedly, to collaborate with people of colour on decolonising work.'

'During one phase, white animals appear in our dreams and waking life. We see white stags, rare albino leopards, and a white dove covered in blood.'

'Last night I dreamt the surface of a face falls away in chunks like white plaster. Whiteness that masks our identity is crumbling.'

Dream

> We live in a community. There is a large drawing room, regency with old brocade curtains. My husband is delighted that this old boardroom will be adapted to teach young people. A young couple appears. The young woman comes to me because writing has appeared on her body overnight, like her whole body is tattooed with paragraphs from a book. The writing creates stories, but all the chapters are mixed up. She doesn't know whether she should share the writing with her partner. And if she does, she doesn't know where to start.

'My voice' in the dream reassures her, 'It doesn't matter where you begin. Just trust the process. Where you will begin will be the right place.'

'It feels like we are following the dreams guidance in how we write this chapter.'

'It's a chaotic and circular processes of discovery rather than following linear or cartesian logic.'

We think about how dreams join up across the sessions.

'The dream about a head in a library contrast with this dream of the woman's body tattooed with the book chapters.'

'Perhaps the two dreams represent the two approaches, indigenous versus colonial, intuitive, and relational versus patronising and hierarchical?'

'I'm slowly reading a book called Riotous Deathscapes by Hugo Ka Canham, proposing Mpondo theory based in Eastern Cape South Africa, as an alternative way of theorising from people and landscapes. Just came across a reference to "collective memories scripted on bodies" which resonates so strongly with the dream of the book written on a woman's body.'

Conclusion: What Is Dead? Or Perhaps 'What Needs to Die?'

Invitation

And once again, we invite you to read the following dream slowly, notice the associations that come to mind.

Dream

> A display case, large, vertical. Inside is a very large orange snake, dead. I am at a wedding reception, with people who are prosperous, considerably more affluent than me and my relatives who could benefit from introductions to these people. I want my mother who has died. I can't cope with all the socialising and I leave the group. One of the well-heeled hosts finds me and tries to persuade me to re-join the gathering. Although I know my children may benefit, I am in too much pain of loss to re-join the group. I wake with enormous pain in my body.

'The sense of obligation to fit in for social gain, in the dream, reflects a social pressure. Snakes are symbolic of transformation and healing. They can also represent treason. Our dream matrix shows how white patriarchal conditioning, betrays us by blocking the expression of a more loving and just society.'

'This huge snake is dead.'

'How would we feel if it was a relative, murdered and on display?'

'It is a large orange snake, not indigenous to the British Isles.'

'This life has been extinguished and contained, just as British museums and old mansions are full of encased dead animals from colonial history.'

'Reminds me of colonial theft of artwork and treasures that have not yet been returned to Indigenous peoples.'

'The snake is killed and taken from their environment, without respect.'

'By the great white hunter.'

'And the colonial practice of taxidermy, displaying creatures under glass domes.'

'Disgusting—animals, insects and birds as curiosities.'

'The Rothschild family museum is full of these stuffed animals. The white coloniser controlling nature.'

'And people, African people taken as slaves, put on display.'

'Modern slavery.'

'Wealthy white cities where people of colour serve in bars and restaurants.'

'My partner, tied to his desk each day, trapped in working hard for a corporate system that he does not agree with.'

'What deadness has the Global North enshrined that we need to let go?'

'The world needs to escape the oppressions, the narrowness, the rigidity, and the disconnectedness of whiteness.'

'Colonial views hasten us towards death. Yet, in the Global North we uphold white, colonial values and cling to outmoded beliefs and business as usual to avoid the pain of racism and the continued ecological disaster that "we" in affluent minority worlds impose on the Global South.'

'The ecological crisis is a continuation of colonialism.'

Our dreams shed light on the misguided beliefs of the Global North. The act of dream-sharing without a pre-determined goal is disruptive. It has created a deep bond between us that strengthens our resolve to address racism and wake up from our whiteness.

Dream

I am in a big kitchen with a sofa bed.

Beside me in the sofa bed is my brother (I feel that he is not my blood brother and I am male). I have a little bit of envy towards my brother, not much, but it is present.

> There is another man nearby who has lots of envy. Right beside our sofa bed is an old sailing ship. I am half asleep but watch this man who is full of envy climb up the sails. As he reaches the top, he pours boiling hot oil on us. I am awake, I escape, my brother dies in the boiling hot oil. I feel guilty, I have done something wrong as I did not save my brother.

'This dream leaves a deep impression. We feel stunned. We did not save our brother—he was killed by the oil! Oil is killing us all!'

'Social dreaming is having a deep impact on all of us. Unconsciously, whiteness is an attempt to split off good from bad and identify with the good. The light is white. The dark is black. Patriarchy is founded on the illusion of control that keeps this split as a universal wounding. Each white individual needs to wake up from the (unconscious) illusion that prejudice will protect us from our own sense of toxic shame and keep us safe from harm.'

The Process of Writing

At times writing about our journey feels inauthentic, like capturing and displaying animals. We try to be respectful, but words evoke a controlling mindset, so we decide that it is healthier to share dreams than concepts.

Whereas excited about translating our experiences into print, we also worry that something may change or get lost. Jennifer says that as a storyteller she does not resonate with writing, preferring the immediacy of the spoken word. Nancy wonders whether in writing, we are colonising our dreams.

Overall, sharing dreams and writing this chapter together has been an experience from which we continue to learn so much:

Els: I have learned to trust the space and whatever emerges; during our sessions it is such a relief to let go of left-brain rationality and play in the large right brain pond with who or whatever swims in there too. It has pivoted me into a new direction that I feel very excited about. Yes, acknowledging my white racialisation is also painful and often embarrassing, but that is no reason not to carry on. In the black reading group, I joined I am learning so much, black and white—we can learn and achieve much more together.

Halina: I feel an inner shift through this dream sharing towards an embodied understanding. Either I can be in control through colonial thinking, or I can be in relationship, embracing the unknown, open to learning and living fully. New layers of rage emerge about racism. Sorrow at the pain caused by the great violations and the daily microaggressions. A new humility to reach out and explore. I feel motivated to form coalition with people of colour. Complacency is not an option. I need to educate myself and work with people of colour to nurture kinship, an alternative system to whiteness.

Nancy: Working with our group in the dream matrix, I experience the wisdom of the collective. This means that I sometimes understand and feel the painful awareness of racism and colonialism in myself. I am now finding it easier to recognise and respond to racism and colonialisation as I encounter them in myself and others in my day-to-day life. This means that I am more able to recognise, to name, and to live in a space where I can live outside the painful and shameful constraints of that conditioning. I am also increasingly able to move into action against racism and colonialism.

Jane: Such a new experience of sharing and connection, experiencing the collective unconscious, dissolving 'inner' and 'outer,' 'individual' and 'collective,' moving out and beyond conventional knowing and expression. I greatly value working with *our* group of white women *who I've come to know in a completely new way*, and would also value shared dreaming with a group with diverse racialisation and heritage. When I participate in black-led groups I often benefit from learning how much my whiteness restricts my experience of living. But then I consider that this work is not (should not be? primarily?) about me, or is that another form of unhelpful/unnecessary white guilt? I reflect on the philosophy of Ubuntu: 'I am because we are,' even as I'm conscious of the risk of cultural appropriation.

Jennifer: I experienced a sense of wonder of how rich our collective dreamworld is and how often it paralleled our collective experience in the outer world. In many of our dreams, the natural world was very present. I was conscious that sometimes we found ourselves thinking that perhaps the animals or plants had a message for us. Maybe they were actually reaching out for help or understanding, as if even in the world of dreams we are colonisers. This has positively affected my relationship with the natural world and the more than human beings that inhabit her.

'Ultimately, this dream work is not about us as individual white women but the broader social systems in which we live. It is a reflection on white supremacy and the systemic racism that exists in society. Social dreaming is an embodied experience of Critical Race Theory' (Delgado & Stefancic, 2012).

'Decolonising work is painful.'

'For white people we take back the projection and grow the strong backbone to speak out against whiteness.'

'As women we strengthen each other and draw on sisterhood, black feminism and social justice.'

'Through sharing dreams we nurture compassion. A desire to act and be transparent about the pain that white supremacy causes people of colour.'

'In every moment the universe offers the opportunity to acknowledge this pain and respond to people with brown and black skin.'

'Each in our own continuing work we work to dismantle whiteness and co-create kinship.'

Social dreaming offers space for complex global issues such as racism and climate emergency that cannot be fully grasped by analytical thinking. The matrix allows a creative flow of dream language and intuited knowledge to emerge. Through dream sharing the threads of connectivity between people and all nature are more available for recognition. In this way, social dreaming nurtures holistic views and respects natural rather than white-man-made laws. At times the intellect may feel dissatisfied with social dreaming as it challenges white thinking and penetrates the sometimes invisible and damaging veneer of colonial domination.

In her recent book, Jennifer Mullan (2023) has stated the need for therapists to acknowledge the oppression and historical trauma of colonialism. Social dreaming is a method that can enhance a politicised practice.

And Finally

As we stated at the beginning, we did not set out to research whiteness, but it happened. We did not set out to share dreams about other species, but they spoke to us. While we are working on this chapter the following dream is shared:

Dream

> I went to the toilet and was surprised at the amount of excrement I had produced. I flushed the toilet and a big part was floating. As I looked closer, it seemed to have the form of a little face on one side. I flushed again and it didn't go away, I realised it could actually be an embryo and I should pick it up and not flush it down the toilet. … I felt resistance, apprehension to picking it up. … The dream ends there.

'Is there an embryo that is waiting to be picked up and cared for properly?'

'What is it an embryo of?'

'Perhaps our waking up from whiteness is still embryonic?'

'But—the dream world has spoken; it wants to talk about shit (on a physical and/or metaphoric level) and what we are doing with it?'

'Luckily, the little embryo could float and was persistent and will now get the attention/care/nutrition it needs to be heard, seen or whatever. What we're exploring is perhaps the beginnings of an embryonic opening for one way of encountering these intersected issues of "race," whiteness, and the climate crisis.'

'The embryo emerging from the shit!'

'Like Blake's line: Pain and joy is woven fine.'

'White patriarchy denies the shit and just wants the joy, but that carves a destructive path, we need to cherish both, sit compassionately with the hate and pain and not deny our own destructiveness.'

'Embrace Kali rage!'[3]

References

Abram, D. (2011). *Becoming Animal.* Vintage Books.

Bale, T. (2017). Retrieved March 31, 2023, from https://theconversation.com/to-me-golliwogs-are-racist-but-a-tearoom-tangle-and-a-new-poll-shows-britain-disagrees-84314

[3] Kali, the Hindu goddess, the creator and destroyer. Kali rage comment is about holding our own anger, destructiveness and shadow and not projecting it onto others, as in racism, or acting destructively, as in Anthropocene ecological damage. When we hold rage wisely it releases power to be constructive.

Dabiri, E. (2021). *What White People Can Do Next. From Allyship to Coalition.* Penguin, Random House.

Delgado, R., & Stefancic, J. (2012). *Critical Race Theory*. NYU Press.

DiAngelo, R. (2019). *White Fragility*. Penguin.

Ghosthorse, T. (2023). Living With Earth Rather Than On Earth. Earth Charter. Retrieved from https://earthcharter.org/podcasts/tiokasin-ghosthorse

Guy, M. (2021). Retrieved March 31, 2023, from https://antiracistcumbria.org/are-gollywogs-really-so-racist/

Hausdoerffer, J., Kimmerer, R. W., & Van Horn, G. (2021). *Kinship Belonging in a World of Relations*. Centre for Nature and Humans Press.

Helms, J. (2019). *A Race is a Nice Thing to Have: A Guide to Being a White Person or Understanding the White Persons in Your Life* (Cognella Series on Advances in Culture, Race and Ethnicity) (3rd ed.). Cognella Academic Publishing.

Jullien, F. (2008/2014). *On the universal: The uniform, the common, and dialogue between cultures* (M. Richardson & K. Fijalkowski, Trans.). Polity Press.

Ka Canham, H. (2023). *Riotous Deathscapes*. Duke University Press.

Kimmerer, R. W. (2015). *Braiding Sweetgrass*. Milkweed Editions.

Lawrence, G. (2005). *Introduction to Social Dreaming*. Routledge.

Manley, J., & Crociani-Windland, L. (2018). *Social Dreaming, Associative Thinking and Intensities of Affect*. Palgrave Macmillan.

Mullan, J. (2023). *Decolonizing Therapy; Oppression, Historical Trauma, and Politicising Your Practice*. Norton.

O'Donohue, J. (2008). *To Bless the Space Between Us*. Doubleday.

Ribbens McCarthy, J. (2012). The Powerful Relational Language of 'Family': Togetherness, Belonging and Personhood. *Sociological Review, 60*(1), 68–90.

Ribbens McCarthy, J., Woodthorpe, K., & Almack, K. (2023). The Aftermath of Death in the Continuing Lives of the Living: Extending 'Bereavement' Paradigms Through Family and Relational Perspectives. *Sociology (Early Access), 57*(6), 1356–1374. https://doi.org/10.1177/00380385221142490

Shawanda, A., & Manitowabi, J. (2023). Anishinaabe Dream Methodology. https://doi.org/10.33137/tijih.vi13.385566

Topa, W., & Narvaez, D. (2022). *Restoring the Kinship Worldview*. North Atlantic Books.

Ward, L. (2020). *America's Radical Karma*. Parallax Press.

Wellesley, M. (2018). Dream Visions, Discovering Literature, Medieval, British Library website. Retrieved from https://www.bl.uk/medieval-literature/articles/dream-visions, https://en.wikipedia.org/wiki/Ethics_of_care

15

Collaborative Fragmentation: Matrixial Experiments in *Writing-as-Encounter*

Clau Di Gianfrancesco and Elena Gkivisi

What Do You Mean *Collaboration*?

The first time I took part in academic collaboration, I was writing an essay with a close friend of mine. We were doing a master's degree and had requested that the department grant us the right to complete our term assignment collaboratively—we were eventually given permission to do so. We had already come up with an issue we both desired to explore and we agreed that there were two major arguments that demanded attention and exploration within the field. Each of us would deal with one side of the argument. We went on to study a lot and do a lot of reading—individually. Eventually, when everything each of us wanted to write was ready and adequately supported, we met and started putting the texts together. Our idea had been from the beginning that our text would have the structure of a dialogue: one or two paragraphs, that had their author's name in the beginning, would lay out an argument and the

C. Di Gianfrancesco • E. Gkivisi (✉)
Birkbeck University, London, UK
e-mail: cdigia02@mail.bbk.ac.uk; e.gkivisi@bbk.ac.uk

G. Kinouani et al. (eds.), *Creative Disruption*, Studies in the Psychosocial,
https://doi.org/10.1007/978-3-031-63661-5_15

next one or two, carrying the other author's name, would complement or contradict the first argument and so on.

We ended up producing and submitting a very good piece of work: we got a good grade and some extra praise for our 'originality of thinking'.[1] However, I didn't enjoy this collaborative process. I found that complex issues of my personality—of our personalities—played out in the process of working together—inevitably. My friend is much more vocal in addressing critique than I am; I often felt hurt by her open dislike of what I had written; I often thought that I was not able to address her writing in the same terms. When we were creating the cover page of our common essay, I wrote the title, followed by our names alphabetically. By the alphabetic order, my name should go first. When my friend checked the cover page, she decided to change the order and write her name first, without consulting me. I found this gesture rather aggressive, but I didn't say anything about it: I didn't want to be petty.

This incident happened many years ago, and through various events and circumstances of life, irrelevant to our writing collaboration, I eventually came to question some of the bases upon which my relationship with this person had been structured. I realised that many aspects of our interaction have always been dominated by antagonism; I am not aware of whether she might have had similar thoughts and feelings as we haven't discussed any of these issues openly. As I am writing about our friendship and our collaborative, academic writing, I feel deeply uncomfortable in a way that makes itself apparent in my body: a straining pain appears in the middle of my back. I feel as if I'm betraying her.

I have chosen to embark on this act of sharing, as a point of departure, for examining enriching and rewarding ways of collaborative work: this has been the topic of discussion with you as we have undertaken to write an academic piece on undoing, fragmentation, 'otherwise' and ways of re-thinking subjectivity and subjectivities. It must have served some purpose: I already feel undone in my academic credibility by having shared this personal information. I already feel fragmented, in-between my

---

[1] On the issues of originality in collaboration, see Di Gianfransesco, C. & Gkivisi, E. (2023). We/I: Reflections on the Process of Collaborative Thinking. *The Psychologist*, January–February 2023. https://www.bps.org.uk/psychologist/wei-reflections-process-collaborative-thinking

aching back, a psychosomatic manifestation of my long-festered guilt and sadness, and my structured academic thinking, my organised methods of putting things together. Is this academic text about *my* sense of fragmentation? Is *this* what I have to offer the academic bibliography?

Furthermore, I have chosen to share this story as a provisional example of what I have been attempting to share with you, as an idea of how we can think about *disruption*. We have been discussing at length how exactly 'novelty' is defined within and without academia—often exploited as a notion that dismisses the prior contributions of thinkers that may have belonged to marginalised and minoritised groups; whether we have something *original* to offer the field; whether we actually *need* to offer something original. This questioning has been closely related to the fact that we are, both of us, writing as female-read, cisgendered and non-binary/trans*, southern European from relatively middle-class backgrounds; we have been concerned with issues about our own compliance to such discourses of productivity and originality in neoliberal academic spaces. I have been enjoying our meetings and our sharing messed-up-free-associative thoughts during the process of writing this piece, so much so that I have come to hope that, perhaps, we have found a good *novel* way of being friends and colleagues who collaborate within and without academia. This way may not be original, in the sense that *being friends* is not really original, but it definitely is a novel experience—a deep sense of trust, co-exposure, co-creating, togetherness. The story of my collaboration with my friend in our assignment, in combination with thinking about trust as a relational process driving collaboration, is then shared here to show that things are not (only) about what you think they are. Academic collaboration can be, in fact, about friendship; rigid theses can be about personal fragmentation; organised thinking and doing may have to do with dispelling, undoing emotions, thoughts and feelings of being undone. Creative writing can be about theory and theory can be about ways in which one can experience everyday life.

In our conversations on different modes of *undoing*, we work closely with concepts and terms such as *fragilisation* and *(co)-response-ability*, both representing a pulsion towards a *sympoietic* becoming—and 'making-with' by communi*caring*. As Donna Haraway writes, this 'making-with' (i.e. sympoiesis) highlights how 'nothing makes itself; nothing is really autopoietic or self-organising. […] It is a word for worlding-with, in company. Sympoiesis enfolds autopoiesis and generatively unfurls and extends it' (Haraway, 2016, p. 58). In your writing, your opening up with me and our readers, I learn something about you but also about myself, something about us and our shared experience of pain. Your autopoietic retelling of an event is, inevitably, a sympoietic act, a willingness to share and be fragile, to open possible routes for coming together, scrutinising and thinking/writing in concert. In reading about your 'decision' to have a textual 'conversation' with your friend, I wonder how in *trusting* another (a colleague, a friend) we allow for the possibility of worlding-with while simultaneously also rendering ourselves vulnerable—running the risk of encountering pain, because through self-fragilisation 'you are reaching compassion-beyond-empathy and a com-passion that is often hard to tolerate on the level of an individual that seeks mental security and needs to withdraw inside its habits' (Ettinger, 2009, p. 9). Yet, doing-things-with, collaborating, or forming bonds is not—as your example shows—intrinsically a revolutionary and/or an emancipatory act. Rather, there are requirements of love and care, of co-response-ability and communi*caring* that must be present in the enactment of sympoietic and copoietic[2] creations. For Bracha Ettinger (2011), love may also intertwine with resistance, moving away from sentimentality and towards senses of worrying and wonder that communicate a compassionate sharing of self-fragilisation. In *The Feminist Killjoy Handbook* (2023), Sara Ahmed questions those 'feelings of unity' in feminist groups that operate especially through the removal and exclusion of black women, women of colour and trans* people, further writing that:

> […] sustaining a bond might mean not saying certain things, not doing certain things, not noticing them, even. So even if you did not aim to snap a bond, when a bond snaps as a consequence of what you say or do, snap-

[2] While at times, we use these two terms interchangeably, as concepts arising from a dissatisfaction with previously defined theories of *autopoiesis*, sympoieis and copoiesis come from different theoretical traditions and may hold diverse connotations. While we relate *sympoiesis* to Haraway's work—as a 'making-with' that is inevitably done 'in company'—we understand *copoiesis*, as a particular kind of knowledge in transformation, an 'aesthetical and ethical creative potentiality of borderlinking and of metramorphic weaving' (Ettinger, 2005, p. 705).

> ping can teach you why you needed to snap; you snap, you get out of the room, you can breathe. (p. 36)

I am wondering whether we can disrupt textuality, from an extratextual position of *messing-up with its authorship*, its authority, the nature of it; I'm wondering whether I can use the space of academic writing to share my worry about my frustrated friendship and whether I can use the space of academic collaboration to create trust, friendship and love (Bryan, see Chap. 5); whether I can use my friendship and trust with you, the shared care between us, to disrupt the established meaning of what academic collaboration is expected to be. I keep imagining a written and writing space that can bring together strands of psychoanalytic theory, literary criticism, queer theory, post/anti-colonial thinking, *with the acknowledged realities of friendship, love, relating*; I optimistically envision this space as disruptive: an *otherwise* of copoiesis and co-habitation.

Otherwise

In trying to *grasp* the otherwise I am left empty-handed. Maybe it is because the otherwise is not some*thing*, rather it is some*where*. A place that I feel has lately been morphing into a new academic buzzword,[3] emptied out of its many histories and of its many meanings. Yet, the otherwise has always been there, offering another space—call it utopia, revolution, opposition—for all those beings who have been too quickly and violently defined, gendered, racialised in ways that have no other aim than to divide, subjugate, exploit, categorise, violate for personal gains and accumulations of wealth.

Lola Olufemi (2021) opens the first part of her book *Experiments in Imagining Otherwise* with the following passage:

> I hold, like those before me, that experiments can and do fail. I am trying to make an argument for the *otherwise*. Not *otherwise* as in>>>>> over

[3] Here, we would like to acknowledge a series of exchanges and conversations that we had with our friend and colleague Rebekka Hölzle.

here!>>>>> come find me, or a small black dot that recedes as I approach. Not that thing that is obscured and needs to be unobscured. Not a smudge, or an absence, or an entity to be owned or conquered. The future is no one's property; no need to shackle it. Not *otherwise* as in, the political horizon awaits; *otherwise* as in, a firm embrace of the unknowable; the unknowable as in, a well of infinity I want us to fall down together. (p. 7, original emphases)

Olufemi's opening invitation to 'fall down *together*' as a possible path to experiment in imagining *otherwise* recurs throughout the book and reflects how thinking and being otherwise take the 'form of re-working how we engage with one another' (Ashtekar, 2022). By purposely leaving blank pages and open questions throughout the book, Olufemi encourages us, her readers, to think and experiment with her. For Olufemi, imagining otherwise is not an individual endeavour, but a collective one. It is not, as we read above, located in an ungraspable future, rather it is 'that thing that keeps you alive or the ferocity with which you detest this world'; a *thing,* a *ferocity,* that is up to us as readers to 'substitute' the otherwise with (Olufemi, 2021, p. 3). Thus, as Avani Ashtekar (2022) writes in her review of the book, 'Olufemi's otherwise is not a pre-determined entity. Rather, it is a cluster of open-ended possibilities', possibilities that arise by *imagining* together. Olufemi calls us to 'take imagination seriously', linking it with affect, political action and our ability to 'act and resist' (Olufemi & Khan, 2022). For her, 'imagination is connected to our emotional being in the world [... and] it has some effects on our ability to being with each other, to being in *relation* with each other' which, if downplayed, leads to feelings of being 'stuck', unable to 'escape the drawn-out present' (ibid.). Olufemi incites us to imagine together and 'feel across all of these [oppressive] structures, and across how the world is organised to siphon us off and isolate' (ibid.)—not solely to imagine better futures but more importantly, to struggle in the present moment and 'extricate oneself from multiple oppressions enacted by patriarchy, capitalism and colonialism' (Ashtekar, 2022). Her rigorous and playful experiments are grounded in and inspired by black feminist thought and political organising (indicatively, Audre Lorde, Gail Lewis, Claudia Jones, the Brixton Black Women's Group, Sisters Uncut).

Like Olufemi, I see the *otherwise* arising from imaginative and collective practices of resistance that are elaborated in response to violent and oppressive systems—offering alternative modalities of being with ourselves and others, creating sanctuaries and spaces to rebel and revolt in and from.

Inspired by Olufemi, I turn to you, my friend, confidant, colleague and thoughtful interlocutor, to see how between gossip, theory and pleasure we might undo those discourses that have brought, and continue to bring us, pain.

Undoing, Unbecoming and Utopia

> In a sense black feminism has always been about saying *what is gender?* It is not this thing that white middle-class women think it is, or at least that's not all it is; there are all sorts of other ways in which gender is produced and unproduced. When as enslaved women we were beaten, beaten and beaten we weren't beaten as gendered subjects, we were beaten as property. [...] In other words, within black feminism, there has always been a critique of gender, the category [...]. (Lewis in *Radicals in Conversation*, 2020)

In encountering the words of Olufemi and Lewis—but also those of other queer and anti-racist thinkers such as Gloria Anzaldúa and Jack Halberstam—I understand the otherwise as this place in which alternative formulations of being and relating can be imagined and actuated together. Through these otherwise modalities of being and relating language gets reinvented shifting away from the colonial 'godlike function of naming'—through which people, animals and plants were catalogued and collected in the name of 'rational and scientific project[s]' (Halberstam, 2011, p. 5)—and towards new grammars of possibilities. The language articulated in and through the otherwise is a language that *germinates* through *cross-pollination* in the *borderlands* (Anzaldúa, 1987) and that opts for 'none of the above' (Alabanza, 2022).

Undoing, unbecoming and utopia, for me, are three companions that travel together, wondering in the meanders of the otherwise.

In our work and interaction, we aim to entwine our efforts and intentions to cross paths, intellectually and affectively, with this tantalising trio.

Border-Thinking, Border-Writing

Subjectivity in psychoanalysis, as in many other disciplines and practices—academic or not—has usually been thought of in binary terms (self/other, man/woman, subject/object), taking a male subject as the norm. Post-modern, feminist, queer and trans* scholars have challenged such binarisms, as well as 'Man' as the universal bearer of the 'self'[4]—where 'Man' must be read as white, cisheterosexual, able-bodied and, in most cases, wealthy and well educated. The critiques cultivated by anti-racist, queer and feminist thinkers and practitioners have always been accompanied by diverse proposals for other ontologies and epistemologies, which offer *alternative* vocabularies and modalities of knowing. Gloria Anzaldúa (1987) speaks of a knowledge that is produced at the 'border' (*border-thinking*), at the 'juncture of cultures' where 'languages cross-pollinate, and are revitalized' (p., *preface*). Careful not to 'glorify' pre-colonial 'culture's values' that have 'injured' her (ibid., p. 22), Anzaldúa speaks against the 'white rationality' that has taught her to 'not deem [her] psychic experiences real' leading her to deny 'their occurrences and let [her] inner senses atrophy'—further bringing her to believe 'that the existence of the "other world" was mere pagan superstition' (p. 36). Anzaldúa tells us how the '"primitive" and therefore deficient minds' white anthropologists attribute to Indians and Mexicans are considered with a mixture of superiority—as unable to 'think in the higher mode of consciousness-rationality'—and '"fascination"—as "magical" and "savage"' (ibid., p. 37). In *Borderlands*, Anzaldúa also speaks of how the Catholic religion brought by the colonisers '[taught them] that the body is an ignorant animal; intelligence dwells only in the head. But the body is smart. It does not discern between external stimuli and stimuli for the imagination. It reacts equally viscerally to events from the

[4] As indicative examples of the richness of this field, see, for instance, Irigaray (1985); Haraway (1985); Battersby (1998); Halberstam (2011); Preciado (2020).

imagination as it does to "real" events' (ibid., pp. 37–38). Yet, while describing the violence of cisheteropatriarchal and colonial epistemologies and ontologies, Anzaldúa's *Borderlands*, as María Lugones writes, further 'creat[es] a theoretical space for resistance' (1992, p. 32). In articulating the 'work of the *mestiza* consciousness', Anzaldúa (1987) speaks of how this consists of

> break[ing] down the subject-object duality that keeps her a prisoner and to show in the flesh and through the images in her work *how duality is transcended.* The answer to the problem between the white race and the colored, between males and females, lies in healing the split that originates in the very foundation of our lives, our culture, our languages, our thoughts. A *massive uprooting of dualistic thinking* in the individual and collective consciousness is the beginning of a long struggle, but one that could, in our best hopes, bring us to the end of rape, of violence, of war. (p. 80, our emphasis)

This 'feminist border thinking' is not simply 'critical of [a] "categorical"/essentialist logic of modernity'—and its erection of dichotomies and dimorphisms (human/non-human; man/woman; male/female, etc.)—rather, it stresses how such logic is also fundamentally predicated on whiteness, capitalism and modernity/coloniality. Such border thinking thus is 'not just a split, not an infinite repetition of dichotomous hierarchies among de-souled spectres of the human', rather it is 'a ground, a space, a borderlands [...]' (Lugones, 2010, p. 753). For these reasons, border thinking practices can be understood as forms 'of knowing otherwise' (Icaza, 2017, p. 33)—that is, as knowledges that are *ecological, embodied, spiritual, erotic, sensual, more-than-rational.* This knowledge is thus premised on a vulnerability that is deeply political and which requires the coming together of multiple beings, offering 'coalitions, and coalitions selves as a necessary step out' (Icaza, 2017, p. 34) and 'rebellion and creation as processes rather than acts' (ibid., 33). Yet, these forms of knowing, imagining and acting *otherwise* 'are not just different' as Lugones reminds us: '[t]hey include affirmation of life over profit, communalism over individualism, "estar" over enterprise, being in relation rather than dichotomously split over and over in hierarchically and violently ordered fragments' (Lugones, 2010, p. 755). The thinkers that accompany us in our work, those that we spoke of and who continue to populate the remaining pages of this chapter, craft alternative modalities of knowing and speaking the self/subject—always and necessarily in relational terms and not with the intention of recreating hierarchies by establishing themselves as better, fuller, deeper modalities for understanding the self/other/cosmos/ecology.[5]

Recent autofictional and autotheoretical life-writing testifies to and challenges the persisting predominance of phallocentric binary perceptions of subjectivity that replicate stereotypes, violence and discrimination. In the past two decades, women's life-writing has become major site for exploring the relationship between gender, writing and the self. Indicatively, Chris Kraus's autofictional epistolary novel *I Love Dick* (2016/1997) has exposed and questioned women's passivity in heterosexual relations as well as the biased gender standards in academia and the art world; Annie Ernaux's collective autobiography *The Years* (2020) narrates the formation of a subjectivity at the same time private and communal, personal and impersonal; Alison Bechdel's graphic memoir *Are You My Mother?* (2012) explores family relationships through psychoanalytic theory and alongside the depiction of lesbian subjectivities and relations; Claudia Rankine's book-length poem *Citizen* (2014) is a lyrical examination of everyday racism and the illusions of justice. Departing from existing auto/biographical and life writing practices, these works represent an intervention in the representation and conceptualisation of subjectivity and selfhood. Sharing a concern with formal innovation, they attempt to reconfigure the limits between subject/object, public/private, self/other and thereby undermine such binary categorisations.

This departure can be read as coterminous with Bracha L. Ettinger's increasingly influential notion of the 'matrixial', which itself departs from typical psychoanalytic theorisations of gendered subjectivity. The 'matrixial' constitutes a radically different model of subject formation, in which traditional binary logics of 'self' and 'other', as corporeal, cognitive and

---

[5] In this chapter, we do not intend to collapse or equate the different traditions of thinking and acting against racist, cisheterosexual, ableist, and classist modalities of thinking/theorising the self/subjectivity. Rather, our wish is to acknowledge the long history preceding and inform our understanding and use of the conceptual vocabulary we employ.

psychic entities, are questioned and re-thought in terms of co-construction. The 'matrix' is conceptually based on the womb and signifies an encounter of sharing and responsiveness between self and non-self. Matrixial subjectivity is asymmetrical, plural and fragmented and is not defined by its difference from another: it is marked by the co-emergence and co-existence of self and other, subject and object, that takes place in prenatality within the archaically feminine space of the womb. This new conceptual framework navigates away from dominant patriarchal constructions of sexual subject formation, epitomised in existing canonical frameworks by Freud and Lacan, amongst others.

Based largely on the Lacanian theory of subjectivity as well as on its critique by feminist philosophers and theorists, Ettinger engages with ethical philosophy as well as with contemporary art and its confrontation with transgenerational trauma, taking the late prenatal conditions of human becoming as a psychological and corporeal start of rich aesthetic imprints and affects. The conceptual matrixial co-emergence and co-existence of 'I' and 'not-I' focuses on jointness in space and time. It thus supplements and shifts phallocentric, post-Freudian or non-Freudian theories of intersubjectivity and relationality that invariably pose the separation of the 'I' from its other (parent, world, object, etc.) as the primary condition of subjectivity (Pollock, 2022). The Ettingerian matrix is not essentialising; it signifies processes and dynamics of relationality and relatedness. In affording us with a dimension of subjectivity, affect and identity that would go beyond oppositional separation, it does not link pregnancy to reproduction and heteronormativity,[6] but it argues for a model of ontological co-existence that would stand beyond the gender of its subjects. A study of the interaction between Ettinger's psycho-philosophical model of subjectivity, and female, feminist and queer life-writing and scholarship challenging dualistic perceptions, can offer grounding for an ethical reflection of self, other, gender, alterity and difference that would be based on co-emergence and shareability.[7]

[6] On this point, see also Pollock (2020) and Gutiérrez-Albilla (2022).

[7] Substituting the antagonistic differentiation between I and not-I, with a model of co-emergence between subject and other, could also, according to Griselda Pollock (2020), undermine separative, socio-psychic processes of racism and disrupt the fixed and oppressive connotations resulting in discrimination and inequality.

In the epistolary autofictional novel *I Love Dick*, Chris is writing letters to Dick, a man with whom she has fallen passionately in love, even though he is at best indifferent, if not hostile, to her efforts at communication. Through this process, she realises that even though she had tried to write for years, she can only do it by inhabiting her specificity: 'For years I tried to write but the compromises of my life made it impossible to inhabit a position. And "who" "am" "I"? Embracing you & *failure's* changed all that 'cause now I know I'm *no one*. And there's a lot to say..." (ibid., p. 205, emphasis added) and later,

> Back to the 1st person: I'd even made up art stories about my inability to use it. (...) That in order to write 1st Person narrative there needs to be a fixed self or persona and by refusing to believe in this I was merging with the *fragmented* reality of the time. But now I think okay, that's right, there's no fixed point of self but it exists & by writing you can somehow chart that movement. That maybe 1st Person writing's just as *fragmentary* as more a personal collage, it's just more serious: bringing change & *fragmentation* closer, bringing it down to where you really are. (2016, pp. 122–123, emphasis added)

Ettinger talks of fragmentation, characteristically suggesting that 'fragment' is not the right word and that it should be replaced by the word 'grain' as '[g]rains are not the result of a process of fragmentation; on the contrary—each grain is *not one* from the beginning' (2020, p. 120, emphasis in the original). From the angle of a matrixial subjective re-orientation of the phallic economy, it seems that 'being a no one', being a 'non-I', is inextricably linked to being able to have access to the 'I'. For Chris, being a 'non-I' has been a prerequisite of being an 'I', in the same way as for Ettinger 'I' and 'non-I' are always inhabited by one another, inhabiting one another, *co/in-habit(u)ating*, witnessing with one another or *wit(h)nessing*. They remain in this inter and intra subjective logical exchangeability by being subjects *of* and *to* change and fragmentation, the two being actually linked as in the metramorphic processes of fragmentation towards pluralisation, 'into *severality* and not endless multiplicity' (Ettinger, 2020, p. 250, emphasis in original). In the Ettingerian model of subjectivity, 'being no one' is a borderspace from which the subject is crossing the thresholds in between the 'auto' (linguistically originating from the Greek reflexive pronoun 'eauton' that denotes a tautology between the subject who is acting and the subject bearing the act), and the 'fiction' that is created by this same subject—in between desire and phantasy. Within a given phallic economy, 'being no one' is the *limit* while it is the borderlink within the matrixial one. The two planes co-exist and alternate, but whilst the phallic configuration of no-one-ness seems to expel the subject towards some irredeemable 'outside', the matrixial '*non-one-ness*' resides on the ever-transforming borderlink in-between outside and inside, being the surface that cannot be touched without touching and from which the subject is not only not expelled but she can actually re-find a subjective voice of multiplicity.

In *The Queer Art of Failure* (2011) Jack Halberstam attempts to re-approach notions of failure, removing them from their capitalistic, cisheteronormative requirements and dependencies. Via Halberstam's re-reading of failure as a path to disordering and undoing traditional narratives that associate success with reproduction and wealth accumulation, Chris's state of passivity in which she finds herself to be embracing 'failure' can foreground that there is 'something powerful in being wrong, in losing, in failing, and that our failures combined might just be enough, if we practice them well, to bring down the winners' (Halberstam, 2011, p. 120). Halberstam suggests that refusal, passivity or failure may be the best way for feminisms to refuse to succumb to liberal demands, expectations and definitions of 'freedom' that keep using the language of 'success', of constantly active momentum of emancipation in terms of capitalistic assimilation and productivity, aligning with fantasies of an autonomous, self-contained female individual. As Claudia Rankine—another writer of autotheory—has written, '[t]the state of emergency is also always a state of emergence' (2014, p. 126).

With growing cultural relevance due to the popularisation of the memoir, auto/biographical writing has always been a space for the exploration and negotiation of subjectivity.[8] Challenging standard life-writing

[8] For a more detailed overview about the rich field of autobiographical writing and how it has been shaped and informed by as well as shaping and informing feminist, queer and anti-colonial writing practices, see, amongst others, Miller (1991); Anderson (2001); and Smith and Watson (2010).

forms and norms, recent autotheory and autofiction foreground affect, embodiment, fragmentation and plurality as well as the dissolvable borders between self and other, truth and fiction, writing and written subject. They constitute textual attempts to entwine narratives of the self to critical theory (Fournier, 2021); explore shame and its link to gender (Mitchell, 2020); expose and exhibit audacity (Cooke, 2020); re-appropriate parasitism (Watkins, 2012) and 'oversharing' (Sykes, 2017). Recent literary approaches insist that, more than a concrete genre, the autofictional mode of writing refers to a 'sense of self and approach to self-presentation' (Effe & Lawlor, 2022), thereby re-examining the traditional perceptions of selfhood and subjectivity within literary writing, theory and everyday life.

Rankine, in her poetic negotiation of racism, ingrained in systemic aggression but also in 'little' everyday events, disguised as jokes or absent-mindedness, attempts to re-appropriate the use of personal pronouns to convey the unspeakable but unmistakable shared-ness of trauma: 'I they he she we you were too concluded yesterday to know whatever was done could also be done, was also done, was never done' (2014, p. 146). The matrixial concept of subjectivity as an encounter on a borderspace of co-existence can be enriched by and with Rankine's lyrical negotiation of the powerlessness of the 'I' as a stand-alone entity:

> Sometimes "I" is supposed to hold what is not there until it
> is. Then *what is* comes apart the closer you are to it.
> This makes the first person a symbol for something.
> The pronoun barely holding the person together.
> (…)
> You said "I" has so much power; it's insane.
> (Ibid., p. 71, emphasis in original)

On the other hand, an exploration and re-configuration of the boundaries and borders between singular existence and co-existence can perhaps allow us to think of writing in general but also life-writing more specifically, as a space of undoing of stable identities and ontologies. The act of self-narrativisation within autofictional writing can lead to a disentanglement of the self of its previous properties, a re-visiting of what has been fundamentally lost, a re-appropriation of non-existence. In her autofictional memoir *Reverse Cowgirl* (2020), McKenzie Wark questions the very process of writing herself, bringing her past into a moment of ungraspable present:

> Who is this I in my head that thinks it's me? Who is this me that thinks it is the recap of a series of phases, adventures, quests, events that carved it into its given form? This I, in this now, remembers all of the past iterations of itself that culminates in this (…) plot-point. This I, in this now—forgets all of other pasts that don't fit this dramedy. (2020, p. 172)

Through the writing of this 'I' that contains and re-contains its past as multiple 'non-I's that can never be radically separated from the 'I', co-inhabiting the self in *difference-in-jointness*, being *neither separated nor fused*, Wark attempts to re-visit the non-existence that has inhabited her existence. Towards the end of the memoir, reminiscing about the narration in the beginning of it where she starts with the death of her mother and later describes her memories of her ex-lover Glen—an Aboriginal communist—she writes that writing *Reverse Cowgirl* has been a way for her to negotiate with non-existence: '(…) my need to go back there, in that place of non-existence, the place where my mother isn't, where Glen's language isn't. The place where all lost language goes: the communism of non-existence' (p. 179).

I want to turn again to the words of Gail Lewis, who when asked to share her thoughts on the concept and project of *futurity* in a recent conversation with Lola Olufemi and Jade Bentil answered with the following:

> I will be swimming in the blue, blue ocean, but my swimming in the blue, blue ocean will be as such that my body, your body and the bodies of everybody around us will be *totally unintelligible* in terms of the normativities that make them intelligible now. That it will make no sense to talk about gender, and race (and racism), and sexuality and all those things as positionalities, as identities, as subjectivities—that they would be unintelligible. And I know that this is a speculation beyond our horizons but that is what I think the project is…. (Lewis in *Radicals in Conversation*, 2020)

In our recent departmental PhD seminar meeting, we have been discussing around writing as a form of loss. In our *matrixial experiments* we are encountering-and-(re)encountering this loss, this self-fragilisation actuated through response-ability—to respond to one another in a way that might prevent us from doing more harm. A response-able shared-fragilisation that requires us to get undone and lose some of the *stuff* we have learned throughout our lives:

losing mastery,
losing authorship,
losing properness in our (academic) writing,
but also…
loosing each-other
into one-another's
words
getting lost,
together.
I keep going back to these words,
to this *blue,*
blue ocean.

Acknowledgements We would like to thank our friends, colleagues and supervisors who guided our thinking and conversations in this chapter. Specifically, we would like to thank Jonathan Clark for his careful reading and insightful comments on this piece. We would also like to thank Silvia Posocco and Margarita Aragon for holding space for the Psychosocial PhD group, enabling some of the ideas discussed in this chapter to flourish. Finally, we would like to thank the series editors, Guilaine Kinouani and Hannah Reeves, for all of their work and for the opportunity to publish our work in this collection.

References

Ahmed, S. (2023). *The Feminist Killjoy Handbook*. Allen Lane.
Alabanza, T. (2022). *None of the Above: Reflections on Life Beyond the Binary*. Canongate Books.

Anderson, L. (2001). *Autobiography*. New York: Routledge.

Anzaldúa, G. (1987). *Borderlands/La Frontera: The New Mestiza*. Aunt Lute Books.

Ashtekar, A. (2022). *Book Review: Experiments in Imagining Otherwise by Lola Olufemi*. Retrieved from https://blogs.lse.ac.uk/lsereviewofbooks/2022/07/15/book-review-experiments-in-imagining-otherwise-by-lola-olufemi/

Battersby, C. (1998). *The Phenomenal Woman: Feminist metaphysics and the patterns of identity*. Cambridge: Polity Press.

Bechdel, A. (2012). *Are you my mother? A Comic Drama*. Boston: Houghton Mifflin.

Cooke, J. (2020). *Contemporary Feminist Life-Writing: The New Audacity*. Cambridge: Cambridge University Press.

Effe, A., & Lawlor, H. (Eds.). (2022). *The Autofictional, Approaches, Affordances, Forms*. Palgrave Macmillan.

Ernaux, A. (2020). *The Years* (A. L. Strayer, Trans.). Fitzcarraldo Editions.

Ettinger, B. (2005). Copoiesis. *Ephemera, 5*(X), 703–713.

Ettinger, B. (2009). 'Fragilization and Resistance' and 'Neighborhood and Shechina'. *Studies in the Maternal, 1*(2), 1–31. https://doi.org/10.16995/sim.141

Ettinger, B. (2011). Uncanny Awe, Uncanny Compassion and Matrixial Transjectivity beyond Uncanny Anxiety. In *Psychoanalysis in French and Francophone Literature and Film*. Brill. https://doi.org/10.1163/9789401207591_002

Ettinger, B. (2020). *Matrixial Subjectivity, Aesthetics, Ethics, Volume I 1990–2000*. Palgrave Macmillan.

Fournier, L. (2021). *Autotheory as Feminist Practice in Art, Writing, and Criticism*. Cambridge Massachusetts: The MIT Press.

Gutiérrez-Albilla, J. D. (2022). Introduction: The Primary Event of Peace: Femininity, Com-passionate Hospitality, and Aesthetic Wit(h)nessing in Bracha L. Ettinger's Matrixial Psychoanalysis. *Psychoanalysis Culture & Society, 27*, 466–484.

Halberstam, J. (2011). *The Queer Art of Failure*. Duke University Press.

Haraway, D. H. (1985). *A Cyborg Manifesto*. Macat Library.

Haraway, D. (2016). *Staying with the Trouble: Making Kin in the Chthulucene*. Duke University Press.

Icaza, R. (2017). Decolonial Feminism and Global Politics: Border Thinking and Vulnerability as a Knowing Otherwise. In M. Woons & S. Wier (Eds.), *Critical Epistemologies of Global Politics* (pp. 26–45). Bristol.

Irigaray, L. (1985). *Speculum of the Other Woman* (trans. G. C. Gill). Ithaca: Cornell University Press.

Kraus, C. (2016). *I Love Dick*. Serpent's Tail. (Original work published 1997).

Lugones, M. (1992). On Borderhnds/~Frontera: An Interpretive Essay. *Hypatia, 7*(4), 31–37.

Lugones, M. (2010). Toward a Decolonial Feminism. *Hypatia, 25*(4), 742–759.

Miller, N. K. (1991). *Getting Personal*. London and New York: Routledge.

Mitchell, K. (2020). *Writing Shame: Contemporary Literature, Gender and Negative Affect*. Edinburgh University Press.

Olufemi, L. (2021). *Experiments in Imagining Otherwise*. Hajar Press.

Olufemi, L., & Khan, A. (2022). *Experiments in Imagining Otherwise with Lola Olufemi and Abeera Khan*. Interview retrieved from https://www.youtube.com/watch?v=wLKgypHOA_g

Preciado, P. (2020). *Can the Monster Speak?* (trans. F. Wynne). London: Fitzcarraldo Editions.

Pollock, G. (2020). Editor's Introduction. In G. Pollock (Ed.), *Matrixial Subjectivity, Aesthetics, Ethics, Volume I 1990–2000* (pp. 1–93). Palgrave Macmillan.

Pollock, G. (2022). Looking Back in Fascinance and Wonder: Reading and Thinking with Ettingerian Concepts. *Psychoanalysis Culture & Society, 27*, 439–465.

Radicals in Conversation (Host.). (2020, March 16). 'Feminism, Interrupted' with Lola Olufemi, Jade Bentil and Gail Lewis. [Audio podcast episode]. In *Pluto Press Podcast*. Retrieved from https://plutopress.podbean.com/e/feminism-interrupted-with-lola-olufemi-jade-bentil-and-gail-lewis/

Rankine, C. (2014). *American Citizen*. Graywolf Press.

Smith, S., & Watson, J. (2010). *Reading Autobiography: A Guide for Interpreting Life Narratives*. Minneapolis: University of Minnesota Press.

Sykes, R. (2017). "Who Gets to Speak and Why?"' Oversharing in Contemporary North American Women's Writing. *Journal of Women in Culture and Society, 43*(1), 151–174.

Wark, M. (2020). *Reverse Cowgirl*. Semiotext(e).

Watkins, F. A. (2012). Manic Impositions: The Parasitical Art of Chris Kraus and Sophie Calle. *WSQ: Women's Studies Quarterly, 40*(1 & 2), 223–235.

16

Afterwords: Epistemic Disruption, the Creative and Liberation

Guilaine Kinouani

> 'Why do you write?
>
> We write for various reasons. I write to honour. Honour the stories of my body. And the stories that were never witnessed.
>
> We write to resist.
>
> We resist to write.
>
> Silence has never been an option for some of us.
>
> Writing is resisting silencing.
>
> Writing is speaking.
>
> We write I feel sometimes because we carry heavy loads […]

Some believe storytellers are chosen by their ancestors to keep their stories alive in our collective memory. I write to secretly prove to myself that I am not mad…There is no glory in adapting to dysfunction, so I write' (Kinouani, 2020).

The afterwords were written as part of the explorations first carried out during my PhD (Kinouani, 2024) and may form part of my doctoral thesis.

G. Kinouani (✉)
Birkbeck University, London, UK

G. Kinouani et al. (eds.), *Creative Disruption*, Studies in the Psychosocial,
https://doi.org/10.1007/978-3-031-63661-5_16

In the opening reflections of the introduction, I named the amputatory fantasies which have led me to this book as I reflect on how for me the psychosocial became evocative of hybridity, of displacement and of *re*placement. But also of boldness, of transgression and of rebelliousness, acts or attributes which not so long ago were indeed punishable by amputation. Ancestral baggage, we might say. Blood memories. Inheritance, perhaps activated along my academic journey, turned into onto-epistemic fuel for the manuscript. I too introduced a note of caution about the risks of idealisation.

Frosh and Baraitser (2008) describe the psychosocial as a critical approach interested in articulating a place of 'suture' between elements whose contributions to the production of the human subject are normally theorised separately. It is at these points of suture that its transgressive and oppositional scholarship finds its genesis.

Sutures…another term which is perhaps reminiscent of the haunting imagery of colonial mutilations. A powerful reminder that the practice of sadistically separating limbs and body parts from black bodies is not separate from epistemic practices. The amputation of limbs, and the dispossession of lands, is also the dispossession of indigenous knowledge systems and their attempts to endure and survive (Berenstain et al., 2022). The erasing and perverting of indigenous traditions, beliefs, language and worldviews and the constitution of the colonial subject as other, we have long known, are part of the same 'two-handed machine' and lay at the centre of epistemic violence (Spivak, 1988, p. 25).

What was violently cut off thus split from the body and discarded under the paradox of colonial projection and colonial extraction later merged into normative assumptions. Assumptions that continue to reify what can be discarded which is necessarily also *who* can be discarded. Form of knowing which inexorably 'continues to constrict Blackness, queerness, womanhood and how these intersecting realities are lived, theorised and archived, often outside of their very body' (Berenstain et al., 2022 p. 284).

In other words, who was brutalised, erased, forgotten in the 'there and then' is who is brutalised, erased, forgotten in 'here and now'. As Sara Ahmed may say, bodies that don't count don't get counted. And bodies that don't get counted do not get remembered as the lives we lost to the flames of Grenfell have shown us, as the lies which were told about the flames of Grenfell have taught us. But as I say in *White Minds* (Kinouani, 2023, p. xiv), 'remembering is resisting'. And as such, reclaiming who and what was discarded and holding it in our mind and in our heart, sacred, is a practice of resistance.

A practice with a long black feminist history (Hill Collins, 2000). A practice too which sits at the core of the psychosocial's 'temporal drag' and its habit of seeking, regenerating, transforming concepts and ideas deemed obsolete, unfashionable, unsavoury, and re-introducing them into the present in 'new' forms (Baraitser, 2017). An attempt we might say, at refusing to forget. At not letting go of that which so many want to forget and let go of.

Beyond personal idiosyncrasies and our varying positionality as co-editors—one white British cis, queer and neurodivergent woman; one white Italian, assigned-female-at-birth, non-binary trans person, and one French African descended migrant woman—it is clear that painful stories punctuated our journeys through dominant structures. These experiences forced us to encounter the 'otherwise' which left us 'fragmented', 'disrupted' or 'undone' in our sense of selves, our very subjectivities as we attempted to theorise the material realities of the human subject. Framing the collection autoethnographically is an ethical and conceptual imperative: it sutures theory to the lived realities of our bodies and the responsibilities and possibilities that they carry.

It is fundamentally these encounters with this very ontological disturbance which united us and brought us to the field of the psychosocial and the manuscript. A disturbance which was unspoken until it was spoken on the journey to writing the book. A disturbance from which therefore sprung the impulse to create and the determination to disrupt, perhaps in a way we had been left disturbed. Containing this collective yet largely disavowed disturbance, bearing witness to it, transforming it into the words that form the chapters of this book, is consequently an act of resistance too.

I take epistemic resistance to refer to '[t]he use of our epistemic resources and abilities to undermine and change oppressive normative structures and the complacent cognitive-affective functioning that sustains those structures' (Medina, 2013, p. 3).

It is, we could say, about using what we know or what we have at our disposal to trouble what refuses to be troubled. What stands still, often idle, safe in the notions of 'this is this way things are' and 'this is the way we do things'. Engaging in epistemic resistance is an active process, we are reminded. A process which necessitates being conscious of what we are reproducing as we participate in knowledge production.

But more than that, it is about purposefully supporting oppositional epistemic practices with the aim of dismantling epistemic injustice and supporting liberation (Medina, 2013). It is thus about refusing to do things in the way that they are purportedly done, 'here'.

This is the only way to disrupt structures of power reified in the onto-epistemic domain. The only way to uphold practices which make possible the articulation of the previously non-articulatable, practices that speak to socially (dis)ordered realities, that speak of 'the walking dead' and from zones, as Fanon may say, of 'non-being' (Asani & Kinouani, 2021).

The psychosocial has thus provided this site for us. A site to do things as they tend not to be done within academia at least. A site to aspire to nurture this freedom impulse, this disruptive aspiration not only to us but to the contributors. And so, all chapters form a freedom dance individually and collectively. They move in the direction of liberation. All contributors in some way dared to be free, if only momentarily.

Dared to speak the unspeakable. Dared to know differently. And dared us all to think and rethink, to feel and 're-feel' what we take for granted when it comes to knowing and feeling, when it comes to the body, to subjectivity, when it comes to the inaccessible terrain of the ever so fiercely resisted moments of uncertainty.

Often asking us to sit in the cracks of not knowing, and to bear that friction, perhaps of 'the real' the Lacanians might say or of the Beta, Bionians might retort; without instantaneously resorting to symbolisation, whether through language or through conceptualisation; acts of cerebral colonisation, I might argue from an Afro-analytic lens (Kinouani, 2024). Paradoxically, the pre-symbolic, the pre-verbal, the so-called unintelligible, as forms of illumination.

Hence you have been invited to witness: intuitive ways of knowing, 'embodied ways of knowing, spiritual ways of knowing, and land-based ways of knowing—these are all forms of knowledge that are violently foreclosed in the name of settler futurity. Dispossessive practices create and are reinforced by settler knowledge systems that generate epistemic oppression as a matter of course' (Berenstain et al., p. 284).

Specifically, provocations to be free from what has been have come in many daring forms. They have included an invitation to use the theatrical to produce knowledge about the politics of Brexit. Autoethnographic considerations on remembrance and memorialisation at the intersections of the body, the land and neurodivergence. The use of play in the Winnicottian sense, to explore tests as scientific formations and objects. Engaging with the creative potential of 'stupidity' as a source of wisdom in the clinic.

Employing love as a methodological paradigm or being guided by the heart as a path to truth. Exploring embodied moments of undoing and unbecoming that unfold within collaborative encounters. Neurodivergifying the masses to achieve liberation. Communicating with ancestral entities to fuel decolonial activism. Doing dreamwork to intimately encounter and dismantle whiteness. Trusting corporeal materialities and the power of the erotic as a way to know and simply, as a way to be.

These varied invitations and provocations perfectly demonstrate that beyond the twists and turns of my 'personal story', the psychosocial analytics do present to us a multitude of opportunities to engage with creativity. Our imagining of knowledge production as disruption has unapologetically centred the body, the flesh, the lived, the felt, the way we move in space, the way space moves into us. The way we encounter one another. The way we come into being through the meeting of our hearts, the moving of our hips, the freeing of our dreams.

Musing that is of critical importance to psychosocial enquiry whose existence as an oppositional force to scholarly territoriality is central. Musing that supports the breaking of boundaries and the crossing of borders. Indeed, the psychosocial as a terrain, as we have introduced, is founded on its oddness with psychology and sociology's formations of the subject and occupies a theoretical juncture which is a combination of 'trans' disciplinary spaces. These include postcolonial theory, psychoanalytic thinking, feminism and queer theory (Frosh, 2013). Or at least, it so aspires. Domains each arguably engaged in the queering of space.

Whilst it may be argued that epistemic resistance and disruption are the precursors to epistemic liberation, we know that it is not enough to dismantle the master's house. Creative energies must also be employed to build, transform, edifice new worlds, or so the thinking goes. Lest we are deemed to exist to simply oppose that which is and in doing so keep it in existence as: 'a destructive force that inevitably retains ties to, and gains definition from, the very system or traditions that are the object of the resistance' (Sharpe, 2016, p. 175).

The volume has been invested, in both sets of preoccupations as it has moved back and forth between attempting to dismantle and attempting to build, evoking the rumba of the Congo and its inherent paradoxical core: the synchrony of life and death energies, the merging of vitality and mortality. A musical tradition so close to death and dying, it compels the body to reconnect to life.

Still, as I read Sharpe's words and I let them sink in my head and in my heart, I am rethinking the possibility of the new as the path to liberation since 'every radicalisation is always indebted to the very thing it radicalises' (Derrida, 1994, p. 116). I ponder upon these ties and whether they too will refuse to die. And I wonder whether the old, the known, the familiar is forever bound to interfere in our imaginaries and relational potentialities and therefore whether the meaning of the 'transformed' needs a new conceptualisation. Whether freedom from what has been, as we so long for and imagine, is an illusion spoken through the aspiration of the new.

Whether, thus, the psychosocial pursuit of the transdisciplinary is a defensive posture which is potentially dangerous. Another aspiration of a view from nowhere, albeit a more sophisticated one—a field from nowhere, one might say. One which so strongly echoes that familiar omnipotent fantasy of the a-spatial, the atemporal, the disembodied.

The re-embodiment of white, masculinist narcissism and its attempt to flee its own body, its own flesh and all the ways in which it becomes acted out in real spaces and in real time. And … all the ways in which it is experienced, often violently by others. Those same discarded others or rather those others we attempt to discard but who, we now know, remain.

As again, beyond personal idiosyncrasies, varying positionalities and experiences of marginality as co-editors and me as the project initiator, and the only black body, I was positioned within the whiteness of my co-editors, within the whiteness of the book 'matrix' and consequently within a terrain which is predominantly white. A white space thus perhaps, despite itself, disrupted, in some intangible yet felt ways by my blackness. Or perhaps more precisely Lewis Gordon might say, by my black consciousness. At a time in history group analysts may observe, censorship in all its guises is rife as mass atrocities are normalised and violent currents of misogynoir are seemingly overtaking all aspects of public life.

As I write this, I must return to my opening question. Why do we write? Why do *I* write? And my response remains unchanged.

I write to honour the stories of my body. And I write to honour the stories that were not witnessed. And so, I ask myself what stories were not witnessed as part of this *creative disruption* story? What new painful stories this black body of mine will now carry? What was discarded on this journey of writing about the discarded? What was split-off, discharged? Ushered out and whispered away, in private, echoes of which leave my body achy?

Were there moments which left me more 'undone', 'fragmented', 'disrupted', 'disturbed'?

Undoubtedly.

These moments have reminded me of the precarity of our connections. Of the inescapability of my blackness. Of the vulnerability and permanent conditionality, it imposes on my humanity. Of how easily it can pervert my womanhood. Of how liberatory intentions can quickly crumble at the intersections.

And so, as I celebrate the completion of the book, the collective efforts it took to give shape to our vision, the perseverance and the passion which fed the project, I will too mourn the emergence of these familiar reenactments. Testament to the permeability and penetrability of the interpersonal by the sociopolitical. Testament too to how easily we can edify the borders we seek to dismantle, reproduce politics of othering and marginalisation as we consciously partake in resistance and turn into the objects whose existence we claim we object to.

Further evidence that what continues to be (de)posited (on)to belong to the racialised object and to find its genesis in their sick and dark thus 'primitive' minds is hardly likely to originate from there. It is indeed not black psyches who rely on repression or forgetting when it comes to the 'past' and associated sanctions for black transgression. This is not theoretically tenable since we are forced to remember or we refuse to forget. And we have been taught that it is those who forget who are 'obliged to repeat the repressed material as a contemporary experience, instead of … remembering it as something belonging to the past' (Freud, 1920, p. 12).

Beyond the individualised repetition compulsion hypothesis, or its corresponding group analytic formulation of *equivalences*—the process by which groups are similarly believed to 'repeat' compulsorily trauma loaded past group dynamic or dysfunctional social configurations through the workings of the social unconscious (Hopper, 2006)—remembering is an ecological and environmental process too. One which can, it has been argued, be sustained in the absence of human subjectivity.

Twahirwa (2021) summarises, drawing from Sharpe's work on 'residence time'—the amount of time it takes for a substance to enter the sea and leave it (for blood residence time is 260 million years)—when it comes to the dwelling in the water, of decomposed enslaved African bodies thrown overboard dead or alive, during the middle passage; that the seas and the oceans remember. These discarded bodies were most likely eaten by fish and other organisms which were then in turn eaten by other organisms. 'It is likely that the flesh, bones, organs and muscles not only of the 132 passengers that were thrown overboard from the Zong, but also the estimated two million Africans who died during the crossing of the Middle Passage are still with us today. The water has a memory' (Twahirwa, 2021).

Blood's 'residence time' provides, a potent illustration of the inseparability of body, subjectivity, water and land/earth when it comes to memory, particularly when it comes to black consciousness and thus when it comes to the work of liberation.

Beyond the temporal interrogation, the dissipation of African flesh and blood, of African DNA into the oceans and surrounding land, speaks too of ecological trauma. Of the elements being helpless witnesses to that suffering, of processes of transference and transformation of the human bodies, even after such genocidal death. In the same vein, the first law of thermodynamics in physics provides that no new energy can ever get created and that no energy can get destroyed either.

All remains.

In some forms. Repurposed, redistributed, re-expressed, at times creatively. This is the way the planet operates. Denying this is an attack on reality. The insistence on a separated new, here too a new 'from nowhere' we may say, is a denial of the laws of physics which some of us believe often overlap with the domain of the spirits, the laws of transcendence, we might say. In the Bionian sense, this disconnection is an 'attack on linking'. An obstinate refusal to link objects.

How fragile we are thus in the face of the psychosocial's predictable eruption into and disruption of our communicational field as we are engaged in the scholarly endeavour of psychosocial disruption. And how tragic to have the epistemic tools to observe and conceptualise these reenactments but not the means to stop the machinery in its ontological or indeed life course.

For those of us who do remember, who are often the same people who are alert to and literate in the critical potentialities of the visceral and the truth it holds, the energy it responds to, we feel the reverberations of injustice in our bones, almost at cellular level. And we can with our heart astutely recognise the patterns of what has been, however, repurposed, redistributed, re-expressed. For us, who are often the writers or, in other words, the storytellers, the Griots and Nzonzis of our communities, those designated to be the memory bearers, who carry the burden of inheritance and whose bodily archives link the living to the dead, the work of mourning is never done because the work of witnessing is never done.

The stories need to be told.
The dead must be remembered.
Hence, the violence shall be confronted.

No one 'heals' from acts of injustice. They too remain and find residence in the sea of our body, I have learnt. However small the injustices, they change you. However small the change.

We grieve. Sometimes we bleed.

Our backs know how to carry collective disturbances, which are discharged onto and into our bodies, again and again. Like the literal toxic waste Western nations dispose of, by (de)positing it onto the land of African nations, as it continues dispossessive practices and, in doing so, furthers that projection-extraction paradox which characterises colonial relations... But unlike our mutilated ancestors whose hands were cut, those who were thrown overboard whether they were still breathing or not and those who today are gasping for air at sea 'in the wake' of those atrocities…

We can hand what is put into us, back.
 We can theorise.
 We can write.

We can escape the prison of the inescapable as we choose to remember those murdered and those whose limbs were brutally amputated, when we make meaning and when we stand in power in the meaningless, when we dance in the mist of it all, when we come together in community, when we insist on living life through the meeting of our hearts, the moving of our hips, the freeing of our dreams. And this is why the creative must be central to our liberatory praxis.

So once more, we write to resist. We resist to write. Silence is never an option for me. Sheeshi and Sheeshi (2022) poignantly remind us that 'resistance keeps us sane' (p. 204). Staying sane in a mad-making world, that too, is an act of disruption. Perhaps even the greatest evidence of creativity. I, in turn, often remind readers that black lives are not theoretical (Kinouani, 2021).

I hope these last few words helped to demonstrate what is at stake. Why this collection is so much more than a collection. I also hope ending the book on this disturbance or rather transferring it back—as I have had to learn to do for my own liberation and as part of my analytic training—allows readers to encounter the 'otherwise' so that more of you are left 'undone', fragmented, disrupted, disturbed.

Acknowledgements A note of gratitude to those who helped to make this project possible, chiefly my co-editors, Clau and Hannah, the contributors, those who reviewed the manuscript, particularly Prof. Frosh, Birkbeck College for giving me space and a scholarship to grow intellectually, and all those who have provided support behind the scenes.

References

Asani, F., & Kinouani, G. (2021). Migration, Homelessness and Internalised Displacement. *Social and Health Sciences, 19*(2). https://doi.org/10.25159/2957-3645/10496

Baraitser, L. (2017). *Enduring Time*. Bloomsbury.

Berenstain, N., Dotson, K., Paredes, J., Ruíz, E., & Noenoe, K. S. (2022). Epistemic Oppression, Resistance, and Resurgence. *Contemporary Political Theory, 21*(2), 283–314.

Derrida, J. (1994). *Specters of Marx: The State of the Debt and the New International*. Routledge.

Freud, S. (1920). *Beyond the Pleasure Principle* (Translated and edited by Strachey J). WW Norton, 1961.

Frosh, S. (2013). Transdisciplinary Tensions and Psychosocial Studies. *Enquire, 6*(1), 1–15.

Frosh, S., & Baraitser, L. (2008). Psychoanalysis and Psychosocial Studies. *Psychoanalysis, Culture & Society, 13*(4), 346–365. https://doi.org/10.1057/pcs.2008.8

Hill Collins, P. (2000). *Black Feminist Thought: Knowledge Consciousness and the Politics of Empowerment* (Rev. 10th anniversary). Routledge. Retrieved December 5, 2023, from http://site.ebrary.com/id/10054558

Hopper, E. (2006). Theoretical and conceptual notes concerning transference and countertransference in groups and by groups, and the social unconscious: Part I' Group Analysis, 39, 549–559.

Kinouani, G. (2020). *Writing and the Fear of Power*. Race Reflections. Retrieved December 5, 2023, from https://racereflections.co.uk/writing-and-the-fear-of-power/

Kinouani, G. (2021). *Living While Black: The Ultimate Guide to Overcoming Racial Trauma*. Ebury, Penguin Random Penguin House.

Kinouani, G. (2023). *White Minds: Everyday Performance, Violence, Resistance*. Policy Press, Bristol University Press.

Kinouani, G. (2024). *Whiteness as Iatrogenic and Traumatogenic: An Afro-analytic Exploration and Reformulation of Racial Trauma in the Clinic and Beyond* [Unpublished dissertation]. Birkbeck College, University of London.

Medina, J. (2013). *The Epistemology of Resistance: Gender and Racial Oppression Epistemic Injustice and Resistant Imaginations*. Oxford University Press.

Sharpe, C. E. (2016). *In the Wake: On Blackness and Being*. Duke University Press.

Sheeshi, S., & Sheeshi, S. (2022). *Psychoanalysis under Occupation: Practising Resistance in Palestine*. Routledge.

Spivak, G. C. (1988). Can the Subaltern Speak? In C. Nelson & L. Grossberg (Eds.), *Marxism and the Interpretation of Culture*. University of Illinois Press.

Twahirwa, R. (2021). *Haunted Memory, Haunted Waters*. University of Oxford. Border Criminologies Blog. Retrieved from https://blogs.law.ox.ac.uk/research-subject-groups/centre-criminology/centreborder-criminologies/blog/2021/09/haunted-memory

Index[1]

[1] Note: Page numbers followed by 'n' refer to notes.

G. Kinouani et al. (eds.), *Creative Disruption*, Studies in the Psychosocial,
https://doi.org/10.1007/978-3-031-63661-5

FSC
www.fsc.org
MIX
Papier | Fördert gute Waldnutzung
FSC® C083411

Kolibri 360 GmbH
Ferdinand-Jühlke-Straße 7
99095 Erfurt, Deutschland
produktsicherheit@kolibri360.de